Educating for Moral Action:
A Sourcebook in Health and Rehabilitation Ethics

Educating for Moral Action:
A Sourcebook in Health and Rehabilitation Ethics

Ruth B. Purtilo, PhD, FAPTA
Director and Dr. C.C. and Mabel L. Criss Professor of Ethics
Creighton University Medical Center
Center for Health Policy and Ethics
Omaha, Nebraska

Gail M. Jensen, PhD, PT, FAPTA
Associate Dean for Faculty Development and Assessment
Professor of Physical Therapy
School of Pharmacy and Health Professions
Creighton University Medical Center
Omaha, Nebraska

Charlotte Brasic Royeen, PhD, OTR/L, FAOTA
Dean, Doisy School of Allied Health Professions
Professor in Occupational Therapy
Saint Louis University
St. Louis, Missouri

F.A. DAVIS COMPANY • Philadelphia

F. A. Davis Company
1915 Arch Street
Philadelphia, PA 19103
www.fadavis.com

Printed in the United States of America

Last digit indicates print number: 10 9 8 7 6 5 4 3 2 1

Acquisition Editor: Margaret Biblis
Developmental Editor: Melissa Reed
Design Manager: Joan Wendt

As new scientific information becomes available through basic and clinical research, recommended treatments and drug therapies undergo changes. The author(s) and publisher have done everything possible to make this book accurate, up to date, and in accord with accepted standards at the time of publication. The author(s), editors, and publisher are not responsible for errors or omissions or for consequences from application of the book, and make no warranty, expressed or implied, in regard to the contents of the book. Any practice described in this book should be applied by the reader in accordance with professional standards of care used in regard to the unique circumstances that may apply in each situation. The reader is advised always to check product information (package inserts) for changes and new information regarding dose and contraindications before administering any drug. Caution is especially urged when using new or infrequently ordered drugs.

Library of Congress Cataloging-in-Publication Data

Educating for moral action : a sourcebook in health and rehabilitation ethics / [edited by] Ruth B. Purtilo, Gail M. Jensen, Charlotte Brasic Royeen.
   p. ; cm.
  Includes bibliographical references and index.
  ISBN 0-8036-1261-3 (hardcover : alk. paper)
  1. Medical ethics. 2. Physical therapists—Professional ethics. 3. Occupational therapists—Professional ethics.
  [DNLM: 1. Physical Therapy (Specialty)—ethics. 2. Bioethics. 3. Occupational Therapy—education. 4. Occupational Therapy—ethics. 5. Physical Therapy (Specialty)—education. WB 460 E24 2005] I. Purtilo, Ruth B. II. Jensen, Gail M. III. Royeen, Charlotte Brasic.
  R724 . E325 2005
  174.2—dc22
                                                     2004021213

To the communities we have the privilege to serve and with whom we share common goals for a more healthful society.

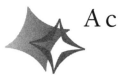

Acknowledgments

The editors and contributors gratefully acknowledge:

Ms. Carol Peters, Creighton University School of Pharmacy and Health Professions, for her outstanding work on the "front end" of the manuscript preparation process.

Ms. Helen Shew, Creighton University Center for Health Policy and Ethics, for her good humor and exceptionally fine skill required for coordinating the many details of the working conference associated with the development of these chapters and for her ongoing editorial and administrative support in bringing the chapters to publication as a book.

Ms. Melissa Reed, Assistant Editor, Development, Health Professions and Medicine, for her able assistance, working with the many contributors, the three editors, and Carol Peters and Helen Shew in the production process of the book

And a special thanks to Margaret M. Biblis, Publisher, Health Professions and Medicine, for her confidence in this project from its inception.

A Note from the Editors

It began over morning coffee and the task of putting together a major grant with an imminent deadline staring us in the face. We shared the conviction that intentional action can emerge from dialogue and the belief that seldom do physical therapists and occupational therapists have an opportunity to enjoy the stimulation of a sustained exchange of shared ideas and concerns. Right then and there we began to dream. Why not create the occasion for such an opportunity?

For all of our planning, even our high expectations were exceeded when the 24-member Dreamcatchers ethics education working group convened for almost 3 days—each member equipped with a working paper he or she had created for the event, plenty of food and wine, four carefully selected ethics consultants from fields outside our own, and a large measure of goodwill and enthusiasm.

The group of contributing authors came together for a working conference on Leadership in Ethics Education for Physical Therapy and Occupational Therapy. This conference was, in part, supported by a Health Resources Services Administration, Allied Health project grant (HRSA Grant #D37 HP 00824), entitled Dreamcatchers and the Common Good: Allied Health Leadership in Generational Health and Ethics. One of the project goals of the grant was to develop and implement innovative leadership in ethics education for allied health. The Leadership in Ethics Institute was held at the Center for Health Policy and Ethics at Creighton University in September 2003. The institute itself was the combined effort of the grant initiative, Center for Health Policy and Ethics, and the School of Pharmacy and Health Professions. We are indebted to all for the support of such a creative project for physical therapy and occupational therapy.

What made this event different from other initiatives that we and many other therapists engage in as committed members of our professional organizations? First, we were an independent think tank, not an "official" group of our professional organizations or institutions. Although several members already are recognized leaders in their organizations, each came as an individual scholar/teacher/clinician. Second, we all were—and are—committed to offering leadership as our professional organizations and institutions develop their ethics curricula and refine their ethical practices and policies. Third, we agreed that not only the classroom but also the clinical, administrative, policy, and research environments must be taken into account in the shaping of ethical issues. Fourth, we agreed that we want to be participants in activities that affirm the common ground in occupational therapy and physical therapy. Fifth, we agreed that all ideas were welcomed and would be respected, acknowledging that we have obviously been informed by what we and other professions have adopted as ethical approaches and relevant topics but that we should not be bound by them. We wanted the freedom to traverse a new path, if necessary, that accurately shows who we were and are and that takes us where we want to go. Finally, we hypothesized that as agents in the larger health care system, our working group materials could be used by ourselves and others to influence the direction ethics education and practice could take to improve ethics educational approaches in other health profession curricula.

At the conclusion of the conference, 10 markers for our (and others') continued work together in our professions emerged. We offer them here for your reflection:

1. Wisdom and continued flourishing counsel toward learning from each other across our professions.
2. Ethics pedagogy should focus learning on both reflection and action.

3. Ethics education and practice must involve assessment of stakeholder values at individual, institutional, and societal levels. Currently the individual realm has a hold on our moral thinking and action.

4. Evidence-based practice pervades all three levels of ethical concern.

5. Moral courage is required in order to tackle sensitive topics and content areas.

6. Professional ethics approaches focused on considerations of "care" and virtue theory are highly compatible with the actual functions assumed by therapists, although expanded understandings are needed to ensure institutional and societal levels are included. Duties, rights, and responsibility also have their place in an overall ethical framework.

7. Use of metaphor as pedagogical tools enhances vision and understanding.

8. Any ethics approach that separates classroom from clinical realities warrants ferreting out of our curricula.

9. We must successfully meet the "just right" challenge of not over- or underestimating students' experience, development, and motivations for entering the professions: the demographics of our student populations are changing.

10. All pedagogy today must be directed to continuing competence and compatible with adult, lifelong learning.

Our goal was not to gather all the important or expert voices, to be exhaustive in our delineation of markers, or to utilize every tool that our respective professions have brought to bear on ethics education to date. Rather, we began somewhere, calling upon colleagues with whom we have had informal conversations, with whom we have worked, or whose writings and teaching we have held in high regard. Even as this book goes to press, the working group members are preparing to bring even more people into the conversation.

We invite you to join the conversation, first through reading this book, which is designed to be a book of resources, not the final path itself. For some, it will be the first broad exposure to various clinicians, academics, ethicists, and policymakers. Others will fall into step with us somewhere along the path, bringing their own experience, disciplinary expertise, and ideas that will help create a better course. Indeed, each of us, as forgers of the path, have an opportunity to work on this "labor of love" together.

The Editors
Ruth Purtilo
Gail Jensen
Charlotte Royeen

Overview Chapter

Ruth B. Purtilo, PhD, FAPTA

A foray into the *Oxford English Dictionary* reveals that "source" comes from ancient roots meaning "a fountainhead or point of origin." As usage often sculpts meaning, over time this term has also become shaped to mean "a generative force or stimulus, an instigator." The authors of this sourcebook designed it to serve as both point of origin and instigator for the reader who ventures along the path of its chapters. Although it will be of most interest to ethics educators in the health professions, the work will stimulate all who are invested in working toward the realization of an ethical environment and an understanding of the behaviors and dispositions that support it.

The authors themselves went back to draw from the origins of their own considered reflection, fields of study, and professional experience. Readers who have been exposed to even basic bioethics approaches and methodologies will recognize that familiar ethical theories and methods are incorporated into many of the authors' contributions. Basic tenets of professionalism, too, some traditionally conceived and others adapted to fit modern characteristics of the professions in society, can be found. Moreover, authors drank deeply from the foundational work of scholars in many disciplines whose insights enrich the understanding of ethics.

As important as the return to foundational origins is, the authors' primary goal from the beginning was to think broadly, imaginatively, to reach and risk. The result is a sourcebook that is a generative force able to stimulate further thought, discussion, debate, and considered action. It is the instigator function that gives this sourcebook its vitality and margin of value among the many other good ethics writings in the health professions, bioethics, and related disciplines.

A significant point of difference distinguishing this sourcebook from other valuable sources is the contributors' collective skill in paring away extraneous material to reveal foundational ethical concepts, a meaningful context, and relevant concerns in today's rehabilitation and other health professions environments where physical therapists and occupational therapists work. I take special delight in this volume because it offers a promising break in the silence that has often ensued in professional, bioethics, and health policy discussions when colleagues are asked to devote their attention to concerns in these settings. We who work there are aware that the well-being of the population of persons seeking services from rehabilitation, community-based, and other professionals can be seriously compromised when there is a failure to give considered attention to key quality-of-life issues, institutional injustices, and damaging attitudes and behaviors encountered by persons with persistent functional impairments. At the same time, the authors of this sourcebook often step back from the usual ethical approaches to patient or client, institutional, and societal challenges to ask "Do the usual approaches and concepts fit? If not, what can we do to improve the situation for students and others faced with real-life everyday challenges in rehabilitation, long-term care, community, and other nonhospital settings?" I am hopeful that the book's success will be just one sign that the health professions, the field of bioethics, and society more generally are committed to preparing the path to answers along with the authors and others who already have taken up this task.

My guess is that many readers of this volume will have come to the point of wanting to explore the topics in this book along a path similar to my own. Most started out on their professional venture with exactly the enthusiasm for their professional choice as I, although many will not have started as many years ago. At first, I had a narrowly construed idea of my role, and it had to do with modalities, skills, and an earnest conviction that I was going to help people in need. Very little self-consciousness was devoted to "ethical" issues.

When I graduated with my physical therapy degree, the scourge of the U.S. polio epidemic was finally receding, thanks to the introduction of a vaccine, but in its place new challenges had washed up on the societal shore. With all the verve of a new therapist, I energetically "rehabbed" patients faced with the functional challenges of spinal cord injuries, burns, strokes, and other common conditions. And when the opportunity to work in Africa was presented, I pulled my ponytail into a bun and went to work with patients who presented with nutritional deficiency–induced impairments, spinal TB, Hansen's disease, and yes, unfortunately, polio. But it was not long before I learned that every patient's "condition," wherever found on the globe, was only a part of the person's story, and it was to the larger story that I was inexplicably drawn over time.

The patient's story seemed to account for so much: who among patients had the courage and stamina, resiliency, and insight to survive amidst challenges that I am sure to this day would overcome my own resolve; which values seemed to support— or undermine—the human will under the extreme circumstances of persistent impairment from injury or illness; when, how, and why did patients' relationships with loved ones and others endure or crumble over the course of my professional encounter with them; and, perhaps, most perplexing, what could I *really* do to make a difference when the very life from which these people had been catapulted had to be transformed into something new and useful for their days, months, and years ahead. My wonder at the larger human questions I faced in the rehabilitation environment followed me from the clinic into the classroom and administrative offices. It was well summed up by a 6-year-old boy who, upon seeing a young man with quadriplegia whom I was treating early in my clinical career asked, awestruck, "You been in a *wreck* or something?" To which David, the patient, replied, "Yeah. Or something."

Looking back, it is not surprising that I stumbled into the study of ethics as a way to try to get at that "or something." I wanted answers to deal with the bigger questions of meaning and value as they presented themselves in the lived experiences of men, women, and children in the institutions of health care where I worked alongside other members of the rehabilitation team. But often I found that the issues I thought pressing did not have the "excitement value" among fellow bioethicists that transplantation and intensive care units, or even "death and dying" issues, held for them. Today, with the changing demographics of our society, where more are living longer but with quality of life challenges as their walking mates and bedfellows, the issues that long have compelled rehabilitation professionals are becoming everyone's concern.

Whatever your own professional journey that leads you to this moment, what can you, the reader/searcher, expect to find in this sourcebook? For one thing, you will find that the authors are writing in a professional and social environment that in some promising regards is dramatically changed from the days when I first started struggling with the bigger questions that accompanied me on my professional path to becoming a physical therapist–ethicist. Let me name some:

Today there is *a dramatic increase in the number of therapists committed to the exploration of the larger questions of value and meaning* through the study of ethics, the social sciences, and other fields while continuing to contribute in their roles of clinician, educator, researcher, and/or administrator. I am no longer by any means one of a scant few rehabilitation professional-ethicists. Several contributors to this

volume include just some of the leaders in the study and application of ethics in rehabilitation and other key settings where therapists apply their skills.

Indeed, today *the range of health-related settings in which physical therapists and
occupational therapists apply their skills has increased dramatically.* They span the continuum from prevention and health maintenance, to acute care settings and the more
traditional rehabilitation context, to home care and hospice. Physical therapists and
occupational therapists also are deeply involved in community (including industry,
school, and public health) settings as reflected in many of the contributors' chapters.
This change not only increases the scope of practice but also of ethical questions
encountered daily. This, in turn, requires therapists to understand and earnestly engage
with a wider range of professional colleagues as solutions to ethical quandaries are
sought. The richness of an enlarged circle of dialogue is reflected in the authors' fram-
ing of the questions and proposed approaches and strategies found in this volume. The
four consultant contributions from the fields of philosophical ethics, nursing, pharmacy, and moral theology further bring home my point.

There is a *dramatically increased awareness in professional education programs that
ethics and human values must be deeply integrated into students' professional preparation
and formation.* This reflects, in part, a trend from the late 1960s onward in academic
health profession programs generally toward a recognition that base competencies must
include ethics knowledge, dispositions, and skills of ethical decision making. The trend
to demand such competencies slowly is changing the face of professional curricula in
both the classroom and clinical settings of rehabilitation and other therapy-oriented
programs. The authors of this volume draw heavily on the good work being done
nationally by their professional associations and in their local institutions.

There is also *a dramatic loss of public confidence in the authority, sincerity, and
authenticity of the health professions as useful partners in societal efforts to improve the
well-being of all persons,* especially those who are socially marginalized. In some
regards, one can hardly call this a positive change. However, a positive outcome from
this negative state of affairs is that the traditional "bedside ethic" that dominated the
growth of bioethics in the United States and the Western world during the past half
century is gradually being replaced by a more accurate conception of ethics as including interrelated individual, institutional, *and* societal dimensions. Consultant contributor John Glaser's framework of the "Three Realms of Ethics" fits well with the lived
experiences of health professionals. The interdependence of clients, professionals, policy makers, and stakeholders in the larger society is no secret to therapists, and the task
of finding a framework and the concepts and issues that highlight it is taken up by
several authors in this book.

In short, overall the path is better laid out today and the overall environment is
more inviting for adding such dimensions as rehabilitation, mental health, and community health concerns to the active bioethics and professionalism discussions than
when I began my professional venture. More therapists are contributing to the discourse; a wider range of professions has increased and refined the areas of professional
contribution and cross-professional collaboration; ethics teaching is finding its way into
various aspects of formal professional preparation, and the necessity of including institutional and larger societal stakes in ethical analysis is saving the professions from ethical obsolescence, which would result if the focus of ethical concern remained solely at
the traditional level of the professional-client relationship.

However, I daresay that in the final analysis, it is not these changes, important as
they are, that will compel the reader to absorb, reflect on, and respond to the contributions in this book. The contributors were able to take advantage of the present environment and the benefit of each others' support and critique to expand upon the

boundaries of their own thinking to date as well as to think collectively about the concepts, context, and pedagogies that will help enrich ethics education in the health professions generally and provide some important markers for it in the rehabilitation fields more specifically.

The book is divided into three major sections focused, respectively, on **concepts**, **context**, and **pedagogy**, each with physical therapists' and occupational therapists' contributions as well as one or more consultant offering. What follows is a brief synopsis of each chapter. My hope is that it will bring some measure of readiness to you, the reader, about what to expect. The surprise will be how much more you will find in these actual chapters!

Section 1, "Broadening Our Worldview of Ethics," contains pieces by seven contributors who chose to explore basic ethics (or ethics-relevant) **concepts** that might warrant consideration or rethinking because of insights from the environments where physical therapists and occupational therapists primarily are employed. Contributors examined ideas not often found in professional ethics texts or that are present but used in a different way. In Chapter 1, I offer commentary and reflection on the basic concept of *respect*, suggesting that by adding insights from modern psychology and law to more traditional interpretations, a professional ethic will give more attention to the role of the professional's *self respect* as well as increase the parameters of traditional expressions of respect for others. Suzanne Peloquin in Chapter 2 asks and addresses the provocative question of whether *empathy*, commonly viewed as a centerpiece of professional interaction, should be interpreted as having a moral dimension in the form of a moral disposition or attitude. (The theme of empathy arises again when Carol Davis addresses it in Section Three, which focuses on ethics education.) The next two chapters shift the reader's attention from the individual virtues of respect and empathy to what one might call a *"group moral virtue" of competence* applied to the entire professional enterprise. Penelope Moyers (Chapter 3) proposes that the moral justification for occupational therapy and physical therapy practice is the development and maintenance of *competence*, tying it to client-centered care; in Chapter 4, Shirley Wells highlights shortcomings in traditional bioethics approaches occasioned by a paucity of *cultural competence* to adequately account for the complexities of race, ethnicity, culture, and religion as well as to shape models of morality and moral reasoning. She outlines *an ethics of diversity* that would move the professions toward redressing these shortcomings. Jeffrey Crabtree (Chapter 5) and Charles Christiansen (Chapter 6) emphasize *moral dimensions of the professional-in-community.* Crabtree's exploration of assumptions about the self as understood in Western mainstream society (with its reliance on individual autonomy) picks up and expands on some of Wells' concerns. His analysis is set against the changing demographics of persons who seek the services of physical therapy and occupational therapy, proposing that they are more consistent with collective conceptions of the self. He provides supportive arguments for *collectivistic approaches and democratic (shared) forms of institutional decision making involving patients and clients.* Christiansen picks up on the theme of communitarian decision making as the appropriate mode for therapists to employ, emphasizing that the health care professions' institutional, especially educational, moral function is to create an environment that helps students appreciate *the special obligation of professionals to assume civic responsibilities.* To flourish, educators must emphasize *an ethics of social responsibility and leadership.*

Section One ends with a consultant contribution by nurse-ethicist Patricia Benner (Chapter 7). She presents the nurse's challenge in the identification and care of persons with chronic disease, taking into account the stigma involved in chronic illness. She walks the reader through several moral dimensions of chronic illness and the caretaker's own coping and proposes a means of gaining a clearer understanding of chronic illness in terms of the lived, social, and cultural experience of patients. The remainder of the chapter describes a framework of how *clinicians move from advanced beginner to expert status through reflective experience and the ethical insights and challenges* at each developmental step.

Section 2, "Health Care Environment: Contextualizing Ethics," contains 10 chapters focused on the larger professional and social **context** in which the professions function. The authors include both important barriers to effective ethical functioning and supports for incorporating ethical concerns perceived from the standpoint of occupational therapy and physical therapy settings and activity.

Charlotte Royeen (Chapter 8) sets out a broad framework for this section. In her engaging analysis of our professions, she critiques some key strengths and weaknesses of evidence-based medicine in the rehabilitation professions setting, concluding that a TRIO model of ethics is appropriate for best practices in interventions involving physical therapy and occupational therapy. The TRIO model includes *habits of the mind, heart, and art.* Six factors therapists can use to ensure best practices are embodied in the form of a mnemonic, ETHICS.

Do therapists in any work setting perceive themselves as moral agents? In Chapter 9, Herman Triezenberg shares observations gleaned from his own research that suggest the answer is "yes." When queried about the interpretation of their moral role and what it entails, physical therapists responded that *there is a moral component to their role (presumably in any work setting)*, some aspects of which are defined by characteristics of the relationship between the individual therapist and patient and others that involve moral obligations to future patients, physical therapy peers, professional organizations, social agencies, and society at large. Adding to the theme of moral agency, Lee Nelson creates a blueprint for change and *the moral role of therapists as change agents in society* (Chapter 11). Taking the case of a lack of lymphedema services, she describes how one state's group of therapists, working with other health professionals, client groups, government officials, and others, was able to develop a plan for the provision and implementation of lymphedema services. This group's experience highlights professional responsibility, advocacy, access to care for chronic conditions, and other justice issues and concerns related to evidence-based medicine.

Two chapters address ethical implications of the exciting and ever-changing health care environment, one from the standpoint of complex technologies, the other from new discoveries related to the brain's functioning. Regina Doherty (Chapter 10) tackles *ethical questions arising from our technology-intensive health care environment.* She skillfully uses a series of case studies to exemplify why occupational therapists and physical therapists are morally obligated to become knowledgeable and competent regarding health-related technologies generally, not just with those they use. The context of her concern focuses primarily on the individual patient-therapist relationship, but with a steady eye she also considers the ethical effects of technology on professional practice and vice-versa. Later, Ivelisse Lazzarini (Chapter 14) takes the reader into a realm where past science fiction has become current scientific reality. Advances in neuroscience help us to understand how the brain works and can be manipulated. The enormous potential for clinical progress in the treatment of neurological conditions carries with it serious ethical and legal implications. She believes that rehabilitation professionals have *a moral obligation to become aware of the ethical dilemmas occasioned by neuroscience advances*, be prepared to respond to them, and include them in the ethics curricula of our students.

In Chapter 12, Laurita Hack *underscores the impact of institutional practices and policies on the behavior of professionals* by analyzing three disparities that face the physical and occupational therapy professions relative to ethical practice and moral behavior: the disparity between reflective and reflexive action, the seeming reversal of some attitudes and values once students become practicing clinicians, and the impact of an organization on the performance of therapists. She makes a persuasive case that to decrease this problem, educators and others must focus attention on the effects of institutional practices and policies.

Mary Ann Wharton (Chapter 13) uses her study of *the mission and role of the American Physical Therapy Association's Chapter Ethics Committees* to examine the current functioning of those committees. She emphasizes ways the Chapter Ethics Committees are similar to (and different from) such committees in the American Occupational Therapy Association. She urges educators to emphasize the importance of using ethics committees for education about ethics, case consultation, and policy development.

An *in-depth comparison of widely used "client-centered care" models* provides the focus of Panelpha Kyler's contribution (Chapter 15). Using examples of the interpretive model and deliberative model in the medical literature, she poses questions about their applicability to occupational therapy's and physical therapy's concepts of client-centered care and family-centered care and provides ethical considerations to support her conclusions.

This section ends with two consultant contributions (Chapters 16 and 17) by John Glaser and Karen Gervais. John Glaser, Vice President for Theology and Ethics in the St. Joseph Health System, describes a foundation of human dignity upon which ethical decisions must rest. There are *three realms of ethics (individual, organizational, and societal)* in which professionals and others must face hard choices. Traditional bioethics focuses primarily on the individual, a shortcoming Glaser sees as devastating to the appropriate work of ethics, since lives are lived within organizations and individual lives are influenced by (as well as influence) organizations and the larger society. He reflects on how a "community of concern" would look, whereby like-minded persons could acknowledge their deep interdependence (such as that described by Crabtree and Christianson in earlier chapters of this book) and in so doing be able to make decisions focused on organizational and societal considerations without unduly compromising their individual well-being.

Philosopher Karen Gervais provides *a process model for ethical decision making.* This straightforward model shows that background knowledge, case analysis, and self-assessment are three types of preparation essential to ethical decision making and describes each. An important point distinguishing this model from many others is its emphasis not only on the clinical but also on the organizational and societal factors (reflective of Glaser's three realms) affecting knowledge acquisition, case analysis, and self-assessment prior to actual decision making.

Section 3, "Transforming Ethics Education: Strategies for Student Learning," beams attention squarely on the educator and learner. Authors in this section make explicit suggestions for ethics education, although every chapter in the book was written with the goal of improving ethics education. These final chapters are not designed to be a template for one approach but rather to provide tools and ideas to guide the ethics educator to her or his own goals.

To begin this section, Gail Jensen (Chapter 18) introduces the reader to the idea of *mindfulness as an instrument enabling health professionals to engage in lifelong learning and continue to gain expertise.* She includes the key concepts found in the literature, applications of them to clinical cases, and a critical self-reflection on her own teaching of ethics, particularly her own exploration of evidence that students are learning mindfulness.

What are the *implications for ethics education of the growing interest in spirituality* within the health professions? In Chapter 19, Linda Gabriel reflects on this from the standpoint of "a nagging feeling that some important affective learning element or ingredient is missing from my [ethics] course." After a descriptive section regarding terms often associated with spirituality, she suggests the concept of "spiritual intelligence" as a conceptual link between spirituality and ethics, the goal being to explore *the possible link between spiritual self-awareness and the teaching and learning of ethics.*

Carol Davis' goal in Chapter 20 is to provide the reader with *suggestions how to best educate and inspire students to exercise moral courage.* She begins with the question of how we develop our moral consciousness and conscience as adults. The chapter reviews components of moral action, including thought, emotion, and social interaction, and then highlights two common emotions, sympathy and empathy, for their links to altruistic behavior. She also contrasts moral sensitivity and judgment with moral courage and action.

Laura Lee Swisher (Chapter 21) offers a *framework for designing appropriate content of an ethics curriculum:* an appreciation of the field's social and environmental context; the necessity of addressing the multidimensional nature of moral behavior; the use of intermediate concepts (e.g., confidentiality, autonomy) for teaching and evaluation of moral judgment; moral motivation based on the professional role and moral obligations of professionalism; and ongoing research and scholarship focused on professional identity within the environmental context. For each of these recommendations, Swisher assigns the ethics educator a role—as organizational construction worker, curriculum architect, everyday philosopher, midwife, and scholar.

Returning to a focus on the adult learner that Gail Jensen, Carol Davis, and others emphasize in other parts of Section Three, Susan Sisola (Chapter 22) addresses barriers that create challenges to developing and implementing ethics education She suggests insights from *three adult education models as direction for overall curricular design and specific educational strategies* in ethics education.

In his "Reflections on Student Learning," Ernest Nalette (Chapter 23) takes the reader through *four foundational concepts to guide pedagogy:* concreteness, objectivity, analysis, and skepticism of convention. He proposes that the goal of ethics education is to help professionals "break the moral silence," a silence he views as a contributing factor to the detriment of patients' and professionals' well-being.

Drawing on her more than 20 years of research, Elizabeth Mostrom focuses Chapter 24 on a description of *student learning and development about ethical and humanistic dimensions of care during their clinical education experiences.* She divides the chapter into what students tell us (the voice of students) and lessons learned from clinical instructors and other colleagues. She ends the chapter with suggestions how academic and clinical faculty can expand and enhance opportunities for teaching and learning about the ethical and human dimensions of care in clinical settings.

Using the innovative pedagogical device of a moot court simulation in Chapter 25, Jan Bruckner illustrates *the effective use of a teaching case and importance of including research ethics in the ethics curriculum.* She describes the process by which informed consent is learned and assessed by students and presents a model of community consent developed by Thomasma based on the principle of beneficence with the claim that every person has the obligation to improve society.

In the penultimate Chapter 26, Aimee Luebben moves the reader's attention from the teaching of ethics to *a focus on the ethics of teaching.* She draws primarily on the ideas of Dewey and Schön, both of whom have "extolled the value of reflection to resolve complex issues" and suggests mechanisms for reflection on this important dimension of the larger picture of ethics education.

Chapter 27 is contributed by consultant ethicist Amy Haddad. A nurse by training and a recent national Carnegie Scholar of the Carnegie Foundation for the Advancement of Teaching, Amy suggests means of applying the scholarship of teaching and learning to critical inquiry about ethics education. As a fitting ending to this ethics sourcebook, she leaves the reader with the challenge of determining what works in ethics education, what is possible, and what is really happening when students learn.

Taken together, the contributors' highest hopes will have been met if, in the reading of these chapters, you bump up against ideas that resonate with not only the best of what ethics education is offering today but also with generative ways to improve our mutual goals in this arena. We hope we have raised some more questions for your own exploration and that you will enthusiastically add to the discourse.

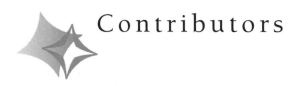

Contributors

Patricia Benner, PhD, RN, FAAN
Thelma Shobe Endowed Professor, Chair of Social and
  Behavioral Sciences
School of Nursing
University of California San Francisco
San Francisco, California

Jan Bruckner, PhD, PT
Associate Professor
Institute for Physical Therapy
Widener University
Chester, Pennsylvania

Charles Christiansen, EdD, OTR, OT(C), FAOTA
Dean, School of Allied Health Sciences and George T.
  Bryan Distinguished Professor
The University of Texas Medical Branch at Galveston
Galveston, Texas

Jeffrey L. Crabtree, OTD, MS, OTR, FAOTA
Associate Professor
Department of Occupational Therapy
School of Health and Rehabilitation Sciences
Indiana University
Indianapolis, Indiana
This work was completed while at the University of
  Texas at El Paso.

Carol M. Davis, EdD, PT, FAPTA
Professor and Associate Director for Curriculum
University of Miami School of Medicine
Department of Physical Therapy
Coral Gables, Florida

Regina F. Doherty MS, OTR/L
Clinical Specialist, Occupational Therapy Services
Massachusetts General Hospital
Boston, Massachusetts

Linda Gabriel, PhD, OTR/L
Assistant Professor
Department of Occupational Therapy
School of Pharmacy and Health Professions
Creighton University Medical Center
Omaha, Nebraska

Karen G. Gervais, PhD
Director
Minnesota Center for Health Care Ethics
Minneapolis, Minnesota

John W. Glaser, STD
Director, Center for Healthcare Reform
Senior Vice President
Theology and Ethics
St. Joseph Health System
Orange, California

Laurita (Laurie) M. Hack, PhD, MBA, PT, FAPTA
Professor and Chair
Department of Physical Therapy
Temple University
Philadelphia, Pennsylvania

Amy Marie Haddad, PhD, RN
Professor in the Creighton University
School of Pharmacy and Health Professions
Assistant Director of the Center for Health Policy
  and Ethics
Creighton University Medical Center
Omaha, Nebraska

Gail M. Jensen, PhD, PT, FAPTA
Professor, Department of Physical Therapy
Associate Dean for Faculty Development and
  Assessment
School of Pharmacy and Health Professions
Creighton University Medical Center
Omaha, Nebraska

Panelpha (Penny) L. Kyler, MA, OTR, FAOTA
Public Health Analyst
Genetic Services Branch
Maternal and Child Health Bureau
Health Resources and Services Administration
Department of Health and Human Services
  Rockville, Maryland

Ivelisse Lazzarini, OTD, OTR/L
Assistant Professor, Department of Occupational
    Therapy
School of Pharmacy and Health Professions
Creighton University Medical Cener
Omaha, Nebraska.
This work was completed under a postdoctoral fel-
    lowship at Saint Louis University.

Aimee J. Luebben, EdD, OTR, FAOTA
Professor and Director, Occupational Therapy
    Program
University of Southern Indiana
Evansville, Indiana

Elizabeth Mostrom, PhD, PT
Professor and Director of Clinical Education
Program in Physical Therapy
School of Rehabilitation and Medical Sciences
Central Michigan University
Mount Pleasant, Michigan

Penelope A. Moyers, EdD, OTR
Dean
School of Occupational Therapy
University of Indianapolis
Indianapolis, Indiana

Ernest Nalette, EdD, PT
Associate Professor
Chair of Graduate Studies in Physical Therapy
Ithaca College
Ithaca, New York

Lee B. Nelson PT, DPT
Clinical Professor
Department of Physical Therapy
University of Vermont
Burlington, Vermont

Suzanne Marie Peloquin, PhD, OTR, FAOTA
Professor
Department of Occupational Therapy
School of Allied Health Sciences
The University of Texas Medical Branch at Galveston
Galveston, Texas

Ruth B. Purtilo, PhD, FAPTA
Director, Center for Health Policy and Ethics
Dr. C.C. and Mabel L. Criss Professor of Ethics
Creighton University Medical Center
Omaha, Nebraska

Charlotte Brasic Royeen, PhD, OTR/L, FAOTA
Dean, Edward and Margaret Doisy School of Allied
    Health Professions
Saint Louis University
Saint Louis, Missouri

Susan W. Sisola, PhD, PT
Associate Professor
Doctor of Physical Therapy Program
College of St. Catherine
Minneapolis, Minnesota

Laura Lee (Dolly) Swisher, PhD, PT
Assistant Professor
College of Medicine
School of Physical Therapy
University of South Florida
Tampa, Florida

Herman L. Triezenberg, PhD, PT
Professor and Chair, School of Rehabilitation and
    Medical Sciences
Director, Graduate Program in Physical Therapy
Central Michigan University
Mt. Pleasant, Michigan

Shirley A. Wells, MPH, OTR, FAOTA
Assistant Professor
Department of Occupational Therapy
University of Texas Pan American
Edinburg, Texas

Mary Ann Wharton, MS, PT
Associate Professor and Curriculum Coordinator
Department of Physical Therapy
Saint Francis University
Loretto, Pennsylvania

Contents

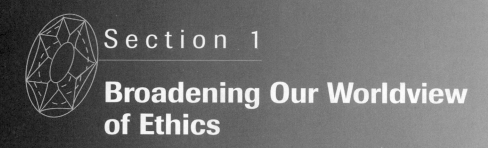

Section 1

Broadening Our Worldview of Ethics

1

New Respect for Respect in Ethics Education

RUTH B. PURTILO, PHD, FAPTA

Abstract

In this chapter I examine the virtue of respect and the role it has played in the development of professional ethics and, more importantly, the role it might now play in everyday practice.

Drawing on the etiology of the term "profession," I propose that our task is to assist students in understanding what it means to become a "professing person." Respect serves as a resource to increase the person's chances of achieving this goal.

Traditionally respect has been treated primarily as an "other-regarding" virtue, serving the professional well in the societal expectation of putting the patient's interests first. Upon analysis I conclude that the moral role respect plays in this context is to give concrete expression to the belief that humans have an inherent dignity that must be honored. The roots of this idea, its strengths, and some concerns about it are addressed.

I then turn to insights about respect gleaned from the modern Western idea of agency and moral psychology. A major contribution of these interpretations of respect is to add self regard/respect into the mix.

In the final section I reflect on the analysis, concluding that ethics educators should be reflective about how this virtue is presented within occupational therapy and physical therapy ethics education. I make tentative recommendations regarding one useful approach, including those incorporating the principles for gaining cultural competence.

From the time I was a small child I have been intrigued by the story of the little shoemaker who, when given the opportunity, realized he wanted to be somewhere/someone else. He was granted three wishes and took the first two to become rich and famous. But, the story goes, when he had one wish left he wished himself back into shoemaking. As a child I was envious of the incredible good luck of the shoemaker to have encountered a means to become instantly rich and famous. But another part of the shoemaker's narrative also was introduced into my thinking, this time in a graduate school course entitled "Conceptions of Identity and Selfhood," and that part of the narrative, too, has stuck with me. In a new twist, the professor used my childhood hero as one example of a self transformed by his journey. The shoemaker went after resources, she said, that he thought would be the most useful and gratifying but learned they were not central to his becoming fully who he wanted to be. Through his journey, his original self-identity ("I am a skilled shoemaker but stuck in a wee shop putting soles on shoes") became transformed ("I am a person with incredible power which I can use to contribute to society's resources through my shoemaking"). His journey made all the difference. For reasons I hope become clear in this chapter, I believe he learned to prize what really mattered most fundamentally, respect in all its forms, including self respect.

The purpose of this chapter is to explore how respect figures in the journey I believe each physical therapy and occupational therapy student must take in their transformation from being a layperson to becoming a highly skilled technologist to becoming a fully and authentically professing person. (This phrase, "professing person," sounds awkward, but the term "professional," literally translated, means "a person who professes" or promises certain benefits in exchange for other benefits or "license."[1] I submit that too often today our educational programs stop at creating highly skilled technologists, mistaking it for what a professional, or more accurately, a professing person is. I submit, further, that a basic cause of this mistake by educators is that, as a whole, we have failed to fully traverse the journey of learning to understand *how* to appropriately show respect to ourselves, so we do not bother to instill it in students. Respect-fullness makes the difference between being a professional narrowly interpreted, (i.e., a "shoemaker") and becoming a person equipped with the inner resources to make a significant contribution. The inner resources are essential if the professional is to fulfill the highest societal ideals of what professionals can contribute, namely, to improve the human condition in ways not otherwise likely to be realized.[2]

✧ WHY US?

Why give *ethics* educators the task of digging into the concept of respect? First of all, I believe that we tend to be journeyers ourselves. Many of the chapters in this volume support that assumption. We are among those not satisfied with merely gaining certain technical tools of our craft, equipping us to work as professionals—in the narrow sense often applied to that term. We are occupational therapists and physical therapists who are among the most compelled by the journey it takes to become fully and authentically professing persons.

Secondly, we are ethics educators. We appreciate that students come into our programs with the legitimate desire to earn a living and gain some measure of recognition for their contribution to society. But we are also aware that their core curriculum all too often fails to offer an adequate opportunity for them to go beyond becoming "shoemakers." In other words, curricular and other pressures contribute to compromising as persons the activities geared to their intentional reflection on who they are becoming and integrating their insights into resources for fulfilling what their professional role reasonably expects of them. We—and usually they—know they are being transformed from laypeople into something else that means that they will never again be able to look at some things the way they did before completing their program of study. But the scholarly and lay literature is strewn with evidence that professional education actually can be a deterrent to preparing students to assume the applaudable goals associated with the provision of health care.[3] We count ourselves among occupational therapy and physical therapy educators who want that transformation to include the means by which students will gain the requisite resources to meet the true challenges and realize the true benefits of their chosen role in society. We believe that doing so will augment the success of their societal role over the lifetime of their career, providing one hedge against the curses of disillusionment, boredom, or burnout.[4]

That being said, I summarize by suggesting that we are invested in the portion of the journey focused on the person's development in ways essential to leading a good life. This cannot be limited to only self-actualization in the individual, important as that is. It must also include resources to respond whole-heartedly to societal expectations associated with the role of being a professional. Philosophers and others who have given a good deal of thought to what constitutes "a good life" are cognizant that, for the majority of humans, a good life must include self-fulfillment but of a type that also contributes to supporting a healthful society. After all, they live in that society, so even an egotistic ideal would include some regard for their society. Characteristics that individuals summon and cultivate for this purpose are called virtues, and the ethics based on them, virtue ethics. Many of our colleagues, including some in this volume, continue to enrich our understanding of the place of various virtues in the development of what I am calling a professing person. More specifically, in the next (and major) section of this chapter, I examine the virtue of respect and the expression of respect toward self and others as a foundational characteristic. In the final section, I offer some directions we as educators might take, all the while inviting your response.

✧ RESPECT

"Respect" comes from the Latin root, "respicere." The verb form "to respect" means that one's approach to a person, idea, or object is from a posture or disposition of holding him/it in high regard. The person or idea is deemed "worth the trouble." Respect traditionally was treated as an "other-regarding" attitude, a self-sacrificing posture focused on the well-being of the other person. Fortunately in more recent times, and due in large part to the contributions of modern psychology, the companion idea of "self respect" has gained equal attention. It follows that the good life governed by respect will include paying attention to one's own quality of living as well as the quality one can help others enjoy. At first glance this may seem at odds with the idea that a professional always should put the patient's interests first, but I will attempt to show that this apparent dichotomy is false.

Respect and Its Relation to Dignity

Respect for persons is almost always associated with the idea that humans have dignity. In professional ethics writings, the usually unspoken assumption or passing comment is that when we show respect we do so as an acknowledgment that we recognize the patient's, family's, teammate's, or other's dignity.

Pullman points out two interpretations of dignity in the health professions context, personal dignity and inherent dignity.[5] Personal dignity associates a client's dignity with a particular characteristic, such as privacy. The woman whose hospital gown is left to flap open during a standing transfer is said to have lost her dignity due to the health professional's carelessness. The breach of a patient's confidence is a reproach to his expectation that you would protect his dignity in his compromised situation of having to blurt out things he would rather have kept to himself. Conversely, your attention to their privacy needs is seen as upholding their dignity. Loss of personal dignity also can be affected by events outside both the patient's and health professional's control. A debilitating disease, for example, might be viewed by the patient and by others as robbing the patient of his dignity.

Most professional ethics writings, even many of those described above, ultimately go beyond the idea of personal dignity associated with remaining in control of one's modesty, embarrassing or shameful information, or former body image. Instead, the virtue of showing respect to persons arises from a deeper claim, namely, that persons possess inherent dignity.[5] Inherent dignity has a certain ring to it, raising the suspicion that a show of respect is more than a polite gesture that can be taken or left, can be bestowed on some and not on others on the basis of a specific characteristic they have or do not have. If it is inherent dignity we are dealing with, we may not only show but must pay respect. Something (i.e., respect!) is due the other, and this respect makes very concrete claims on us. For example, the Preamble to the *United Nations Universal Declaration of Human Rights* appeals to the "inherent dignity" of every human. Several very concrete rights follow, each of which requires governments and citizens to arrange their communities, institutions, and daily lives so that everyone can enjoy these rights.[6] If dignity is universal and inalienable it pushes respect over the edge of professional manners into the deeper realm of professional morality. It shoves respect out of the domain of aesthetic virtue only (i.e., something that looks good) into the terrain of moral virtue (i.e., something that has positive relevance to the basic fabric of society). It cannot be treated as etiquette without also recognizing that it is ethics.

Where has the demanding idea of inherent dignity come from? (I do not claim to be a scholar in this area so I beg your forbearance in tapping what seem to be some especially promising avenues of exploration.) The premise of inherent dignity and the major line of thinking that linked respect to inherent dignity traditionally came from religious and anthropological ideas about the nature of human beings, as well as philosophical reflection on these ideas. The most common Western religious interpretation of why human dignity is "inherent" relies on the argument that humans are created in the likeness of God and so, in this one fundamental aspect of having one element of the sacred or divine in us, are equal. There is not a specific set of external characteristics (i.e., wealth, beauty, culture, accomplishments, personal habits) that makes one person more deserving of respect than anyone else, and because of the privilege of being God-like in our sacredness, each person should be approached with similar high regard.[7]

At the same time, the idea of inherent dignity is not only a religious concept. One interesting historical-anthropological story that attempts to get at the same idea is the ancient Greek myth of the phoenix. The myth says that only one phoenix lived at a time, but after about 500 years the phoenix set its nest on fire, killing itself. From the burning nest a new phoenix arose. The new phoenix then was both the same and different from the one who died and eventually became a symbol of the continuity of all individuals in the form of the one. In other words, the fundamental "essence" of each individual creature was the same as that of the others.[8] But how did belief about humans' shared essence lead to the conclusion that it was

an essence worthy of high regard? Philosophers such as Paul Rabinow and others who have thought about this conclude that the Western religious notion previously described and similar philosophically rooted thinking combined with politically motivated democratic ideas had to become integrated with the anthropology of the phoenix-type myths to ascribe inherent dignity to everyone.[9] From these ideas it is possible to see how humans became deemed worthy of respect on both the individual and the species level.

What should we, physical and occupational therapy ethics educators just over the threshold of the 21st century, make of these narratives? They certainly do not prove (or disprove) the existence of inherent dignity; however, that is not my purpose in sharing them. We can appreciate them as examples of thinking that have worked their way deeply into modern Western, and some forms of Eastern, thought, giving support to the idea of a shared essential human dignity. Everyone has to marvel at the creative juices that flowed to describe the feeling, intuition, and/or hope that we individuals share a deep common humanity worthy of everyone else's regard. There is the collective wisdom of the ages to suggest that we are intricately connected in ways that should engender high regard.

Today, myths are sometimes interpreted and dismissed as untruths, but the accurate understanding of the idea is that they are the deepest truths that come down to us across the ages, incorporating knowledge and understandings of the world current at that time.[10] They are the essential human narratives. So I have no difficulty drawing on them to try to understand what, if anything, is "essentially human."

However, there's a rub. This inquiry into dignity began for us with the concern that in professional ethics writings and practice there seems to be the idea of an inherent dignity, and it is that inherent dignity to which the command of respect attaches in the tradition of the health professions. What if inherent dignity does not exist? Since it is largely derived from the realm of ideas, what about peoples or societies who do not subscribe to those particular beliefs, myths or philosophical assumptions?

Does the concept and role of respect then also fall fallow?

The answer to the latter question is "not necessarily." The weight of intuition is on the side of continuing to understand respect as a pivotal moral resource in the health professions, fostering development of fulfilled and authentic professing persons. We use it in commonsensical ways all the time to ascribe meaning to what we are doing. Fortunately, all peoples continue to create stories about the deep truths that affect their lives, some affirming or refining the old myths, and others critiquing or adding to them. In the future, historians will surely look on our modern understandings of the world as fanciful myths, along with those of the ancient Greeks and other groups who have left behind profound stories. And because we have both the benefit of and the blinders from being steeped in modern Western understandings of ourselves, as individuals in relationship, I invite you to consider some insights about the connection of respect to human flourishing that sidesteps the focus on inherent human dignity while maintaining the view that respect is more than an expression of good manners. More specifically, I will outline key aspects of the kind of thinking that informs such a position, illustrating them with various thoughts from the contemporary idea of moral agency and from modern moral psychology.

Respect and Its Relation to Human Flourishing Today

In my introduction I suggested that the concept of respect traditionally was viewed only as an other-regarding virtue. It is no wonder that from Hippocratic times onward respect has been seen as a good fit with the highest ideals of a line of work where service to others characterizes everyday activity. It is also no wonder that these thoughtful writers searched diligently for what in the other person professionals should hold in high regard and lit on the good idea of dignity.

But these early formative periods, and many centuries thereafter, lacked a fully integrated idea of how a professional's own well-being and interests factor into the societal role she/he willingly agrees to assume. In fact, any discussion of fulfillment is cast in the context of giving, helping, and service to others—an ideal heralded to this day. Anything else is treated as a potential threat to this self-less ideal.

I believe a rich idea of respect that does take the self into account, and as a being not only dedicated to the well-being of others, can be discerned from insights provided by the idea of moral agency and modern moral psychology. In these approaches, respect as a moral virtue is not replaced. Rather some commonsense individual and social reasons for showing respect to others *and oneself* are highlighted. The basic thesis is that only when respect is exercised toward everyone, including the self, can humans flourish.

So far these modern insights could be packaged in the ancient wrapper of inherent human dignity: when one shows respect for everyone's dignity (including the professional's) there is an increased chance for human flourishing. This is important to note because nothing that modern moral agency ideas or modern moral psychology adds necessarily dumps out the older narratives based on inherent dignity.

At the same time, the idea of human flourishing plays a different part in the scheme of moral thought. Dignity is treated as a characteristic attributed to humans that commands a certain kind of virtuous response from others, which in common parlance is termed "respect." In contrast, human flourishing is treated as an individual and societal outcome (or consequence) of a certain kind of virtuous response, which in common parlance is termed respect. The outcome takes a myriad of legitimate forms at the level of individual human flourishing. Although inherent dignity rests on the assumption of our equality, human flourishing focuses on the relevant differences among us. But the idea of human flourishing suggests that it, too, is both an individual and species flourishing. One individual's flourishing cannot be bought at the unjust price of another's. It is this diversity in individual manifestations of human flourishing that allows respect for the health professional's own interests and well-being to be added to the account, suggesting that it too must in fact be boldly brought into the equation. Respect is both a self-regarding and other-regarding virtue.

Insights from the Idea of Agency

The modern idea of moral agency is a philosophical contribution that has emerged as Western cultures have become more secular and individualized. An agent of any kind (e.g., a legal agent, moral agent) is one who has both the responsibility and the authority to "call the shots" in a certain domain delegated to him or her. Responsibility simply means that the buck stops with the agent. Authority means the person has the power to affect certain consequences and if she or he chooses to do so, it cannot legitimately be blamed on someone else when the effort fails. Conversely, if it succeeds, the agent has the prerogative of taking all the credit if she or he chooses. Sometimes society confers authority on the basis of "office" so that one becomes the person "in authority" simply by one's accidental position in society. Parenting, royal succession to the throne, and becoming the new chief executive officer by virtue of inheritance in a family-owned company are examples that could have both moral and legal bases in Western societies. At other times conferring of authority rests on the judgment that the person is "an authority" by virtue of her skill, knowledge or other attributes. Health professionals, of course, fall into the second category. A moral agent is one who has been given responsibility and authority for decisions affecting society's deep moral fabric.

Drawing on the way Western laws have interpreted this individualistic idea, there are two kinds of agency relationships; the latter is relevant to the discussion here: In contract relationships each party is assumed to have equal authority and responsibility to get the agreement right to the benefit of both (thus the entreaty to "read the fine print"). In fiduciary ("fides" [L], meaning faithfulness) relationships the idea is that a person or group is required to put well-placed trust in the agent and the agent is obliged to be trust-worthy. The underlying assumption is that there is responsibility on the part of the agent to act with care for the other's best interests because the latter cannot do that alone. American agency law treats the health professional and patient relationship as a fiduciary relationship, suggesting that society gets the point of its own vulnerability and requires the health professional agent to assume the moral characteristic of trust-worthiness.[11]

At least two conditions are necessary for a person who is "an authority" to garner the necessary confidence and courage that taking responsibility for an outcome requires:

First, she must be capable of making such decisions. One hears echoes of what professional education strives to do, namely to create a cadre of people in society who are competent to assume appropriate responsibility for outcomes related to others' health care–related needs.

Second, in order to sustain her responsibility effectively, she must be able to live with herself when she goes home at the end of the day. Living with herself at the end of the day requires that she be able to face inevitable mistakes, deal with guilt when corners are necessarily cut in order to balance competing claims, call on support when she needs it, and find the inner strength to go on. It also means being able to say, "I did my best," "I am doing an important job," "My contributions matter." In other words, she needs the wherewithal to conclude what any *self respecting* person would conclude, namely, "I take my professional, including its moral, obligations extremely seriously and as a person-who-professes I am playing out my professional role as diligently as I can." So self respect plays center stage as a necessary component of doing one's job well over the course, and in the context, of living a good life.

Insights from Psychology

How does a health professional gain this necessary self respect? It cannot be accomplished in isolation. Here I call on an analysis of modern moral psychology that relies less (or not at all) on an idea that moral claims spring from the fact that another has human dignity and, therefore, one must show respect to him/her. It relies, in addition, or instead, on an understanding of humans in relationships with each other who respond to claims on the judgment that oneself as an individual and as a member of the species is more likely to flourish. John Rawls, the recently deceased (2002)

American moral philosopher, uses this understanding of moral psychology as an underpinning for his approach to human flourishing. I choose him because he has often been called the most influential Western moral philosopher of modern times. His theories reflect assumptions consistent with postmodern, scientific, highly individualistic, and secularized societies. No medieval myths dominate his thought. His basic approach falls within the school of "social contract" philosophy, the basic psychological premises of which are that members of a society simply "contract" a set of agreements that work well for them. In a well-working society each individual is psychologically motivated to act out of self interest, but this self interest will, in fact, push them to agree to certain social arrangements that help ensure some common-good goals are met in the process. There is nothing more than that to call upon in determining what human flourishing involves.

The idea of inherent human dignity does not figure in his scheme, but it is noteworthy that respect plays a central role. Unlike older analyses that make respect solely an other-regarding virtue, directed toward honoring the other's dignity, Rawls makes *self* respect the engine that drives the whole system toward human flourishing. However, this is not the kind of self respect that might be confused today with self satisfaction in an egotistic sense. Although he ties self respect to the psychological notion of self esteem, he is not concerned only with "self actualization." Self esteem, he argues, is a resource that buoys up self respect in very particular ways in modern societies: The person with high self esteem is more likely to make choices of societal arrangements that are not good only for himself but for everyone, and that in turn will bolster self respect because he has become a force to help assure human species flourishing (not the least of which is his own flourishing). Neither self esteem nor its result, self respect, is gained in a social vacuum. Rawls describes the process accordingly: "Self esteem grows as a result of positive feedback from others that one 'is somebody.' This understanding of one's own worth within the larger societal context allows one to have high regard for the societal tasks one assumes. The point is

crucial because strong self respect positions a person psychologically to lay claim to societal resources." When self respect is dealt a blow by society's negative treatment, the person tends to internalize it as shame and his confidence in his value suffers. Moreover, the shame takes on a moral dimension: "In such a society we are liable to moral shame when we lack characteristics that our own identity depends on for a feeling of worth and fulfillment and which society encourages us to realize."[12]

The burden of moral shame is not just a private one when a person has assumed a societal role that requires advocacy for others. "In moral shame we focus on our infringement of what we have come to believe are the just claims of others and the injury we have done to them and on their probable (deserved) resentment or indignation towards us."[12]

It requires no imagination to make the connection between an occupational therapist's or physical therapist's self respect and her ability to go home at night knowing she did what any person could and should do to fulfill the just claims of others on her regarding her societal role, in other words, to do her fair share in fostering human flourishing.

An understanding at the outset of her career that she deserves self respect because of her willingness to uphold the other-regarding values required by her special societal role will have several very practical positive effects: She will appreciate that one great price of not having self respect is that it will psychologically undermine her very ability to demand the necessary conditions to do her job successfully. She will be less tempted than generations before her have been to think that society's indignation is warranted when there is resistance to increased support for her services (e.g., resistance to an increase in reimbursement rates for physical therapy or occupational therapy services) or that the devaluing of her skills in relation to, say, a physician's is understandable. She will be better prepared psychologically than many of her predecessors to resist internalizing shame and guilt when she fails against all odds to do what is in the best interest of the patient or client. Her self respect should help her seek out colleagues, and with them, make it clear that they expect/demand policies and practice guidelines that prevent them from being stripped of their appropriate moral role in society. She will be better prepared to boldly fix her gaze on the moral goals of care and thereby recognize that her moral/ethical distress is caused by institutional injustices imposed on physical therapists and occupational therapists when they are being held responsible as moral agents but barriers to their success are being thrown into their path.[13] These are just a few of the benefits of becoming fully cognizant of and empowered by the view that society itself has given "the professional" an important moral role to play in human flourishing and, therefore, society must help meet the expectations of that role.

In short, the insights gained from moral psychology help to highlight how a professionally prepared person's inner resources in the form of self respect and his experience of social support and belongingness work to create the appropriate role for the professions. Self respect and a person's respect for the conditions that support everyone's flourishing are deeply interrelated. A self concept characterized by low self respect, as one who has "defects," becomes the occasion for moral shame because she does not, then, have the courage to do what should be done such as effectively advocate on behalf of patients for their fair share of society's resources. Obviously professional educational experiences that clothe the person in self respect help to counter this tragedy. One can conclude with confidence that the modern psychological understanding of how self respect becomes a source of social empowerment, combined with the notion of moral agency, provide a convincing contemporary narrative for ways that respect is relevant for professional ethics today. The respect can only be deepened by the added notion of human dignity.

✧ RESPECT IN THE DETAILS

You might conclude with me that respect as both an other-regarding and self-regarding moral concept has utility within the health professions ethos and still not know fully how it

should be expressed in the everyday lives of professing persons.

At the outset of this chapter, I suggested some examples (e.g., maintaining a person's modesty or privacy) of common indicators that the person is being shown respect. There is an intuitive seed of truth in those examples insofar as it is difficult to launch a convincing argument against them, and I, for one, have been persistent in advocating for them. But the writers who wanted to go deeper (to an idea of inherent dignity) were right in judging that those kinds of details taken alone are weak building blocks for creating a robust marker of respect because they (and others such as autonomous individual decision-making) stand the chance of being based on nothing more than manners or personal biases conceived in mainstream American life. Professionals in occupational therapy and physical therapy, still overwhelmingly Anglo-white, English-speaking, middle-to-upper–middle-class adults, can impose polite conduct without the slightest reflection on what it means to other persons or groups and get by with appearing as if respect were being shown. In Wells' insightful contribution to this volume, she highlights the challenge before us by taking the dominant moral principle of autonomy as an example of how showing respect for individual decision-making may not always be a show of respect: "Currently the principle of autonomy is at the center of medical decision-making .... Yet much of the world, if not most, embraces a value system that places the family, the community or the society as a whole above that of the individual ... conflicts around issues, such as autonomy, have raised questions about whether principles of autonomy and veracity are truly respectful of all people in all cultures."[14]

Philosophers often look for "middle principles" or "middle axioms" to connect a concept with the real life challenge. I suggest that for the concept of respect such principles can be found in current approaches to incorporating cultural competency into the everyday expectations of the health professions. Cultural competence has been defined as "a set of congruent behaviors, attitudes and policies that come together to work effectively in cross-cultural situations."[15]

Although attaining a command of cultural competence during one's professional preparation does not ensure that one will internalize an attitude of respect that fosters human flourishing in its myriad of forms, at least the professing person will have had the opportunity to undergo a formal learning and reflection process on what is at stake in honoring diversity.

There are several methods available for instilling cultural competency into educational curricula. It goes beyond the scope of my analysis (and ability) to fully examine the educational experiences that might help prepare students to become authentic professing persons by gaining competence in an area that strikes to the heart of values, meaning, and beliefs of the people who seek their services. However, I offer one example of what each student could have an opportunity to think about and master. The Cultural Competency Instrument is designed to identify levels of cultural competence and proficiency of health care providers. Exercises are designed to take each student through his or her own level until competence is attained:

Level 1. Cultural destructiveness

Level 2. Cultural incapacity

Level 3. Cultural blindness

Level 4. Cultural pre-competence

Level 5. Cultural competence

The last three levels focus on communication, indicating that the listener attempts to understand the beliefs, attitudes, and practices of the other.[15] Both self respect for the job to be accomplished and respect for cultural and other differences in the variety of patients or clients could be enhanced by students who completed their physical therapy or occupational therapy professional preparation with this kind of competence.

✧ RESPECT FOR RESPECT— A CONCLUDING PERSONAL NOTE

When we began the Dreamcatchers project my original abstract for my contribution simply declared that "respect and moral courage" were solid building blocks for a modern professional ethic. But I confess that as I began to write, and reflect on my several years of writing on the topic of respect, I became less confident of my own premise. Thus, this chapter has given me an opportunity to take the idea out of the drawer and examine respect itself.

Probing critiques on my initial draft by members of the working group added to my thinking, and to the extent I did not benefit thoroughly from their input, it is to your detriment as well as my own. In any case, I have emerged with a new respect for respect as a virtue that can serve us and others well, especially as it allows health professionals to more fully understand their role as contributors to the well-being of society and the self respect required for sustaining their contributions. I am more than ever convinced that it—and all of the moral concepts upon which we rely for our professional ethic—need to be shaken out and taken apart for examination as situations change, but that we seldom do so. I remain convinced that respect is not the only virtue, and that, if idolized, any of them will create the same kind of dilemmas we have created by allowing "autonomy" to have a monopoly on our moral attention in modern health care ethics. In a word, I have a new respect for some of the origins, the potentials, and the limitations of respect in ethics education. I invite you, the reader, to continue to explore these ideas with me.

References

1. Pellegrino ED, and Thomasma DC: The Virtues in Medical Practice. Oxford University Press, New York, 1993.
2. Purtilo R, and Haddad A: Respect: The difference it makes. In Purtilo R (ed): Health Professional and Patient Interaction. WB Saunders, Philadelphia, 2002, pp 3–18.
3. Wear D, and Bickel J (eds): Educating for Professionalism: Creating a Culture of Humanism in Medical Education. University of Iowa Press, Iowa City, IA, 2000.
4. Aiken LH, et al: Hospital nurse staffing and patient mortality, nurse burnout and job dissatisfaction. JAMA 288(16):1987–1993, 1986.
5. Pullman D: Human dignity and the ethics and aesthetics of pain and suffering. Theor Med Bioeth 23:75–94, 2002.
6. United Nations General Assembly. Universal Declaration of Human Rights. 1948.

7. Lammers SE, and Verhay A (eds): On Moral Medicine: Theological Perspectives in Medical Ethics. ed 2. William B. Eerdmans, Grand Rapids, MI, 1998.

8. Kantorowitz E: The King's Two Bodies: A Study of Medieval Political Theology. Princeton University Press, Princeton, NJ, 1957.

9. Rabinow P: Essays on the Anthropology of Reason. Princeton University Press, Princeton, NJ, 1996.

10. Frazer JG: The Golden Bough: A Study in Magic and Religion. Macmillan, New York, 1922.

11. Garner BA (ed): Black's Law Dictionary. ed 7. West Group, St. Paul, MN, 2001.

12. Rawls J: A Theory of Justice. Harvard University Press, Cambridge, MA, 1971.

13. Purtilo R: Ethical Dimensions in the Health Professions. ed 4. WB Saunders, Philadelphia, 2004.

14. Wells SA, and Black RM: Cultural Competency for Health Professionals. American Occupational Therapy Association, Bethesda, MD, 2000.

15. Cross TL, et al: Towards a culturally competent system of care, vol 1. Georgetown University Child Development Center, Washington, DC and CASSP Technical Assistance Center, Washington, DC, 1989.

2

Affirming Empathy as a Moral Disposition

SUZANNE MARIE PELOQUIN, PHD, OTR, FAOTA

Abstract

In the health care literature, empathy has been discussed as a capacity that disposes individuals toward effective communication and helping. One common theme in occupational therapy and physical therapy is that empathy is foundational to therapeutic relationships and compassionate helping. The aim of this reflective piece is to explore the conceptual dimensions of a related but distinct question: Might empathy be considered, more radically, as a *moral* disposition for practice?

The meaning of morality is multidimensional. Moral behavior is commonly understood as conformity with standards of right and wrong, with terms like "ethical," "virtuous," "righteous," and "noble" termed synonymous. Each of the synonyms casts a different spin on moral behavior. Ethical behavior, for example, is thought to be the enactment of ethical principles in health care, such as autonomy, justice, beneficence, nonmaleficence, fidelity, veracity, and confidentiality. Virtuous behavior, by contrast, is associated with virtue, understood as excellence and efficaciousness. Righteous behavior is behavior that is genuinely good. And noble behavior is thought to be a manifestation of superior character or a possession of outstanding qualities.

Might practitioners in both disciplines be inclined to be ethical, virtuous, righteous, and noble if empathy were openly declared as a radical attitude? Might practitioners grounded in empathy be empowered as moral agents in delivery systems that are perceived as depersonalized? These questions shape this reflection.

Empathy may be described as a tendency toward understanding through which one person apprehends the perspectives and feelings of another. The common dictionary definition of the term empathy is the ability to share in another's thoughts or emotions.[1] Colloquially, the metaphor of walking a mile in another's shoes illustrates the empathic process for most. In the last century, much has been written about the nature, development, and manifestations of empathy. It is not surprising that within this large body of literature that either hypothesizes and postulates, elaborates and illustrates, or researches and educates on empathy, common themes emerge alongside distinct views. In health care disciplines, the construct has been widely discussed as a capacity that disposes individuals toward effective communication and helping.

The aim of this reflection is to explore three interrelated questions: Might empathy be considered a radical moral disposition for occupational and physical therapy practice? Might practitioners in both disciplines be inclined to be ethical, virtuous, righteous, and noble—the many ways of being that are associated with the term moral—if empathy were openly declared a radical or fundamental attitude? Might practitioners grounded in empathy be empowered as moral agents within delivery systems perceived as depersonalized? These questions might be explored in many ways. Within this piece; however, I discuss (1) common themes about empathy that course through occupational therapy and physical therapy literature, (2) less-considered links between the concepts of morality and empathy, and (3) select practical issues related to the affirmation of empathy as a moral disposition.

✧ COMMON THEMES IN PROFESSIONAL PRACTICE

An apt starting point for this discussion is with an understanding of congruent themes related to empathy and found within the occupational and physical therapy literature. One shared theme reflects the belief held across most helping professions that empathy disposes individuals toward effective communication and helping. This belief is broadened and deepened in our literature, with the claim that empathy supports therapeutic relationships and compassionate helping.

Cited in both disciplines, Carl Rogers described empathy as a way of being.[2] He captured the metaphor of walking in another's shoes while intimating empathy's link with relationship and compassion:

The way of being with another person, which is termed empathic, has several facets. It means entering the private perceptual world of the other and becoming thoroughly at home in it. It involves being sensitive, moment to moment, to the changing felt meanings which flow in this other person. … It means temporarily living in his or her life, moving about in it delicately without making judgments. … It includes communicating your sensings of his/her world as you look with fresh and unfrightened eyes at that which the individual is fearful. It means frequently checking with him/her as to the accuracy of your sensing, and being guided by the response you receive.[2]

Because this description occurred within a discussion of helping, Rogers' depiction of empathy might be seen as applied or practical. Rogers argued that some situations called for the empathic way of being: "When the other person is hurting, confused, troubled, anxious, alienated, terrified; or when he or she is doubtful of self-worth, uncertain as to identity."[2] Personal encounters in health care practice seem precisely such situations. Sadly, Rogers noted a rarity of empathy in health care, entitling his discussion "Empathy, an unappreciated way of being."[2]

One aim of this reflection is to ask questions about empathy that are more conceptual. Because conceptual discussions within occupational therapy and physical therapy place empathy in a practice context, practical illustrations emerge alongside conceptual views. The following sampling, if not exhausting the topic of empathy in both professions, captures points salient to this discussion.

In a physical therapy text on developing the art of health care, Davis characterized empathy as a "merging with another person in a unique moment of shared meaning."[3] Turning to interpersonal interactions, she argued the importance of the aspect of empathy thought to be a listening with the "third ear." She recapitulated the early phenomenological work of Edith Stein, agreeing that empathy "happens" to individuals after they have cognitively attended to another person in a self-transposal that is a "cognitive thinking of oneself into the position of the other."[4]

Davis noted that the intersubjective process of empathy happens when a practitioner feels at one with another and the other, in turn, senses a holistic listening.[5] In this way, Davis said, empathy "can unite the therapist with the patient, yet allow the patient and the therapist to remain fully separate in the healing process."[5] Davis agreed with Stein that empathy happens in three stages: self transposal or cognitive attention; identification or crossing over; fellow feeling or sympathy.[4] She argued the merits of empathy for physical therapy practice, saying that "empathy empowers us to listen deeply, to communicate humanistically and therapeutically, thus contributing to helpful helping."[5]

Within a phenomenological research study, Davis examined the views of physical therapists about their experiences with empathy. Each therapist had experienced stages like those described by Stein: (1) a kind of listening and cognitive attempt to understand, (2) an emotional deepening, and (3) a strong feeling of "at one-ness with the other person."[4,5]

Within occupational therapy, theoretician Anne Mosey launched a conceptual discourse on empathy, identifying it as an aspect of the art of practice.[6] She distinguished empathy from a desire to help others, the skilled application of scientific knowledge, or the act of being systematic or sympathetic. She warned that the science of occupational therapy, applied without its art, would occur in a sterile vacuum.[6]

Several years ago, when considering empathy in occupational therapy, I found the wide-ranging and synthetic conceptual work of Robert Katz helpful.[7] Katz said: "A simple way to explain the origins of the empathic skill is to postulate that we are born to understand. Part of our biological heritage is the capacity to visualize and to apprehend the feelings of other members of our species."[7]

Katz reminded readers that the word empathy originated in the psychology of aesthetics in 1897 when Theodore Lipps introduced the term "einfühlung" to explain how a person "feels into" art forms to appreciate them.[7] The term later acquired interpersonal meaning when Titchener identified the act of reading the bodily movements of another as a rendering of einfühlung.[8]

Katz described empathic engagement as a number of constituting actions that I have understood as (a) an expression of being there, (b) a turning of the soul, (c) a recognition in the other of both likeness and uniqueness, (d) an entry into the other's experience, (e) a connection with the other's feelings, (f) a power to recover from that connection, and (g) a personal enrichment that derives from these actions.[7,9] It was easy for me to find illustrations of each of these actions within *The Healing Heart*, a biography of Ora Ruggles, an early reconstruction aide and later occupational therapist who worked in many settings.[9,10] After considering stories of her practice, I observed that "to be present to one's patients empathically is to take a stand from which one participates in their experiences. Such a supportive stance is aptly named an understanding."[9]

Rogers' characterization of empathy as an unappreciated way of being captured is a theme in both professions that frames an ambivalence about making emotional connections that could be troubling or painful.[2] The call for objectivity and level-headedness in practice seems counter to the call for the fellow feeling implicit in empathy. In occupational therapy, this difficulty was reflected in an early mandate to be impersonally personal with patients, a way of being that is hard to envision.[11] Purtilo and Haddad regretted that messages in the health professions about the need to consider respectful boundaries had somehow metamorphosed into a mistaken idea that a dichotomy exists between professional and personal ways of being.[12]

Years ago, I encouraged occupational therapy practitioners to take an empathic stand, to use friendship and covenanting partnership as more helpful guiding images than the image of being impersonally personal.[13] I thought it wise to acknowledge and address the inherent challenges of empathy while emphasizing the gains: "Empathy does not exact a fusion but a connection. It implies an experience not only of the pain of another, but of the integrity and courage that dwell alongside the pain. Empathy, in health care practice, can be seen as an enactment of the conviction that, empowered by someone's willingness to understand, the patient will gather a measure of courage."[9]

Important to mention, perhaps, is the fact that practitioners who empathize say they are not burned out but strengthened by empathic engagements. Ruggles felt that in helping others, she helped herself; she said that with the passing of years, she "felt more than rich."[10] Her words call to mind the empathic enrichment of which Katz spoke.[7]

This quick overview of common themes across occupational therapy and physical therapy literature establishes, in brief, that we see the merits of empathy as relating to therapeutic relationships and compassionate helping. Further reflection that builds on but moves past these themes will address the central question that prompted this overview: Might empathy be considered, conceptually, a moral disposition for occupational and physical therapy practice? The professional and conceptual literature on empathy, examined more deeply with this question in mind, offers connections between empathy and morality that are less often considered.

✧ REFRAMING EMPATHY AS A MORAL DISPOSITION: CONCEPTUAL CONSIDERATIONS

A first step in addressing the question of whether empathy might be conceptualized as a moral disposition is a consideration of what most people understand to be the concept of morality. When one examines dictionary definitions, the meaning of morality emerges as multidimensional.[1] Moral behavior is commonly understood as a rather all-encompassing conformity with standards of right and wrong, synonymous with terms like ethical, virtuous, noble, and righteous. Each synonym casts a slightly different spin on moral behavior. Ethical behavior, for example, is thought to be the enactment of ethical principles, such as autonomy, justice, beneficence, nonmaleficence, fidelity, veracity, and confidentiality. Virtuous behavior, by contrast, is associated with virtue, which is defined as excellence and efficaciousness. Righteous behavior is genuinely good, associating with individuals considered to be upright. And noble behavior is thought to be a manifestation of superior character or a possession of outstanding qualities.

Another term that begs clarification is the term "disposition." A disposition is a tendency or inclination to act in a certain manner.[1] A person disposed toward moral behavior is, thus, inclined to engage in it. A disposition is also understood as a typical orientation, as when one is said to have a sunny disposition. To propose that empathy is a moral disposition is to suggest that a person who typically engages in empathy is disposed to moral action. Another way to frame my question about empathy as a moral disposition is to consider MacIntyre's reasoning about the internal goods of any practice.[14] He argued that a practice is any coherent form of activity within which goods internal to that activity are realized in the course of meeting its standards. From this viewpoint, empathy and morality are practices. MacIntyre's example

might clarify his view: Chess players, or practitioners of chess, can increase their capacity to solve problems—with problem solving seen as a good internal to chess—as they master the game.[14] I am thus asking, conceptually, if it seems reasonable to suggest that empathizers can increase their capacity for moral action—a good internal to empathy, by empathizing.

Interestingly, discussions of the measurement of empathy in the 20th century included a connection with morality. When Hogan described his development of a scale to measure empathy, he noted that empathy might be seen as the capacity to adopt a *moral* point of view, that is, to consider the implications of one's actions for the welfare of others.[15] In addition, historians have made the connection between 19th century compassionate and occupation-based moral treatment practices among mentally ill patients and occupational therapy's reclamation of a similar form of care in the early 20th century.[16,17] Although the term "moral" in the 19th century aligns more with our understanding of the term "affective," the connection is interesting.

One last term that I will clarify is the term "radical." When I suggest that empathy be considered a radical disposition, I mean that it be considered a fundamental and essential disposition for one who would be moral. I am suggesting that empathy seems to be at the root or foundation of morality.[1] I am not suggesting that this connection seems in any way extreme, a more colloquial meaning attached to the term radical.

Back to the question: Can empathy and morality be so conceptually linked that empathy emerges, radically, as a moral disposition? I believe so. I suggest that empathy is a moral disposition because empathic engagement disposes individuals to action that is moral in its many dimensions: ethical, virtuous, righteous, and noble. From MacIntyre's standpoint, I suggest that the practice of empathy can develop the practice of morality.[14] I restrict myself to the four more commonly used and understood dictionary dimensions of morality, realizing that other constructs, such as role virtues and character ethics, elaborated within the bioethics literature and elsewhere, may prompt more reflection later.

Empathy as a Disposition Toward Ethical Behavior

Empathy can be characterized as a radical moral disposition in that it disposes individuals toward ethical behavior, which is understood as an upholding of ethical principles. Ethical behavior is often captured in a familiar proverb cast as the golden rule. Used as a touchstone for moral action, that rule is colloquially stated as "Do unto others as you would have them do unto you." The rule crosses cultures and religions, sometimes as a call not so much to beneficence as to an overarching non-maleficence. Kornblau and Starling shared several rules that they considered equivalents to the golden rule.[18] In Buddhism, for example, the statement is "Hurt not others in ways that you yourself would find hurtful" from Udan-Varga 5:18. And in Islam, there is "No one of you is a believer until he desires for his brother that which he desires for himself" from Sunnah. And from Confucianism, "Surely it is the maxim of loving-kindness: Do not unto others that which you would not have them do unto you" from Analects 15, 23.

How, then, might empathy be seen to dispose individuals toward ethical behavior? Consider the behavioral rule drawn from empathy that reads, "Do unto others as they would have you do unto them." Business visionaries call this mandate the platinum rule, thought a higher standard for interpersonal behavior because the monetary value of platinum exceeds that of gold.[19] Empathy cast as a rule is, thus, a mandate for ethical behavior in its call for the upholding of an overarching beneficence as seen from the other's perspective. Following this "rule of empathy" disposes one toward ethical action.

Katz made a similar point about empathy's ethical nature, saying, "Metaphysically, the basis of empathy is the belief in the brotherhood of man."[7] Katz pressed further, saying that a practitioner better appreciates the "psychological and ethical truth" of being a brother's keeper after taking the role of another. More essentially, Katz argued that "at the core of empathy is ethical concern for the sacredness of the individual."[7] Empathy, seen as a beneficent action based on fellowship, with an ethical good internal to its practice, is a moral disposition toward ethical behavior.

Empathy as a Disposition Toward Virtuous Behavior

Empathy can be characterized as a radical moral disposition in that it disposes individuals toward virtuous behavior, understood as an efficacious practice of excellences. If one examines the excellences ascribed to occupational and physical therapy professions in their broadest articulation, they are the science and art of practice. Efficacious practice requires a confluence of artistry and science, best seen as complementary functions for meeting personal needs.[20] Whether one names the professional excellences (or virtues) more broadly as science and art or less so as competence and caring, the principle of efficacious integration is the same. Collins and Porras likened such dual excellences to a beneficial yin and yang.[21] One would not, they said, "blend yin and yang into a gray indistinguishable circle that is neither highly yin nor highly yang; it aims to be distinctly yin AND distinctly yang—both at the same time, all the time."[21] If this broad professional view of virtue as dual excellences seems to stretch the meaning of the term virtuous for some, an argument can be made that personal virtues (integrity, trustworthiness, fortitude, and prudence, for example) are associated with the professional practice of artistry and science.

How, then, might empathy be seen to dispose individuals toward virtuous behavior? Empathy, itself an integrative process of thinking and feeling, disposes individuals toward the wholeness that integrity in practice implies. Coursing through discussions of empathy is the idea that empathy is a whole-person process. Empathy requires that individuals be cognitively and affectively engaged and, thus, both reflects and disposes individuals toward realizing the "genius of the AND" applauded by Collins and Porras.[21]

The integrative nature of empathy is also clear from its other dualities. The description given earlier by Rogers illustrates activity and passivity, attending and responding, receiving and giving.[2] Both Katz and Stein identified similar complementarities.[4,7] Fundamentally, empathy is grounded in a human paradox: Persons are alike enough that they can grasp their similarities and different enough that they must strive to understand their differences. Ease with the integrative aspects of empathy disposes one to the practice of integrated excellences essential for occupational and physical therapy. Empathy, seen as a whole-person and integrative action, with virtuous good internal to its practice, is a moral disposition toward virtuous behavior.

Empathy as a Disposition Toward Righteous Behavior

Empathy can be characterized as a radical moral disposition in that it disposes individuals toward righteous behavior, understood as behavior that is genuinely good. Within the professions of occupational and physical therapy, one finds a commitment to genuine goodness that transcends goodness of skill or goodness of strategy to include personal attitudes and values that together constitute the ethos of a profession. Generally defined as its essential character, a profession's ethos is colloquially considered its soul. In this light, a professional ethos might be seen as a collective way of being. At personal and professional levels, acts of genuine goodness do, in fact, evoke images of "being a good soul."

Hoping to nudge helpers closer to seeing the inadequacy of mere skills training, Plum cited R.D. Laing, who metaphorically highlighted the need for what I call a goodness of soul in an act of giving:[22,23]

It is not so easy for one person to give another a cup of tea. If a lady gives me a cup of tea, she might be showing off her teapot, or her tea set; she might be trying to put me in a good mood in order to get something out of me; she may be trying to get me to like her; she might be wanting me as an ally for her own purposes against others. She might pour tea from a pot into a cup and shove out her hand with cup and saucer in it, whereupon I am expected to grab them within two seconds before they will become dead weight. The action could be a mechanical one in which there is no recognition of me in it. A cup of tea could be handed me without me being given a cup of tea.[23]

Laing here described actions that seem frivolous and hollow, self-serving or mechanical, without a goodness of soul.[23]

Inquiring into physical therapy, Stiller interviewed therapists who identified the profession's ethos as the enduring traits of caring and helping, warmth and openness, all expressions of goodness.[24] Romanella and Knight-Abowitz described an ethic of care in physical therapy: "Care in the relationship between the physical therapist and the patient often has been seen as that activity that reflects an attitude of sensitivity to the patient's deepest values and concerns and constructively addresses them."[25]

In a review of significant visions promoted within occupational therapy since its founding, I sought the profession's ethos.[26] I found salient references, including these words of Kidner, one of the profession's founders:[27]

In your chosen field, a part of the noblest work of man—the care and relief of weak and suffering humanity—may you realize in increasing measure the value of certain spiritual things which are the real making of life, but which we call by many common names. Kindness, humanity, decency, honor, and good faith—to give these up under any circumstances whatever would be a loss greater than any defeat, or even death itself.[27]

The most elegant and profound vision of the occupational therapy ethos, however, was this: "It is not enough to give a patient something to do with his hands. You must reach for the heart as well as the hands. It's the heart that really does the healing."[10]

How, then, might empathy be seen to dispose individuals toward such righteous, or genuinely good behavior? Rogers' characterization of empathy as a way of being present to another, "sensitive, moment to moment, to the changing felt meanings which flow in the other" comes to mind.[2] When one remembers the nonjudgmental nature of this sensitivity, its righteousness seems clear.[2] Even more notably, one of empathy's actions has been likened to a turning of the soul, not unlike the feeling of at-oneness described by Davis.[5,7] Both depth of regard and goodness inhere in such an action. Neither soul turning nor feeling at-one with another is a superficial attention to problems, mindless use of protocols, or rote application of communication skills. The kind of being-there that is described is a personal presence to another, much like Buber's sense of dialogue in an I-Thou relationship.[28] Empathy, seen as a soul turning or meaningful merging, with real goodness internal to its practice, is a moral disposition toward righteous behavior.

Empathy as a Disposition Toward Noble Behavior

Empathy can be characterized as a radical moral disposition in that it disposes individuals toward noble behavior, understood as a manifestation of superior character and outstanding qualities. Superior moral character attaches to individuals known to have gumption, spirit, or heart. We name noble acts of character brave-hearted and courageous. We see such outstanding acts as inspiring others. Purtilo described moral courage in physical therapy as a superior form of character, explaining it as "a readiness for voluntary, purposive action in situations that engender realistic fear and anxiety in order to uphold something of great moral value."[29] Courageous therapists are those whose outstanding qualities lead them to risk much for noble causes. They may serve in advocacy roles, engage in fearful political action, press practice into global realms, lead public debate over policy decisions, or launch provocative discourse. The call to moral courage invites actions proposed by Davies: engender restlessness through the system; disturb complacency; and insist that rules be broken when there is good and sufficient reason.[30]

One finds such courage in Van Amburg's moral critique of the occupational therapy profession's call for objectivity in therapeutic relationships within an earlier version of the *Occupational Therapy Code of Ethics*.[31,32] Through this code, he said, "The problem of disengaged, depersonalized therapeutic relationships is exacerbated."[31] Van Amburg supported engagement, instead, arguing that an overemphasis on objectivity and autonomy harms patients and practitioners alike.[31] His stand was bold; it took courage to voice his view.

How might empathy dispose individuals toward such noble behavior? When Treizenberg and Davis advocated moral development that transcends the teaching of moral codes to prepare physical therapists as moral agents, they endorsed a confluent cultivation of empathy, skills for action, and personal courage.[33] Certainly, courage is needed for empathy. Katz described the countervailing pull that an empathizer feels:[7] "It is the power which pulls him back from intimacy with the client for fear that something will endanger him. He fears being possessed by the demons who already dominate his patient and who are poised within him too and ready to seize power. He would like to keep the sparks of the client's anxiety from reaching him and kindling."[7]

Rogers' description of empathy also conveys the courage of one who looks "with fresh and unfrightened eyes at that which the individual is fearful."[2] Most agree that several actions within empathy take courage: an expression of being there; a turning of the soul; an entry into the other's experience; a connection with the other's feelings; a crossing over; a fellow feeling.[5,7] Empathy, seen as an expression of courage, with a noble good internal to its practice, is a moral disposition toward noble behavior.

An Overview of the Conceptual Analysis

This conceptual analysis of empathy suggests that it is reasonable to affirm empathy as a radical moral disposition. Seen conceptually as fundamental to morality, empathy might be framed as essential to professional development. Current links made between empathy and either interpersonal relationships or compassionate helping may portray empathy as "soft" or "esoteric," the fluffy periphery rather than solid substance of practice. Instead, professionals might affirm empathy's radical links to ethical, virtuous, righteous, and noble behavior, establishing these four manifestations of morality as cornerstones for practice.

Two related and practical questions already addressed, to some extent within this conceptual analysis, bear repeating here: Might practitioners in both disciplines be inclined to be ethical, virtuous, righteous, or noble if empathy were openly declared as a radical attitude? And might practitioners grounded in empathy be empowered as moral agents in delivery systems that are perceived as depersonalized? It would seem so. Table 2.1 provides a brief recapitulation of the four dimensions of morality and their conceptual links with empathy.

✧ REFRAMING EMPATHY AS A MORAL DISPOSITION: PRACTICAL CONSIDERATIONS

Illustrations of what an empathic practice might look like have already emerged from this analysis of empathy. Select practical concerns that go beyond those already discussed seem important to mention. One of these is the current context created by health care systems.

Empathy and Health Delivery Systems

Presently, most professionals discuss threats to moral practice. Purtilo's image of a shifting health care landscape captures the unsure footing and imbalance felt by practitioners for whom paradigm shifts have challenged priorities and values.[34] The empathic stance, a powerful position based on ethical and holistic principles, may give strong footing and better balance. The shifting landscape is so unsettling that Treizenberg and Davis made a persuasive case for moral agents who are "called to *be* something."[33] Purtilo, remember, named the

Table 2.1 ✧ An Overview of the Suggestion that Empathy is a Radical Moral Disposition for Practice			
MORALITY ARTICULATED IN ITS VARIOUS ASPECTS	MORALITY'S ASPECTS DEFINED	THE POSTULATE	SUPPORT FOR THE POSTULATE
Morality is ethical behavior.	Ethical behavior is the enactment of ethical principles, such as beneficence.	Ethical action can flow from empathy.	Empathy enhances an other-centered beneficence. Empathy grounds practice; is behavior for the sake of fellowship and the sacredness of humanity.
Morality is virtuous action.	Virtuous behavior is the enactment of excellence and efficaciousness.	Virtuous action can flow from empathy.	Empathy's whole-person dynamic is a disposition to personal integrity and holistic practice. Empathy prompts efficacious integration of the art and science (the excellences) of practice.
Morality is righteous action.	Righteous behavior is genuinely good behavior.	Righteous action can flow from empathy.	Empathy calls for a goodness of soul that transforms skilled performances into real giving. Empathy is a way of being that supports a profession's caring ethos.
Morality is noble action.	Noble behavior is a manifestation of superior character and outstanding qualities.	Noble behavior can flow from empathy.	Empathy takes personal character and moral courage. Empathy invites bravehearted behavior and moral agency.

call of the new millennium "a call to courage."[29] Opacich agreed, warning that therapists "must reiterate which philosophical beliefs and ethical commitments they hold dear or risk being defined by cost-controlling strategies that do not accommodate" values.[35] The empathic way of being, good and courageous in its essence, seems an apt response to the call.

Another delivery system concern touches two functions that occupational and physical therapy practitioners commonly link with empathy: therapeutic relationships and compassionate helping. A poignant patient complaint related to these functions emerged in the 1980s from within phenomenological literature: Health care is depersonalized. Patients elaborated on the complaint, criticizing caregiver behaviors such as these: (1) failure to see the personal consequences of illness or disability, (2) establishment of a distance that felt dismissive, (3) harmful withholdings of care and information, (4) the use of discouraging words when encouragement was needed, (5) engagement in brusque and rude behaviors, and (6) a misuse of power that precludes collaborative partnering.[36] Similar complaints can still be heard today. They shape a plea for a morality grounded in fellowship.

Practitioners, also writing during the 1980s, said that influences within health care had so commandeered their high regard that such impersonal behaviors had emerged unbidden. Practitioners named influences that pulled against their caring: (1) emphasis on a rational fixing of problems rather than on the treatment of persons, (2) a reliance on best method and protocol to the exclusion of the patient's view, and (3) a health care system driven by business, efficiency, and profit.[13] Fisher's more recent analysis of health care reform cites similar effects in an ethical context:[37]

As health care professionals are asked by their organization to provide care at the lowest level possible, a myriad of potential ethical dilemmas arise. Such dilemmas include the need to prioritize the care given to patients and the treatment of their problems, the need to provide services faster and more efficiently, the need to utilize less resources and spend less money, and the need to balance the time spent documenting care with the time actually spent caring for patients. Practitioners, experienced and inexperienced alike, are faced with dealing with these ongoing and complex issues on a daily basis.[37]

Given this view of health care contexts, I revisit this question: Might practitioners grounded in empathy be inspired as moral agents in delivery systems that are perceived as depersonalized? I believe so and offer a few more thoughts related to patients' complaints.

Empathic practitioners might remember that treatment in health care has as much to do with persons as with their problems. Empathic practitioners might prize the patient's view of what should be done as much as they value professional protocols. Empathic practitioners might both manage *and* inspire health care systems. Empathic practitioners might disturb complacency, engender restlessness, and break depersonalizing rules that need to be broken. Empathic practitioners might apply the principles of patient-centered care, linking these powerfully with quality-care initiatives in order to humanize practice. Empathic practitioners might be compassionate.

Empathy's Place in Guiding Documents of the Professions

Both occupational therapy and physical therapy professions promulgate guiding documents that aim to shape moral action. Both professions educate practitioners through guidelines that delineate required attitudes and behaviors, grounding these in respect and linking them to ethical principles. But in these documents, empathy is an unappreciated way of being. Present only implicitly, empathy lacks a central place and is not a central construct.

If reframing empathy as a radical moral disposition makes sense conceptually, then a formal affirmation of that belief seems in order in many venues. The conceptual and sometimes visionary nature of the preambles of guiding documents seems a suitable place for beginning such affirmation. I thus end this reflection about provocative questions with one more: What if, as a modest starting point, words like the following graced the preambles of our codes of ethics:

This Code of Ethics springs from vital beliefs and longstanding traditions. Striving to sustain a caring ethos, individuals wrote this code using moral reasoning about practice and empathic reflection about others. They established guidelines that point to moral action. But moral action transcends a rote following of rules or a mindless application of principles. Moral action is a manifestation of moral character. It is sound reasoning about circumstances and a realization of fellowship in practice. The professional call to morality is a call to ethical, virtuous, righteous, and noble action. It is a call to ethical beneficence for the sake of others, to virtuous practice of artistry and science, to genuinely good behaviors, and to noble acts of courage. It is a call to an empathic way of being among others. The call to empathy is made every day, in every circumstance, to every practitioner: Do unto others as they would have you do unto them.

References

1. Merriam Webster's Collegiate Dictionary. Merriam-Webster, Inc. Springfield, MA, 2001.
2. Rogers CR: Empathic: An unappreciated way of being. Couns Psychol 5:2–10, 1975.
3. Davis CM: Patient Practitioner Interaction: An Experimental Manual for Developing the Art of Heath Care. Slack, Thorofare, NJ, 1994.
4. Stein E: On the Problem of Empathy. Stein W, translator. Martinus Nijhoff, The Hague, 1970 (original work published in 1930).
5. Davis CM: What is empathy, and can empathy be taught? Phys Ther 70:32–36, 1990.
6. Mosey AC: Occupational Therapy: Configuration of a Profession. Raven Press, New York, 1981.
7. Katz RL: Empathy: Its Nature and Uses. Free Press of Glencoe, London, 1963.
8. Titchener EB: Lectures on the Experimental Psychology of the Thought Processes: Classics in Psychology. Arno Press, New York, 1973 (original work published in 1909).
9. Peloquin SM: The fullness of empathy: Reflections and illustrations. Am J Occup Ther 49(1):24–31, 1995.
10. Carlova J, and Ruggles O: The Healing Heart. Messner, New York, 1946.
11. Fay EV, and Marsh I: Occupational therapy in general and special hospitals. In Willard HS, and Spackman CS (eds): Principles of Occupational Therapy. JB Lippincott Co, Philadelphia, 1947, pp 118–137.
12. Purtilo R, and Haddad A: Health Professional and Patient Interaction. WB Saunders Co, Philadelphia, 2002.
13. Peloquin SM: The patient-therapist relationship in occupational therapy: Understanding visions and images. Am J Occup Ther 44:13–21, 1990.
14. McIntyre A: After Virtue. A Study in Moral Theory. University of Notre Dame Press, Terre-Haute, IN, 1984.
15. Greif EB, and Hogan R: The theory and measurement of empathy. J Couns Psychol 20:280–284, 1973.
16. Bockoven JS: Moral Treatment in American Psychiatry. Springs Publishing, New York, 1963.
17. Bing RK: Eleanor Clarke Slale Lectureship 1981—Occupational therapy revisited: A paraphrastic journey. Am J Occup Ther 35:499–518, 1981.
18. Kornblau BK, and Starling SP: Ethics in Rehabilitation. Slack, Thorofare, NJ, 2000.
19. Rasmussen T: The ASTD Trainer's Sourcebook: Diversity. McGraw-Hill, Inc. New York, 1996.
20. Peloquin SM: Confluence: Moving forward with affective strength. Am J Occup Ther 56(1):69–77, 2002.
21. Collins JC, and Porras J: Built to Last: Successful Habits of Visionary Companies. Harper and Collins, New York, 1994.
22. Plum A: Communication as skill: A critique and alternate proposal. J Humanist Psychol 21:3–19, 1981.
23. Laing RD: Self and Others. Penguin, London, 1969.
24. Stiller C: Exploring the ethos of the physical therapy profession in the United States: Social, cultural and historical influences and their relationship to education. J Phys Ther Educ 14(3):7–16, 2000.
25. Romanella M, and Knight-Abowitz K: The "Ethic of Care" in physical therapy practice and education: Challenges and opportunities. J Phys Ther Educ 14(3):20–25, 2000.
26. Peloquin SM: Reclaiming the vision of reaching for heart as well as hands. Am J Occup Ther 56:517–526, 2002.
27. Kidner TB: Address to graduates. Occup Ther Rehab 8:379–385, 1929.
28. Buber M: Between Man and Man. Macmillan, New York, 1965.
29. Purtilo RB: A time to harvest, a time to sow: Ethics for a shifting landscape. Phys Ther 80(11):1112–1119, 2000.
30. Davies GK: Teaching and learning: What are the questions. Teaching Educ 4:57–61, 1991.
31. Van Amburg RA: Copernican revolution in clinical ethics: Engagement versus disengagement. Am J Occup Ther 51:186–190, 1996.
32. American Occupational Therapy Association: Occupational therapy code of ethics. Am J Occup Ther 48:1037–1038, 1994.
33. Treizenberg H, and Cipriany-Dacko L: A case study in pro-bono care: Ethical considerations. GeriNotes 8(2):23–26, 2001.
34. Purtilo R: Moral courage in times of change: Visions for the future. J Phys Ther Educ 14(3):4–6, 2000.
35. Opacich KJ: Moral tensions and obligations of occupational therapy practitioners providing home care. Am J Occup Ther 51:430–435, 1997.
36. Peloquin SM: The depersonalization of patients: A profile gleaned from narratives. Am J Occup Ther 47:830–837, 1993.
37. Fisher GS: Health care reform, managed care, and clinical reasoning: Implications for ethics occupational therapy practice. In Fisher GS (ed): Occupational Therapy in Health Care. Vol 11(1). Haworth Press, New Jersey, pp 26–37, 1997.

3

The Ethics of Competence

PENELOPE A. MOYERS EDD, OTR, FAOTA

Abstract

The purpose of this chapter is to examine the ethical issues related to competence raised in the AOTA (American Occupational Therapy Association) (2000) and the APTA (American Physical Therapy Association) (2002) ethical codes. These two professional codes suggest the importance of scientific knowledge in meeting the high moral demands for continuing competence. Rapid advances in technology and working in a health care system that creates barriers to quality of care are common problems in today's practice. Consequently, there is growing importance for therapists to develop and manage a plan for maintaining competency and for engaging in continuing competence. In analyzing the ethical issues of competence, a dynamic model was developed involving such variables as competency characteristics, competencies, abilities, virtues, and principles from a professional code of ethics. The relative importance of these variables to each other in their contribution to continuing competence is influenced by one's job responsibilities and by quality improvement data from the system in which one works. Professional knowledge bases are in a constant state of evolution; therefore, it is necessary for therapists to recognize that improving client care is a continuous process partially resulting from an aggressive program of continuing competence.

The moral justification for implementing the occupational therapy and physical therapy processes arises from the competence of the therapist. The American Occupational Therapy Association (AOTA) and the American Physical Therapy Association (APTA) ethical codes reflect the commitment of therapists to practice in an ethical manner, acting in the best interest of the client.[1,2] Principle 4 of the AOTA Code and Principle 5 of the APTA Code are devoted to the therapist's responsibility for achieving and continually maintaining high standards of competence.[1,2] Because occupational and physical therapists are regularly asked to demonstrate competency, what does it mean to be competent?

The purpose of this chapter is to examine competence as the moral justification for practice. To better understand competence, terms are defined, the relationship to client-centered care is established, the issues involving scientific knowledge are delineated, the challenges in maintaining competence are described, and the importance of quality improvement as a competence building activity is explained. This analysis helped to develop a dynamic model of competence involving competency characteristics, competencies, abilities, virtues, and principles from a professional code of ethics.

✧ COMPETENCE DEFINED

Because a principle in both the occupational and physical therapy codes is devoted to competence, therapists should understand their responsibility in meeting this high moral demand. *Competence* is defined as "an individual's capacity to perform job responsibilities."[3] Improved capacity partly results from formal education, professional training, and experience. Continuing competence is, thus, the ongoing effort to update capacity throughout one's career as a therapist. The process of continuing competence involves the occupational therapist or physical therapist maintaining appropriate credentials, adhering to professional standards and other relevant documents, self-assessing current competence, participating in educational activities necessary to enhance skills and knowledge, critically examining and keeping current with emerging knowledge, and practicing within the scope of one's competence and level of education, training, and experience.[1,2]

The term *competency* is subtly different in that it implies a determination of whether one is currently competent to perform a behavior or task as measured against a specific criterion.[4] Benner emphasized that competency is reflected in one's ability to perform "under the varied circumstances of the real world."[5] Continuing competence (building capacity) and competency (current performance against standards) are both necessary if one is to be adequately prepared for the complex demands of practice over time. The evolving nature of the health care, educational, and social service systems leads to changing roles and responsibilities of occupational therapists and physical therapists; thus, lifelong learning is required to maintain competency and to improve capacity for performance on job tasks in the future.

The issues of continuing competence and competency are well outlined in AOTA's *Standards for Continuing Competence*.[6] These five standards are global in nature in that they address the need for the therapist to remain current in knowledge, performance skills, interpersonal abilities, critical reasoning skills, and ethical reasoning skills. One could view these skills and abilities as forming the underlying requirements upon which competencies are based. *Competencies* are a set of explicit statements necessary for effective job performance.[7] For instance, being able to select the appropriate evaluation instrument and to interpret results are two competencies associated with the client evaluation process. Decker refers to the underlying requirements of knowledge, skills, and abilities as *competency characteristics*.[7] Using the evaluation example of selecting the appropriate evaluation instrument, the therapist must have the competency characteristic of knowledge about the instruments available to measure a specific behavior or performance and must have the competency characteristic of skill in using these instruments.

Both the AOTA and APTA codes require a therapist to examine his or her competency characteristics in relationship to a precise set of competencies. Expert knowledge and skills are the most visible competency characteristics to measure and develop as these characteristics involve particular behaviors or activities and have discrete performance criteria. There are other competency characteristics that most continuing education or training programs fail to address because of their invisible nature. *Threshold competencies* refer to the tasks that must at minimum be performed in order to practice competently and safely. Competencies may also depend upon the therapist's motivation to change performance; may be more conducive to those therapists with specific physical and character traits, such as those with a positive self concept or self image; or may depend upon having certain attitudes or values.[7] Because of their invisible nature, occupational and physical therapists may not realize the ethical issues involving continuing competence and competency related to a negative self concept or to low motivation to remain updated.

✧ COMPETENCE AND CLIENT-CENTERED CARE

Competence also forms the basis for demonstrating concern for the well-being of the client. The Institute of Medicine in its report,

Health Professions Education: A Bridge to Quality, identified a set of competencies that are lacking in the current skill set of most health care professionals, but are required for current and future practice.[8] One of these competencies includes client-centered care. The question is: how well do occupational therapists and physical therapists practice client-centered therapy based on the client's individual characteristics so that services are more likely to meet the real needs of the client?

Cultural competence forms the basis of client-centered occupational therapy and physical therapy, as does the possession of interpersonal skills related to effective communication and respect for the client's values, preferences, and expressed needs.[8,9] Health care systems are problematic in that they are not designed to recognize the individual needs of clients, but instead are designed to recognize the typical or average need, or are restricted to addressing only certain kinds of problems, such as acute disease.[10,11] Likewise, health care research is limited in terms of informing occupational and physical therapists about the reactions to various interventions of persons of different races, ethnic groups, sexual orientation, and socioeconomic groups.[12]

Harm and Client Safety

The Institute of Medicine recently highlighted the problem of medical errors in its 1999 report, *To Err is Human: Building a Safer Health System*, in which medical errors are suggested as the eighth leading cause of death.[13] Medical errors were defined as "the failure of a planned action to be completed as intended (i.e., error of execution) or the use of a wrong plan to achieve an aim (i.e., error of planning)."[13] Errors resulting from skill deficits may be an ethical problem due to the focus of the AOTA and APTA ethical codes on the maintenance of competence.[1,2]

Scheirton, Mu, and Lohman, as well as Anderson and Towell, studied the problem of errors in occupational and physical therapy, respectively.[14,15] These authors recommended training as an important strategy for improving competence and avoiding harm related to medical errors. "Occupational therapists in the

study valued the lessons learned from their errors, an outcome that had positive effects on their practice and important implications for education, training, and current practice."[14] Anderson and Towell likewise concluded that it is important to "use information identified through error analysis and incorporate it in entry-level education and professional training programs."[15] Similar to these studies, lack of knowledge was also one of the causes of error as determined in a survey of nurses.[16]

Competence and Scientific Knowledge

Given the emphasis upon knowledge, it is therefore necessary to evaluate the role and limitations of scientific knowledge in maintaining competency and in engaging in continuing competence. Evidence-based practice requires the therapists to use an ethical, conscientious, and discriminative process for applying the best available evidence when collaborating with the client on evaluation and intervention decisions.[17,18] Although evidence-based practice has been discussed in the therapy literature,[19–27] its practical implementation remains at what Dysart and Tomlin referred to as modest.[28] In their study, 57% of 209 occupational therapists implemented between 1 and 5 new, research-based treatment plans within the year previous to data collection.[28] However, the occupational therapists reported barriers to evidence-based treatment planning related to lack of time at work to access research information, high costs of continuing education, the lack of research analysis skills, and the placement of higher value on clinical experience than on research. In physical therapy, the perceived barriers to continuing education have been studied and included: costs, traveling distance, loss of time with the family, previous experience with programs, lack of information about available courses, and lack of pertinent programs.[29]

In a similar study about the reading patterns and attitudes of occupational therapists, 85% of the 626 therapists from 5 states reported reading the *American Journal of Occupational Therapy* (AJOT).[30] Those who did not read the main journal for occupational therapy in the United States reported impediments comparable to those cited by Dysart and Tomlin.[28] The nonreaders reported that AJOT contained too much scientific information and not enough clinical information. The scientific studies were rated as not being useful to inform clinical practices.

In addition to the barriers related to health care practitioner competence in using evidence-based practice, the availability of high-level evidence is problematic as well.[31] Lack of strong evidence becomes acute if using a hierarchy of evidence that places greater importance on the randomized controlled trial.[10,23,27] Occupational and physical therapy theories rarely capture the intricacies of the therapeutic process. Even when theory approaches significant complexity, there is great difficulty in substantiating the validity of such theories, particularly given most occupational and physical therapists do not exclusively prescribe to one theory, but report themselves as being eclectic.[32,33]

Eclecticism is needed due to the importance of carefully matching the client's occupational and physical performance needs with the best occupational therapy or physical therapy approach and intervention methods.[33–35] Therefore, not only is it tricky to determine the efficacy of interventions in well-controlled research studies, but demonstrating the effectiveness of the intervention in daily practice where conditions are uncontrolled and involve a confluence of theoretical approaches is difficult. As a result, it is likely that interventions found to be efficacious in experimental studies may overestimate their potential effectiveness in a messy practice environment.[32]

✧ CHALLENGE OF REMAINING COMPETENT

A lifelong learning process or continuing competence program should include a wide range of learning and educational activities (e.g., academic course work, continuing education, presentations, publication, research, advanced certification, peer review, work experience, etc.) that enhance the knowledge, skills, and attitudes the person will need to practice competently.[36] AOTA has outlined a continuing competence plan, which an occupational ther-

apist may use to foster current competency to practice in an area of expertise and may use to promote continuing competence for future practice.[37,38] Because AOTA's Continuing Competence Plan for Professional Development is applicable to many disciplines, physical therapists will find this outline of the processes in developing a learning plan to be useful as well.[37,38] APTA states in their guidelines for the Code of Ethics that competence does involve self-assessment and engagement in learning activities.[2] The process of planning one's learning for maintaining competency and engaging in continuing competence is a self-initiated approach that consists of eight components: (1) examining responsibilities, (2) using triggers to determine the need for self-assessment, (3) performing a self-assessment, (4) identifying needs in light of the *Standards for Continuing Competence*, (5) developing a plan for continuing competence, (6) implementing the continuing competence plan, (7) documenting professional development and changes in performance, and (8) implementing changes in the plan and demonstrating continuing competence. Demonstrating continuing competence includes the ethical responsibility to evaluate the impact of the changed performance of the therapist on client outcomes. The American Speech and Hearing Association's Code of Ethics describes this responsibility by stating, "individuals shall evaluate the effectiveness of services rendered."[39]

Self-Assessment Challenges

The key to an effective plan to improve competence is the examination of one's responsibilities in light of triggers that may signal a need for a self-assessment of one's competence. Triggers are events or circumstances in the job setting that necessitate a person examine his or her knowledge, skills, or attitudes. Triggers may include changes in the individual, government regulations, marketplace, or the profession itself. Triggers may be gradual or sudden, and can involve significant events or minor changes in the health care system. The occupational therapist and physical therapist must become adept at recognizing triggers given that change is constant. Self-assessment studies the match between one's competency characteristics (i.e., knowledge, performance skills, critical reasoning, interpersonal abilities, and ethical reasoning) and the ability to satisfactorily implement the competencies involved in one's job tasks. If there is a mismatch because of new technology, for example, the occupational or physical therapist develops a learning plan to gain the knowledge and performance skill needed to use the technology, as well as to acquire the critical reasoning necessary to determine when to use the technology, and if needed, to develop the ethical reasoning required if the technology is too expensive in its use with those without medical insurance.

AOTA has launched a web-based Professional Development Tool (PDT) that includes a self-assessment process, a learning plan, and a portfolio to archive documentation of the competence process and of the outcomes for that process.[40] Self-assessment, however, is not without its pitfalls.[41] The effectiveness of a self-assessment depends upon the ability of the therapist to recognize the key competencies that need improvement as well as the most important competency characteristics on which to focus. Most studies of self-assessment processes indicate that professionals overestimate their abilities and underestimate the demands of the new job task to be learned.[42]

Also to be effective, one needs to be aware of the best methods for learning performance skills, gaining knowledge, developing critical and ethical reasoning, and enhancing interpersonal abilities. For instance, reading may be appropriate for gaining knowledge, but does not compare to role-playing and simulation strategies that may be more effective in enhancing interpersonal abilities. One must also have access to specific resources needed for implementing the learning plan, as well as for obtaining the support from management to implement the newly acquired competencies as a regular component of one's job tasks. Because processes may not exist to adequately support the use of the new competencies, the health care system in which one works may actually prevent the occupational and physical therapist from incorporating the competencies within the job.[43,44]

Self-assessment raises other issues involving the liability of the occupational therapist and physical therapist in admitting that one's performance lacks competence or could benefit from improved competence. Self-assessment is more acceptable when new learning is involved, as in the example of a new technology being implemented as a component of the assigned job tasks.[42] It is quite another matter when the triggers signaling the need for self-assessment involve a negative change in client outcomes that cannot be explained by a change in client characteristics or by other changes within the system.

The question is whether the self-assessment is an admission of incompetence that potentially could be legally discoverable and used against the person if the therapist commits a medical error, or if the person is sued for malpractice or negligence. What is the liability in this circumstance for the employer or for the accrediting body or licensure board if these organizations have accepted the self-assessment as a part of a professional development plan? Is liability a greater problem if the employer does not see a need for additional supervision while the occupational therapist or physical therapist is relearning skills, or the accrediting body or licensure board does not implement corresponding action to suspend the credential or license if the need for relearning is such that threshold competencies cannot be met?

Because the occupational and physical therapy fields continually change and evolve, therapists cannot be expert in every aspect of the profession. A plan for continuing competence is not comprehensive or exhaustive. Most legal authorities would recognize that a plan for continuing competence is simply one source of information about performance and, in fact, is a commonly accepted way for professionals to continue their development. Continuing competence self-assessments and plans do not identify all areas in which improvement may be desirable. There should be understanding that the determination of legal liability or adequacy of professional performance in a given context cannot result from a self-assessment and continuing competence planning process. Doing what is morally right in terms of self-assessing one's state of competence supersedes this concern for protecting the self from potential legal circumstances that may never be realized. It is more likely that self-assessment followed by professional development planning and implementation will prevent errors from occurring because of lack of knowledge or skill.[14,15]

Challenges Due to System Design

The literature about practice errors indicated that the system was a primary factor in the occurrence of errors.[14,15] According to Scheirton, Mu, and Lohman, "system errors can be described as those that are outside of the direct control of the occupational therapist."[14] Examples of system errors include poor technical design, lack of equipment maintenance or faulty equipment installation, organizational barriers, and inappropriate managerial decisions.[14] Anderson and Towell described system errors as occurring because of interactions among the therapist and client, other people, such as the family, reimbursement and regulatory agencies, and the employer.[15]

According to Anderson and Towell, "if there is to be a significant change in the health care attitude and approach to error, there must be a series of behavioral modifications throughout all sections of the health care culture.[15] Accusations of malpractice and acquisitive court decisions must be replaced by an earnest attempt to evaluate and prevent all medical errors."[15] The PROCESS model for approaching error has been proposed in which there is a partnership among all stakeholders to solve the problem, there is reporting of errors without fear of punishment, there are open-ended focus groups used to reduce secrecy and to analyze error, there is a cultural shift from secrecy to open identification of error, there are education and training programs designed to improve competence and to decrease error, there are statistical analyses of error data to support continuous quality improvement, and there is a redesigning of the system based on the information about error and its causes.[15]

Assistance Through Quality Improvement Mechanisms

Continuous quality improvement, or total quality management, fosters ethical behavior because it leads to explicit articulation of organizational commitments and goals, and fosters the development of good listening skills in leaders within the organization.[45] Articulating its goals clarifies the targets upon which the entire organization is focusing, thereby bringing the competency of all employees in line. When leaders and managers possess good listening skills, early identification of problematic behavior, through discussion of problems detracting from the articulated organizational goals, is more likely. Good listening throughout the organization promotes honesty and fair dealing, as well as checks the human tendency to demonize other people in terms of blaming poor performance on a few supposedly incompetent employees. Continuous quality improvement highlights, through mindfulness of all personnel, the ethical dimension of the work processes so that the organization is efficient and effective, thereby preventing the wasting of key assets. Awareness on the part of all employees and management helps facilitate examination of the "big picture" and exploration of the many interconnections involved in producing the desired outcomes or goals.

Continuous quality improvement, however, is not a panacea for an organization to avoid harm and to improve outcomes.[45] Overfocusing on the system ignores crucial ethical issues pertaining to the role played by the individual provider in committing errors that may be underestimated. Consequently, there must be a balance between focusing on the competence of the individual provider and focusing on the efficiency and effectiveness of the system to allow individual providers to engage in competent practices.[46]

✧ THEORY OF COMPETENCE

Johnson's conceptual framework for analyzing the competence needed to mentor inexperienced professional colleagues stimulated my thinking about a comparable model that illustrates the process for developing and maintaining competence for any job task. Figure 3.1 illustrates the model of competence.[47]

In this model, job task competence ranges

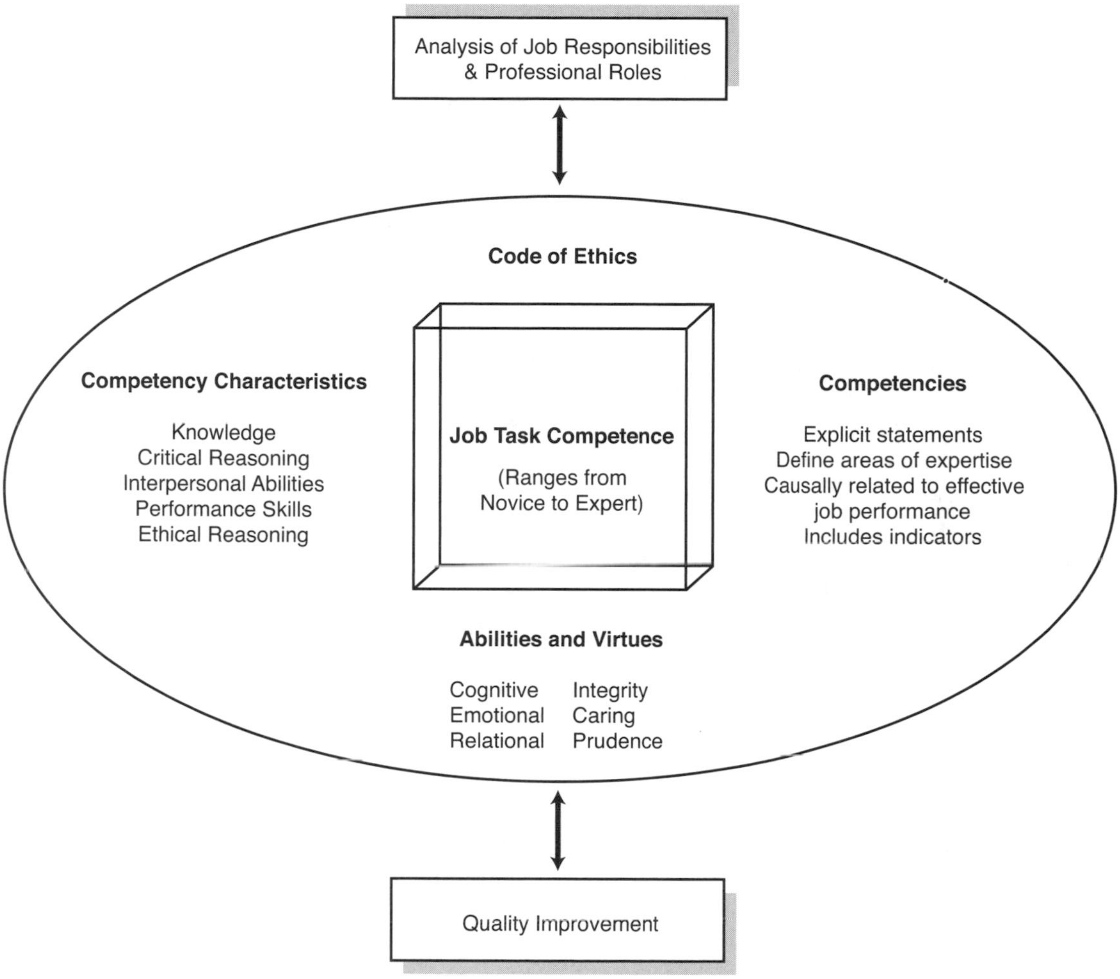

```
            ┌─────────────────────────────┐
            │ Analysis of Job Responsibilities │
            │    & Professional Roles      │
            └─────────────────────────────┘
                         ↕
```

Code of Ethics

Competency Characteristics

Knowledge
Critical Reasoning
Interpersonal Abilities
Performance Skills
Ethical Reasoning

Job Task Competence

(Ranges from
Novice to Expert)

Competencies

Explicit statements
Define areas of expertise
Causally related to effective
job performance
Includes indicators

Abilities and Virtues

Cognitive   Integrity
Emotional   Caring
Relational   Prudence

```
            ┌─────────────────────────────┐
            │      Quality Improvement     │
            └─────────────────────────────┘
```

Figure 3.1 ✧ Competence model.

from being a novice to being an expert.[48,49] Note that an individual may have a lengthy tenure in a particular job but due to new task assignments may be considered a novice for a particular task.

Job task competence is made up of explicit statements or competencies that are causally related to effective job performance. Competencies are developed as a result of an analysis of one's job or professional roles and as a result of quality improvement data. Decker and Strader proposed that once competencies and outcomes are determined for contemporary practice, the next step is to delineate the indicators that define these competencies.[50] For example, the task of client evaluation may

require the occupational and the physical therapist to be able to select the most appropriate evaluation instrument given the client's goals and preferences for specific outcomes (competency statement). The indicators that the therapist meets this competency statement could include evidence that the evaluations selected for specific clients are instruments most likely to: identify important functional problems and the impairments that contribute to these functional problems, delineate the prognosis regarding resolution of the impairments and the functional problems, and determine the relationship of the context in exacerbating problems or in supporting function.

Successful implementation of competencies depends upon the way in which the therapist's competency characteristics match the demands that the competencies make upon these competency characteristics. Selecting the best evaluation instrument requires the occupational and physical therapist to have knowledge of a variety of test instruments and to use critical reasoning to determine which would be the best test given the circumstances involved. If there is a mismatch between the competencies and the competency characteristics, the therapist in this instance must self-assess the limits in knowledge and then must devise a plan to improve his or her knowledge base.

The occupational therapist and physical therapist must also have the ability to learn this new knowledge including the requisite intellectual skill and cognitive complexity to understand and synthesize this new information.[47] Emotional abilities involve balance and personality adjustment (e.g., open-mindedness, flexibility, absence of personality disturbance).[47] Relational abilities include the capacity for intimacy and the ability to use relational skills in establishing rapport with clients.

Given that the competence process is the moral justification for providing occupational and physical therapy, the virtues of the therapist are important to ensure that the therapist engages routinely in competence improvement activities. In other words, following the AOTA and the APTA ethical codes involves procedural ethics in which the question "What should I do?" is answered.[1,2] Virtue ethics, in contrast, calls upon "individual professionals to aspire toward ideals and to develop virtues of character that enable them to achieve those ideals."[47] Virtue ethics answer the question, "What shall I be?"

The therapist must genuinely care for the client, understanding the altruistic responsibility involved. Another important virtue is prudence, or the "ability to govern and discipline oneself through the use of reason."[51] The therapist must also display integrity or the attitudes of honesty and sincerity. Taken together, these virtues motivate competence because of the therapist's caring for the client, or wanting to perform better so that the client has a more satisfactory outcome.[41] Prudence is a virtue that facilitates the disciplined pursuit of competence

in which there is an honest and sincere effort to focus on those competencies and competency characteristics that are most likely to lead to job task competence.

Education and training to improve the competence of the therapist focuses on improving the match between competency characteristics and delineated competencies. Because virtues are defined as "distinctly good or admirable human qualities that denote moral excellence or uprightness in the way one lives," it is clear that the virtues and the abilities of the therapist provide the necessary conditions for the acquisition of competencies and the subsequent expression of job task competence.[47] Given that virtues and abilities are less malleable to training, hiring therapists requires careful selection to ensure the applicant has the necessary virtues and abilities to competently perform the job tasks. Understanding the relationship between virtues and competence also has implications for selecting students into professional educational programs.

Researchers have attempted to determine, for example, what makes a good nurse or a good doctor, with some difficulty in reaching consensus about which are the most important virtues.[52,53] Regardless of this obstacle, the inclusion of virtues as a basis of competence may provide an explanation of how motivation for improved performance is generated. Differences in the possession and expression of virtues may explain why some therapists will readily engage in competence improvement while others wait to be coerced or engage in only the minimum amount of competence improvement activity necessary. Virtues are "an expression of habits that dispose one to act in certain ways."[54] Competence relies heavily on the formation of character, on learning and growth in abilities and competency characteristics, as well as on following ethical principles, such as the AOTA and the APTA ethical codes.[1,2]

✧ SUMMARY

The development of a competence model highlights issues related to ensuring that therapists have the virtues associated with active engagement in continuing competence. In addition, the therapist must have skills needed to judiciously use the best available evidence to support the collaborative client/therapist choices inherent in the therapy process. There is also growing importance for understanding and preventing harm to the client from overuse, underuse, and misuse of professional services. Harm is an ethical issue that clearly delineates the therapist's responsibility for updating competence. Because there is a system component in creating harm, the therapist is obliged to participate in quality improvement activities as an aspect of improving competence.[46]

We cannot afford the luxury of assuming that competence is a fixed state to be achieved. Therefore, the learning processes for meeting the spirit of our ethical principles related to competence should be in a constant state of evolution and development within an ethically conscious community. This constant state of change implies that we must continually craft an ethic to improve the lives of our clients, seeking to create a community that strives to reach its vision of the good.

References

1. American Occupational Therapy Association: Occupational therapy code of ethics. Am J Occup Ther 54:614–16, 2000.
2. American Physical Therapy Association: APTA Code of Ethics and Guide for Professional Conduct. Available at: http://www.apta.org/PT_Practice/ethics_pt/pro_conduct.
3. McConnell EA: Competence vs. competency. Nurs Manage 32(5):14, 2001.
4. Hinojosa J: Implications for occupational therapy of a competency-based orientation. Am J Occup Ther 39:539–541, 1985.
5. Benner P: Issues in competency-based testing. Nurs Outlook 30:303–309, 1982.
6. American Occupational Therapy Association: Standards: Standards for continuing competence. Am J Occup Ther 53:559–560, 1999.
7. Decker PJ: The hidden competencies of healthcare: Why self-esteem, accountability, and professionalism may affect hospital customer satisfaction scores. Hosp Top 77(1):1–14, 1999.
8. Institute of Medicine: Health Professions Education: A Bridge to Quality. National Academy Press, Washington, DC, 2003.
9. Wittman P, and Velde BP: The issue is—attaining cultural competence, critical thinking, and intellectual development: A challenge for occupational therapists. Am J Occup Ther 56:454–456, 2002.
10. Tickle-Degnen L: Evidence-based practice forum—Where is the individual in statistics? Am J Occup Ther 57:112–115, 2003.
11. Finlay L: Holism in occupational therapy: Elusive fiction and ambivalent struggle. Am J Occup Ther 55:268–276, 2000.
12. Hasselkus BR: From the desk of the editor. The use of "race" in research. Am J Occup Ther 56:127–129, 2002.
13. Institute of Medicine: To Err is Human: Building a Safer Health System. National Academy Press, Washington, DC, 1999.
14. Scheirton L, Mu K, and Lohman H: Occupational therapists' responses to practice error in physical rehabilitation settings. Am J Occup Ther 57:307–314, 2003.
15. Anderson JC, and Towell ER: Perspectives on assessment of physical therapy error in the new millennium. J Phys Ther Educ 16:54–60, 2002.
16. Meurier CE, Vincent CA, and Parmar DG: Learning from errors in nursing practice. J Adv Nurs 26:111–119, 1997.
17. Christiansen C, and Lou JQ: Evidenced-based practice forum—Ethical considerations related to evidence-based practice. Am J Occup Ther 55:345–349, 2001.
18. Lloyd-Smith W: Evidence-based practice and occupational therapy. Br J Occup Ther 60:474–478, 1997.
19. Holm MB: Our mandate for the new millennium: Evidence-based practice, 2000 Eleanor Clarke Slagle Lecture. Am J Occup Ther 54:575–585, 2000.
20. Law M (ed): Evidence-Based Rehabilitation: A Guide to Practice. Slack, Thorofare, NJ, 2002.
21. Lee CJ, and Miller LT: Evidence-based practice forum—The process of evidence-based clinical decision making in occupational therapy. Am J Occup Ther 57:473–477, 2003.
22. Ottenbacher KJ, Tickle-Degnen L, and Hasselkus BR: Therapists awake! The challenge of evidence-based occupational therapy. Am J Occup Ther 56:247–249, 2002.
23. Tickle-Degnen L: Evidence-based practice forum—Communicating with clients, family members, and colleagues about research evidence. Am J Occup Ther 54:341–343, 2000.
24. Tickle-Degnen L: Evidence-based practice forum—Gathering current research evidence to enhance clinical reasoning. Am J Occup Ther 54:102–105, 2000.
25. Tickle-Degnen L: Evidence-based practice forum—Monitoring and documenting evidence during assessment and intervention. Am J Occup Ther 54:434–436, 2000.
26. Tickle-Degnen L: Evidence-based practice forum—What is the best evidence to use in practice? Am J Occup Ther 54:218–222, 2000.
27. Tickle-Degnen L, and Bedell G: Evidence-based practice forum—Heterarchy and hierarchy: A critical appraisal of the "levels of evidence" as a tool for clinical decision making. Am J Occup Ther 57:234–237, 2003.
28. Dysart AM, and Tomlin GS: Factors related to evidence-based practice among U.S. occupational therapy clinicians. Am J Occup Ther 56:275–284, 2002.
29. Karp VN: Physical therapy continuing education: Perceived barriers and preferences. Part 1. J Cont Educ Health Prof 12(2):111–120, 1992.
30. Philibert DB, et al: Practitioners' reading patterns, attitudes, and use of research reported in occupational therapy journals. Am J Occup Ther 57:450–458, 2003.
31. DeLisa JA, et al: Evidence-based medicine in physiatry: The experience of one department's faculty and trainees. Am J Phys Med Rehab 78:228–232, 1999.

32. Poortinga YH, and Lunt I: Defining the competence of psychologists with a view to public accountability. Eur Psychol 2:1016–1040, 1997.
33. Reed KL, and Sanderson SN: Concepts of Occupational Therapy, ed 4. Lippincott Williams & Wilkins, Philadelphia, PA, 1999.
34. American Occupational Therapy Association: Occupational therapy practice framework: Domain and process. Am J Occup Ther 56:609–639, 2002.
35. Hooper B, and Wood W: Pragmatism and structuralism in occupational therapy: The long conversation. Am J Occup Ther 56:40–50, 2002.
36. Thomson LK, et al: Developing, maintaining, and updating competency in occupational therapy: A guide to self-appraisal. American Occupational Therapy Association, Bethesda, MD, 1995.
37. Hinojosa J, et al: Self-initiated continuing competence. OT Pract 5(24):CE1–CE8, 2000.
38. Hinojosa J, et al: Professional development for continuing competency. American Occupational Therapy Association, Bethesda, MD, 1999.
39. Mustain W: The ethics of competence. ASHA Leader 8:14, 2003.
40. Case-Smith J: AOTA Continuing Education Article. Using the AOTA professional development tool (PDT). OT Pract 8:CE1–CE7, 2003.
41. Mustard LW: Caring and competency. JONAS Healthc Law Ethics Regul 4:36–43, 2002.
42. Regan-Klich J: Continuing education in dietetics: Present paradoxes and changing paradigms. In Young WH (ed): Continuing Professional Education in Transition: Visions for the Professions and New Strategies for Lifelong Learning. Krieger Publishing Co, Malabar, FL, 1998.
43. Batalden PB: If improvement of the quality and value of health and health care is the goal, why focus on health professional development? Qual Manag Health Care 6:52–61, 1998.
44. Cervero RM: Continuing professional education and behavioral change: A model for research and evaluation. J Cont Educ Nurs 16:85–88, 1985.
45. Nayebpour MR, and Koehn D: The ethics of quality: Problems and preconditions. J Bus Ethics 44:37–48, 2003.
46. Llott I: Evidence-Based Practice Forum—Challenging the rhetoric and reality: Only an individual and systemic approach will work for evidence-based occupational therapy. Am J Occup Ther 57:351–354, 2003.
47. Johnson WB: A framework for conceptualizing competence to mentor. Ethics Behav 13:127–151, 2003.
48. Benner P: From Novice to Expert. Addison-Wesley Publishing Co Inc, Menlo Park, CA, 1984.
49. Slater DY, and Cohn ES: Staff development through analysis of practice. Am J Occup Ther 45:1038–1044, 1991.
50. Decker PJ, and Strader MK: Beyond JCAHO: Using competency models to improve healthcare organizations, Part 1. Hosp Top 75:1–23, 1997.
51. American Occupational Therapy Association: Core values and attitudes of occupational therapy practice. Am J Occup Ther 54:614–616, 1993.
52. Smith KV, and Godfey NS: Being a good nurse and doing the right thing: A qualitative study. Nurs Ethics 9:301–312, 2002.
53. Ashcroft RE: Searching for the good doctor. Br Med J 325:719, 2002.
54. Loewy EH: Developing habits and knowing what habits to develop: A look at the role of virtue in ethics. Camb Q Healthc Ethics 6:347–355, 1997.

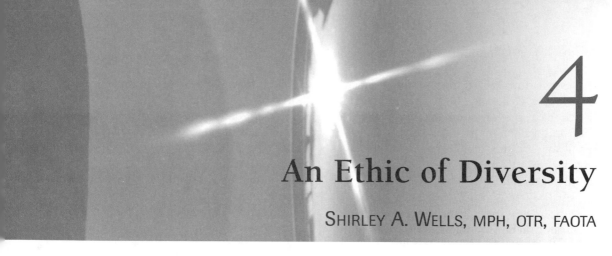

4

An Ethic of Diversity

SHIRLEY A. WELLS, MPH, OTR, FAOTA

Abstract

Contemporary ethical decision making approaches used by physical therapists and occupational therapists are based on bioethical concepts that assume all societies share common moral values and that "reasonable people" will reach the same conclusions when faced with an ethical problem, issue, or dilemma. These concepts of moral deliberation are based on four ethical principles—autonomy, beneficence, nonmaleficence, and justice. Historically, however, these approaches fail to recognize the influences and complexities of race, ethnicity, culture, religion, and other differences in shaping experiences of birth, illness, suffering, aging, loss, and death. In moral reasoning, these approaches do not acknowledge that different cultural and religious traditions might endorse distinctive, substantive principles, or provide resources for interpreting the four "core" principles in markedly divergent ways.

In multicultural settings, patients and their families as well as providers bring many different cultural models of morality and moral reasoning. It is the constant overlapping and interaction of cultures and dialects that are creating the daily conflicts and dilemmas in providing health care services. Yet, present bioethical concepts of moral deliberation offer little insight into developing meaningful responses, frameworks, and public policies to deal with cultural pluralism, religious diversity, and norm conflicts. The task before us is to develop, teach, and promote an ethic of diversity—a moral framework that recognizes diversity as the norm and not the exception. We must devise an ethical framework that addresses cross-cultural communication and cultural competence. We must create a moral construct that will allow occupational and physical therapy students to offer care within a multicultural setting without sacrificing equality, justice, or respect. In response to this need, I present a model for using the principles of an ethic of diversity.

CASE STUDY

Sharon, a therapist, was sitting at her desk after a busy day reviewing her current list of clients. When she reached the name of one client she asked herself, "So, how am I supposed to handle this situation?" This question arose from her encounter earlier that day. Sharon had received a referral to provide therapy to Joan who had recently experienced a right cerebral vascular accident. During the initial interview, Sharon learned that Joan is in a committed lesbian relationship with her lifelong partner and two adopted children. She had not mentioned her uneasiness with this client and family to anyone. She now wonders if she should say something, for this lifestyle is in direct conflict with her religious beliefs. Can Sharon give the client ethical and quality care?

Doing the right thing in clinical practice is always a challenge. In a pluralistic society, health care providers are finding themselves confronting choices that increasingly depend on moral values rather than just on medical knowledge. Sharon's dilemma is not a question of what treatment method to use but how to resolve her personal religious beliefs with an obligation to provide quality care. The interaction between client and therapist embodies a form of multiculturalism in which several cultures—health care profession, institution, family, community, traditional culture, etc.—are merged.[1-4]

Our individual cultural beliefs affect how we approach, speak to, and measure outcomes for our clients. As individuals and professionals, we take a particular action based on our own sense of right and wrong as well as the moral perspectives that frame our professional responsibilities.[5,6] Therefore, it is crucial that physical and occupational therapy students are provided an ethical approach for formulating a response to dilemmas around culture and diversity.

The purpose of this chapter is to describe a framework for ethical analysis and decision making that moves considerations of diversity from the periphery to the center focus of professional decision making. This is important because the responsibility for making ethically sound decisions in the clinical environment rests squarely with the individual practitioner; the professional codes of ethics for each profession demands a level of respect for all clients; and as the demographics of the United States continue to change, physical therapists and occupational therapists can expect to care for clients from varied backgrounds during the course of their career. Educational programs must prepare students of the future for increased competence in areas related to culture and other differences, a goal that cannot be achieved without a framework such as the one that I am proposing. Ethical practice in a multicultural society requires understanding, tolerance, cultural competency, respect, and skills.

✧ NEED FOR AN ETHIC OF DIVERSITY

The need for an ethic of diversity arises in part because of the rapidly changing demographics of not only the United States but also the world. The profile of the United States has undergone significant change over the past years. Ethnic groups constitute a significant and growing percentage of the population. Widespread immigrations have increased population diversity in many communities.[1-3] So, in the course of everyday practice occupational and physical therapists will frequently encounter individuals with different values and belief systems about health, caring, wellness, illness, death, and disabilities. They will be asked to perform evaluations and develop treatment plans with consumers who may not share their language, class, education, ethnicity, and reactions to illness and health. Important differences exist among groups of people related to customs, values, behaviors, and the meaning of abstract concepts, such as benefit and harm.

There are many therapist-patient interac-

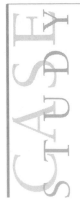

John received a referral to evaluate and treat an elderly client who is Hispanic and recently experienced an increase in episodes of falling and difficulties with walking. The client arrives at the clinic with her daughter who provides the background information about her mother. After completing the evaluation and outlining the therapy treatment approach, the daughter asks to speak to the therapist in private. She says, "I did not tell you everything. My mother has cancer and is receiving treatment. As a family we decided not to tell her about the diagnosis. I feel that you should know this, but please do not tell my mother that she has cancer."

tions in which culture affects health, but the interactions are not perceived as culturally related. Recognizing that cultural differences exist is not the same as respecting and understanding those differences, or using this knowledge to make ethically sound decisions regarding the delivery of care.[3]

Such a request places John in an ethical quandary. Can the patient give an informed consent for therapy? Should he tell her about the diagnosis? Is this request culturally related? A study by Blackhall, Murphy, Frank, and Azen, found that Mexican Americans and Korean Americans tend to have a negative sentiment toward telling a family member that they have a terminal illness.[7] These groups believe that a patient should not be told of a terminal prognosis. They feel that the family and not the patient should make end-of-life decisions.

Another need for an ethic of diversity is centered on the bioethics concepts that guide Western medicine decision making. Current health care providers are trained in bioethics concepts that have ignored multiethnic and religious difference.[5,6,8] Practical ethical issues in medicine and health care all presume the existence of a stable, settled moral order. "The notion of 'common morality' tends to obfuscate the complex realities of providing medical care in multicultural, multifaith societies."[9] Relying upon approaches that presume the existence of shared principles and moral paradigms neglects the cultural and subcultural variations that exist in today's societies.

Diversity and Bioethics Principles

According to Turner contemporary bioethics is based on the principlist model of practical moral reasoning.[6] This model is built on the notion of shared paradigms, common moral norms, and basic intuitions concerning moral practice. The principlist approach assumes that all societies recognize four core moral norms for health professionals—autonomy, beneficence, nonmaleficence, and justice. She found within the writings of moral theorists, "there is little mention of cultural differences, variations in ethnicity, and attitudes toward health, illness, and suffering, or significant distinctions amongst religious understandings of moral

practice."[6] These scholars tend to valorize personal choice and minimize cultural or any other form of social forces. Western philosophy has evolved into a culture preoccupied with the self, focusing on the individual body and embodied personality.[10]

Several authors have identified a number of underlying principles of contemporary bioethics that may be in direct opposition to certain cultural values and beliefs as sources of ethical conflicts and issues.[3,6,10–12]

Autonomy

This principle is at the center of most medical decisions. It refers to the individual's right to self-determination, that is, the right to make decisions. Many cultures embrace a value system that places the family, the community, or society as a whole above that of the individual. Alternative values, such as the good of the community, take precedence over the autonomy of the individual.[13] Solidarity rather than individualism is their highest value. By focusing monistically on the individual, patients can be cut from their families, religious practices, or cultural values.[11,14]

Truth-Telling

The predominant norm of disclosing a diagnosis of serious illness to the patient is not universally accepted. Some cultural groups (i.e., Mexican Americans, Korean Americans, and Native Americans) believe that the family not the patient should make important health care decisions. They tend to place great emphasis on family-centered, as opposed to client-centered, decision making style.[7,15]

Informed Consent

This bioethical concept comes into conflict with the belief that health is maintained and restored through positive ritual language (i.e., Native Americans). When health care providers disclose risks of a treatment in an informed consent discussion, they speak in a negative way, thereby violating the Navajo value that one should think and speak in a positive way. They believe that thought and language have the power to shape and control future events. Therefore, advance care planning and discussion about end-of-life treatment are a dangerous violation of traditional practice and values.[15]

Justice

This principle deals with what is due or owed to an individual, group, or society. A recent study by the Institute of Medicine, *Unequal Treatment: Confronting Racial/Ethnic Disparities in Health Care,* identified well over 175 studies documenting racial/ethnic disparities in the diagnosis and treatment of various conditions, even when analyses were controlled for socioeconomic status, insurance status, site of care, stage of disease, comorbidity, and age.[16] Ethnic minorities are overrepresented among the rolls of the uninsured. "And the prolonged impact of racism has been studied and linked to poor outcomes among African Americans."[17] As we struggle to decide in regard to health care who is entitled to what and who is to pay, questions of race, ethnicity, and cultural beliefs have entered the equation when resources are finite or scarce.

Self-Independence

Contemporary therapy approaches tend to focus on promoting independence for the sick person. Some cultures believe (i.e., Asian, Hispanic) it is their duty to care for its members. The role of the sick person is viewed as dependent and passive. If the sick person is independent in meeting their personal needs, what is the role of the family member? It is believed that a person is ill because of the sins committed by the family and therefore becomes their responsibility.[18] The meaning and values of "occupation" hinge on the local interpretation of human action.[5]

Codes of Ethics

A last reason for an ethic of diversity can be found within the professional Codes of Ethics for both occupational and physical therapy. Principle 1 of the American Physical Therapy Association states, "A physical therapist shall respect the rights and dignity of all individuals and shall provide compassionate care."[19] The American Occupational Therapy Code of Ethics says, "Occupational therapy personnel shall provide services in a fair and equitable manner. They shall recognize and appreciate the cultural components of economics, geography, race, ethnicity, religious and political factors, marital status, sexual orientation, and disability of all recipients of their services."[20] Both associations go on to say that to provide ethical and sound decision making, practitioners need to recognize, respect, and be responsive to differences. They should be able to provide culturally competent services. And their professional judgment should be based on their knowledge, skill, education, training, and experiences. If these practitioners are making decisions based on contemporary bioethical concepts, they may lack a framework for including cultural and religious differences in the moral deliberation of ethical conflicts. This, in turn, will make these practitioners out of compliance with their own Codes of Ethics.

Principle- and case-based approaches to ethical issues and dilemmas are insufficient for culturally complex societies. Contemporary bioethics has not adequately included cultural models of morality in their frameworks or modes of moral thought. Our own Codes of Ethics dictate that clinicians (including occupational therapists and physical therapists) incorporate diversity and culture in their ethical decision making model.

❖ ETHIC CONSTRUCT

Ethics is about how we conduct ourselves. It has been described as the study of the rules of right and wrong. The term comes from the Greek word "ethos," meaning cultural custom or habit.[3] The word moral, which is often used interchangeably with the term ethics, refers to "beliefs, principles, and values about what is right and wrong, which are personal to each and every individual," which also means customs.[21] Both terms focus on how we make judgments. Ethics offers a way to examine moral life.[22] It is a conscious stepping back and reflecting on our beliefs and practices about good and evil.[23] It is concerned with the suffering people cause one another and the corresponding capacity of humans to recognize suffering through the empathetic values of sympathy, compassion, and caring.[24] Ethics is based on human feelings and making judgments from within that humanity. We each experience feelings of pleasure or disgust concerning certain actions and events that occur in our surroundings. Accordingly, "we are the final judges of morality but before making any judgment we must remember that morality is more properly felt than judged."[25] Thus, morality is an emotional response that is culture-based.

Ethics is also grounded in time. It is rooted in the practical belief of closed societies. It is "culturally constructed, embedded in religious and political ideologies that influence individuals and communities at particular biographical and historical moments."[26] Moral standards of behaviors, which are what we believe to be right and wrong, have a personal and social component as well as cultural and time contexts. What is morally right or wrong depends on one's identity and historical events. One's race, gender, and culture are central to that identity.[27]

These dimensions—the personal, social, and cultural context—often come into conflict when making ethical decisions. In all moral choices there is a personal interest at stake in the action performed. There are various social roles and responsibilities, legal or not, that place demands on the action performed. There are moral rights and duties, which are dictated by race, culture, religion, or tradition that command the action performed.[28] This is when moral/ethical principles help the individual harmonize interests and roles, and resolve conflicts. According to Hinman, morality is the first-order set of beliefs and practices about how to live a good life that comes into play.[23] And ethics is a second-order set in which the conscious mind reflects on the adequacy of our moral beliefs. Therefore, the goal of ethical reflection is moral health. We are constantly seeking to determine what will nourish our moral life and what will poison it.

At a basic level, a primary function of ethics is to help one develop a virtuous character by means of which the person will guide his/her behaviors. It represents what ought to be and helps set standards for human behavior. Developing a good character helps us to achieve personal fulfillment. This goodness of character contributes to the goodness of the society in which we are a part.

✧ AN ETHIC OF DIVERSITY

In a diverse society the questions are: On what basis should we make moral decisions? What moral theory is the right one to use? What do we do when duties, rights, and values are in conflict? What rules of conduct should govern our actions and responses when faced with an ethical problem, issue, or dilemma involving diversity and culture? The proposed ethic of diversity presented in this chapter is a conceptual model resulting in a guide for analyzing and designing a decision. It offers the moral principles and rules of human conduct for making a choice in a pluralistic environment. It can assist in making sense out of moral conflicts. This conceptual model is a decision making tool designed to bring consistency rather than arbitrarily reaching a decision about what action to take. It can help the student and therapist use consistent criteria and weigh these criteria in a sound way. An ethic of diversity will help therapists discover means and ways to give care to people who have different values and lifestyles.

In conceptualizing my ethic of diversity, one central tenet is held: diversity is the norm and not the exception. All ethical decision-making requires a recognition, acknowledgment, and consideration of all involved cultures—client, practitioner, setting, profession, and tradition. In pluralistic settings, different interpretive communities can exist, with distinctive understandings of what constitutes moral conduct. This ethic of diversity also necessitates the inclusion of cross-cultural communication, cultural competence, and moral reasoning. The foundation for my ethic of diversity is a combination of moral and ethical theories and principles.

Ethical relativism and ethical pluralism offer several important insights for making practical everyday decisions.

Ethical Relativism

Ethical relativism, generally speaking, holds that moral values are relative to a particular culture or individual and cannot be judged outside of that culture. There are two types of relativism: descriptive ethical relativism, which states that different people have different moral beliefs, and normative ethical relativism, which claims that each moral code is only valid relative to the culture or group in which it exists.[29] As such, no objective standards can be used to judge one societal code better than another. Each society determines what is right in their society.[5,8] Ethical relativism holds that morality is relative to the society in which one is brought up. Relativists hold that moral rightness and wrongness is always relative to and determined by culture.[10,22] In this sense, nothing can be right or wrong without a consideration of the culture and social context.

Ethical relativism also calls for tolerance, understanding, and moral diversity. It maintains that if we cannot make judgments about others, neither can they judge us. It says that judging cultures is mere arrogance and this gives rise to atrocities, such as slavery, the Holocaust, and apartheid. Ethical relativism suggests that we let each culture live as it sees fit.[8,23] But in a multicultural society, it is the constant overlapping and interaction of cultures that are creating the daily conflicts.[30,31] Do we allow others to act in ways they think morally acceptable, even if we think them morally unacceptable? Does respecting another person's opinion or culture's traditions mean allowing them to do anything, even if it harms others? Ethical relativism is not helpful in dealing with the overlapping of cultures—which is precisely where we need help in resolving ethical conflicts.[4,30]

Ethical Pluralism

In health care, at least sometimes, we need to make judgments about some cultural practices and beliefs that are totally unacceptable and intolerable. Ethical pluralism challenges us to find ways to live together with differing and conflicting values. Ethical pluralism is the belief that there are multiple perspectives on an issue.[29] There are many truths, sometimes partial and sometimes conflicting. This does not mean that there is no truth, nor does it mean that all truth is relative. It means that at least in some situations, there is not just a single truth.[6,29,32] According to Hinman, ethical pluralism offers three categories to describe actions:[33]

- ✦ *Prohibited*—those actions that are not seen as permissible
- ✦ *Tolerated*—those actions and values in which legitimate differences are possible
- ✦ *Ideal*—a moral vision of what the ideal society would be like

Each action or policy we make can be placed in one of these categories. As we go through the reasoning process, ethically we move from the prohibited to the ideal.

Principles

As noted earlier, moral principles are the rules used to evaluate the behaviors of individual and groups. Ethical relativism and pluralism propose several ethical principles to guide and evaluate our responses when confronted with moral conflicts based on cultural differences. Hinman endorses four key principles about how we should respond to moral conflicts in a diverse world.[29]

- ✦ *Principle of Understanding*: We seek to understand other cultures before we pass judgment on them.
- ✦ *Principle of Tolerance*: We recognized that there are important areas in which intelligent people of goodwill in fact differ.
- ✦ *Principle of Standing up to Evil*: We recognize that, at some point, we must stand up against evil, even when it is outside of our own bodies.
- ✦ *Principle of Fallibility*: We recognize that, even with the best of intentions, our judgment may be flawed and mistaken.

The literature, however, also suggests other principles that should be a part of an ethic of diversity such as:[1,3,4,10,17,30,31,34]

- ✦ *Principle of Respect*: We recognize that all

human beings are worthy of respect simply because they are human.

✦ *Principle of Cultural Competency*: We seek self-exploration, knowledge, and skills to interact effectively and humanely with people different from ourselves.

✦ *Principle of Justice*: We seek to deal with everyone fairly and equitably in the distribution of goods and services.

✦ *Principle of Care*: We recognize that the needs of others play a part in all ethical decision making.

These principles can be used to protect individuals against harm and to help identify the good of people. These principles collectively assist us in acknowledging differences as the "norms."

Ethical relativism and pluralism suggest that we respect the moral choices made by patients in light of their culture or religious beliefs.[34] Cultural pluralism increases learning opportunities and facilitates cultural competency.[32,35] Cultural competency (a) increases the sense of one's own cultural identity, (b) heightens awareness of one's own cultural perspectives and the effect of those perspectives on individuals from other groups, as well as their interaction, (c) develops knowledge of other cultures, and (d) develops skills in using effective strategies for interaction and interrupting the behaviors of people different from yourself.[3]

This ethic of diversity offers an opportunity to extend human knowledge by finding wisdom in dissimilar cultural practices. It allows therapists to teach what, from a medical point of view, may damage health and to learn more about the rationale for and techniques of many traditional practices.[36] These principles can provide guidance to making responses when faced with an ethical problem, issue, or dilemma.

A Case for Cultural Competence

Health care is a culture that has its own body of knowledge, value system, beliefs, rules, and language.[32] Every clinical interaction involves a variety of cultures—client's culture, client's traditional culture, practitioner's professional culture, practitioner's personal culture, culture of the health care setting, societal culture, and others.[3] With every clinical encounter therapists are speaking across cultural gaps. In order to genuinely understand a client, each therapeutic exchange should be considered a cross-cultural event. The challenge to providing culturally competent care is the diversity of meanings that can be applied to similar concepts and principles.[5] The meaning we assign to various ideas and concepts are culturally based and culturally driven.

Culture can shape our views of illness and well-being in both the physical and spiritual realm and affect our perceptions of health care as well as the outcome of treatment.[4]

This situation can create an ethical problem if the therapist is not aware of or knowledgeable about Feng Shui, which is a Chinese practical technique for manipulating the ch'i

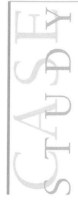

CASE STUDY

Chi-wan, a Chinese American woman, has been transferred to the rehabilitation unit. Upon entering the therapy area she notices that all the mat tables are against a wall so that the foot faces the doorway. She asks if the mat can be turned to face south. The therapist tries to explain that the room could not be rearranged. Chi-wan insists that the mat be changed or she could not attend therapy.

energy to promote health and healing.[37] Some practitioners may be comfortable with the idea of respecting cultural difference when the patient is a competent adult, but when children are involved they may be unwilling to tolerate decisions that result in what they perceive to be compromised care or harm, even when these decisions make sense in the context of a particular culture.[4,30,38] Thus, the principle of cultural competency is key to making sound, ethical, and culturally appropriate decisions.

Cultural competence refers to the process of actively developing and practicing appropriate, relevant, and sensitive strategies and skills in interacting with culturally different people. It is the capacity to respond to the needs of populations whose cultures are different from what might be called dominant or mainstream.[3] "Cultural competence in health care entails understanding the importance of social and cultural influences on patients' health beliefs and behaviors and considering how these factors interact at multiple levels of the health care delivery system."[17] To be culturally competent, therapists need to understand the social, political, and historical forces that constitute the larger context in which individual cross-cultural relationships are embedded.[39] Therapists need to be aware of the value assumptions embodied in biomedical approaches and the culture, power, and ethics of medicine and how they play out in clinical practice.[32]

Cultural competence requires the awareness of one's own biases and attitudes, knowledge about other cultures, and skills in cross-culture communication and intervention. Occupational and physical therapy practitioners need a nonjudgmental attitude toward unfamiliar beliefs and health practices, and must be willing to negotiate and compromise when conflicts arise.[3,39,40] Cultural competence is a reminder to therapists to respect, protect, and advocate for their patient and family.[41]

Interest in cultural competence training has gained momentum as a result of studies that have raised an awareness of health care provider bias and discrimination in medical decision making.[17,42] Attention is also being given by the private health care industry, as well as the government, in view of the overwhelming literature on racial/ethnic disparities in health and health care regarding the education and training of health care providers.[16,17] Therefore, a conceptual model is presented in Figure 4.1, which places culture as the center of ethical decision making, can facilitate culturally appropriate interventions.

The next section of this chapter, "Applying the Ethic of Diversity," will apply the model.

✧ APPLYING THE ETHIC OF DIVERSITY

It is our reflective nature that enables us to engage in moral deliberation. Each day we are faced with deciding: what to do, what kind of person to be, and what to value? Given that the aim of the ethic of diversity is to provide principles that can be used to guide our thought and

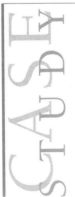

Let us take the case of Wind Wolf, a 5-year-old boy who is Creek Indian. He was born and raised on a reservation. He has black hair, dark brown eyes, and an olive complexion. And like many Indian children his age, he is shy and quiet in the classroom. If you ask him how many months there are in a year, he says 13. He has trouble writing his name on a piece of paper. He does not engage in conversation with the other children or do class activities. He responds only when called upon. When you speak to him, Wind Wolf does not maintain eye contact. Instead he looks down at the floor. He has difficulty grasping the English language. And he is not as fluent in English as the teacher thinks he should be at this age.[3]

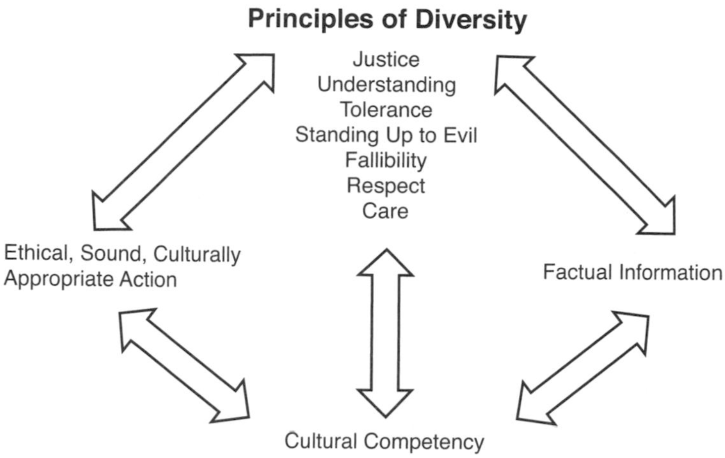

Principles of Diversity

Justice
Understanding
Tolerance
Standing Up to Evil
Fallibility
Respect
Care

Ethical, Sound, Culturally
Appropriate Action

Factual Information

Cultural Competency

Figure 4.1 ✧ Model for using the principles of an ethic of diversity.

action, it is reasonable to ask how we are supposed to use them for this purpose.

Wind Wolf is in kindergarten and has already been labeled a slow learner. You have been asked to evaluate him to collaborate the teacher's assessment and identify his level of developmental delay. Do you carry out the assessment using culturally biased tools that will show Wind Wolf is developmentally delayed? Is his behavior being judged against the dominant culture or his culture? What is your responsibility to the child, teacher, school, and profession? The principles of the ethics of diversity can assist the therapist in deciding on an action in this case as presented in the following guide for interpretation:

Principles + factual information
→ cultural competency =
moral conclusion about the action

Let us use this guide for interpreting the situation. Review the principles of the ethic of diversity—understanding, respect, tolerance, justice, standing up to evil, fallibility, and care. Add the factual information about the situation, such as the child is from a culture that may have different child-rearing practices; standard assessment tools are based largely on the sociocultural norms of the white, middle-class population; and you are being asked to validate another's judgment.[3] Next combine your training in cultural competency to further clarify the situation and seek other information. With all the perspectives considered, choose a course of action that will be ethical, sound, and culturally appropriate.

✧ TEACHING AN ETHIC OF DIVERSITY

The overarching goal of any educational or training intervention must be to equip the student or practitioner with tools and skills to better understand and manage sociocultural issues in the clinical encounter. Occupational and physical therapy students must receive training not only in theories of moral reasoning and bioethical concepts but also on the impact of culture on ethical decisions in health care. They should receive information about the process of cross-cultural communication and social illness and health beliefs that are present in all cultures. The focus should be on using the patient as a teacher and developing attitudes and skills necessary for working with a variety of people. "Some balance of cross-cultural knowledge and communication skills seems to be the best approach to cultural competence education and training."[17]

Course materials can come from sociology, history, literature, poetry, videos, and music. In addition to reading, writing, case discussion, and watching videos, there should be individual speakers, and panels from medical community ethics committees, consumers, and health care providers. Educational sessions in which community members teach by describing their experiences, history, and daily life will create a rich backdrop for students to appreciate the cultural and moral context within which health decisions are made.

Genao and colleagues state that curricula should commit to teaching "(a) understanding patient attitudes toward the health care system and health seeking behaviors, (b) awareness of the different perceptions of health, illness, disabilities, and bereavement by different ethnic and cultural groups, (c) recognition of the validity of the patient belief system regardless of its perceived rationality in the context of Western medical treatment, and (d) understanding the elements that form and define culture as well as their impact on health and illness (p. 139)."[1] Seibert and coworkers advocate using a "Cultural Sensitivity and Awareness Checklist" that focuses on the multidimensional communication that occurs in clinical encounters.[43]

Students need opportunities to learn how to work collaboratively with diverse cultures and values. Experiential learning activities, such as role playing and real patient-therapist interaction, are therefore, essential. All of these activities allow and encourage active participation from which students can construct meaning and skills for resolving ethical problems, issues, and dilemmas.

✦ SUMMARY

Literature and studies have demonstrated that cultures and values serve as a basis for moral decision making and, do indeed, vary with cultural beliefs. Ethics is greatly influenced by the cultural framework in which it is practiced. Yet, current American bioethical principles lack the tools to comprehensively investigate and resolve the social and cultural realities that matter to diverse patient populations. My proposed model to guide ethical analysis rejects moral or cultural imperialism, and instead asks occupational therapy and physical therapy students to engage in moral reasoning and to test their own moral opinions against those of others. It asks for openness

to personal bias that can stimulate them to critically examine the cultural norms of their own practice.[30] By increasing personal self-exploration, knowledge, and skills (cultural competence), ethical decision making will be (a) guided by the ability to communicate appropriately and effectively, (b) culturally framed while remaining aware of individual variances, and (c) based on sound principles of moral reasoning.[3,23,25]

In a multicultural environment good intentions alone are insufficient to guide moral decision making. An ethic of diversity can assist students in finding resolutions. It supports the expectation of "differences" at some level in all clinical interaction. If we are to be consistent and responsible moral agents, we need to engage in open-minded debates. We need to become more open, spontaneous, and flexible in order to appreciate the inner beauty of all persons. Cross-cultural ethical conflicts may not have a single, ethically correct resolution, but many possible resolutions, each with ethical costs and advantages. Which resolution is ultimately adopted will depend on which voices are included in the moral dialogue. Through the principles of cultural competency, understanding, tolerance, fallibility, standing up to evil, respect, justice, and care, therapists have a framework to guide their decisions when conflicts arise.

References

1. Genao I, et al: Building the case for cultural competence. Am J Med Sci 326(3):136–140, 2003.
2. Kundhal KK: Cultural diversity: An evolving challenge to physician-patient communication. JAMA 289(1):94–95, 2003.
3. Wells SA, and Black RM: Cultural Competency for Health Professionals. American Occupational Therapy Association, Bethesda, MD, 2000.
4. Carrese J: Commentary (on culture, healing, and professional obligations). Hastings Cent Rep 23(4):16, 1993.
5. Iwama M: Toward culturally relevant epistemologies in occupational therapy. Am J Occup Ther 57(5):582–588, 2003.
6. Turner L: Biothetics in a multicultural world: Medicine and morality in pluralistic settings. Health Care Anal 11(2):99–117, 2003.
7. Blackhall LJ, et al: Ethnicity and attitudes toward patient autonomy. JAMA 274(10):820–825, 1995.
8. Sheikh A: Dealing with ethics in a multicultural world. West J Med 174:87–88, 2001.
9. Leigh T: Medical ethic in a multicultural society. J R Soc Med 94(1):592–594, 2001.

10. Elliot AC: Health care ethics: Cultural relativity of autonomy. J Transcultural Nurs 12(4):326–330, 2001.
11. Ludwick R, and Silva MC: Nursing around the world: Cultural values and ethical conflicts. Online J Issues Nurs, www.nursingworld.org/ojin/ethicol/ethics_4.htm, 2000.
12. Hyun I: Waver of informed consent, cultural sensitivity, and the problem of unjust families and traditions. Hastings Cent Rep 32(5):14–22, 2002.
13. Kaufert JM, and Putsch RW: Communication through interpreters in health care: Ethical dilemmas arising from differences in class, cultures, languages, and power. J Clin Ethics 8(1):71–87, 1997.
14. Davis AJ: Global influence of American nursing: Some ethical issues. Nurs Ethics: Int J Heath Care Prof 6(2):118–125, 1999.
15. Carrese J, and Rhodes LA: Western bioethics on the Navajo reservation, benefit to harm. JAMA 274(10):826–829, 1995.
16. Institute of Medicine: Unequal Treatment: Confronting Racial and Ethnic Disparities in Health Care. National Academy Press, Washington, DC, 2002.
17. Betancourt JR, et al: Defining cultural competence: A practical framework for addressing racial/ethnic disparities in health and health care. Public Health Rep 118:293–302, 2003.
18. Jang Y: Chinese culture and occupational therapy. Br J Occup Ther 103:106, 1995.
19. American Physical Therapy Association: APTA Code of Ethics and Guide for Professional Conduct. Available at: http://www.apta.org/PT_Practice/ethics_pt/pro_conduct. Accessed November, 2003.
20. American Occupational Therapy Association: Reference Guide to the Occupational Therapy Code of Ethics, AOTA Press, 2000.
21. Scott R: Professional Ethics: A Guide for Rehabilitation Professionals. Mosby, St. Louis, MO, 1998.
22. Edge RS, and Groves JR: Ethics of Health Care: A Guide for Clinical Practice. ed 2. Delmar Publishers, Albany, NY, 1999.
23. Hinman L: The moral point of view. Available at: http://www.ethics.sandiego.edu/values.
24. Lani R: Teaching the ethics of diversity or getting to the heart of the matter. Paper presented at: Values in Higher Education; April 11–13, 1996; University of Tennessee at Knoxville.
25. Hume D: A Treatise of Human Nature. Book 3. Oxford University Press Inc, New York, 2000.
26. Marshall PA, and Koening BA: Bioethics in anthropology: Perspectives on culture, medicine and morality. In Sargent CF, and Johnson TM (eds): Medical Anthropology: Contemporary Theory and Method, Prager, 1996:349–373.
27. Hinman L: What place if any do race, ethnicity, and culture have in moral theory? Available at: http://www.ethics.sandiego.edu/values.
28. Becker GK: Asian and western ethics: Some remarks on a productive tension. Eubios J Asian Int Bioethics 5:31–33, 1995.
29. Hinman LM (ed): Understanding the diversity of moral beliefs: Relativism, absolutism, and pluralism. In Ethics: A Pluralistic Approach to Moral Theory. ed 2. Harcourt, Brace, Fort Worth, 1997.
30. Catherwood JF: An argument for intolerance. J Med Ethics 26:427–443, 2000.
31. Macklin R: Ethical relativism in a multicultural society. Kennedy Inst Ethics J 8(1):1–22, 1998.
32. Coward H, and Hartick G: Perspective on health and cultural pluralism: Ethics in medical education. Clin Invest Med 2000;23(4):261–266, 2000.
33. Hinman LM: Ethical relativism, absolutism, and pluralism. Available at: http://ethics.acusd.edu/relativism.html.
34. Haddad A: Ethics in action. RN 61(3):21–24, 2001.
35. Erlen J: Culture, ethics, and respect: The bottom line is understanding. Orthop Nurs 17(6):79–85, 1998.
36. Brown K, and Jameton A: Commentary on culture, healing, and professional obligations. Hastings Cent Rep 23(4):17, 1993.
37. Skinner S: Guide to Feng Shui. DK Publishing, London, 2001.
38. Pooser P: When clinician and parent disagree (ethics). ASHA Leader 7(21):9, 2002.
39. Carrese J, and Rhodes L: Bridging cultural differences in medical practice: The case of discussing negative information with Navajo patients. J Gen Int Med 15:92–96, 2000.
40. Tucker CM, et al: Cultural sensitivity in physician-patient relationships: Perspectives of an ethnically diverse sample of low-income primary care patients. Med Care 41(7):859–870, 2003.
41. Boulware LE, et al: Race and trust in the health care system. Public Health Rep 118:358–365, 2003.
42. Carrillo JE, Green AR, and Betancourt JR: Cross-cultural primary care: A patient-based approach. Ann Intern Med 130:829–834, 1999.
43. Seibert PS, Stridh-Igo P, and Zimmerman CG: A checklist to facilitate cultural awareness and sensitivity. J Med Ethics 28(3):143–147, 2002.

5

The Self Under Siege: Warring Constructs of Individualism versus Communitarianism and Autocratic versus Democratic Models of Governance in Rehabilitation Settings

JEFFREY L. CRABTREE, OTD, MS, OTR, FAOTA

Abstract

This chapter investigates two overlapping core constructs, or concepts, that have an impact on virtually every aspect of rehabilitation services: the first is the complex notion of the self and what it means to be an individual patient in the context of Western rehabilitation; the second is our notion of appropriate governance as a means of controlling behavior, whether that control be outpatients' follow-through with a treatment regimen, or control of nursing home residents' daily activities. Further, this chapter explores the impact on rehabilitation patients of being caught in moral collisions of conflicting (i.e., individualistic versus community-oriented) notions of what it means to be "an autonomous individual" and conflicting (i.e., autocratic versus shared or democratic) forms of government in health care settings.

The general purpose of this chapter is to explore, not to claim, moral territory. I believe as Johnston said regarding the notion of moral expertise, "Given the nature of the questions [bioethics] deals with, there is no basis for assuming that if we all studied bioethics, we would all come to the same conclusions. There is no guarantee that everyone would agree what the main issues were or which views were worthy of respect (or serious consideration) and which were not."[1] He goes on to identify many other reasons why, in his opinion, there can be no such thing as a moral expert: (a) no bioethical approach or method is accepted by everyone, (b) the bioethicist cannot demonstrate the correctness of what she says, for if someone disagrees with her claim, there is no grounds to believe that by studying bioethics the challenger will change his position, and (c) the status of bioethicists' statements about moral dilemmas is the same as those of anyone else. This may seem a harsh assessment of the status of both bioethics and the bioethicist, but I find that such an assessment forms a useful assumption for a source book on health and rehabilitation, an assumption that hopefully will lead to critical thinking, not a particular brand of ethics.

The more specific purpose of this chapter is to explore the concept of the self and how it can be diminished by forms of health care governance that tend to preempt personal choice, decision making, and the opportunity for self-rule (autonomy), and by Western assumptions about being an individual that often set unrealistic or inappropriate expectations for rehabilitation patients. I first discuss my assumptions about changes in the demographics of rehabilitation patients and the goal of rehabilitation; I then explore the concept of the autonomous self from individualistic and communitarian perspectives; finally I explore notions of governance in a range of applications from the dyadic relationship of the therapist and patient to the institutional governance of hospitals, nursing homes, and the like.

✧ ASSUMPTIONS ABOUT THE GOAL OF REHABILITATION AND REHABILITATION PATIENTS

From the perspective of ethics, and for the purpose of this chapter, I make the following six assumptions. First, the goal of Western rehabilitation is not only to help restore function, but, as Jennings has said, the goal is to help reshape the patient's *self*.[2] "For good therapeutic as well as ethical reasons, rehabilitation must be individually oriented because the patient must be treated as a subject, an active participant and partner in the process of his or her own recovery."[2] Second, as Jennings also asserts, a paradox arises in our liberal culture in that "an important part of the socially defined good is the idea that there is no socially defined conception of the good that should be imposed on individuals."[2] Third, most rehabilitation practitioners are oriented to the above Western beliefs about rehabilitation. Fourth, those receiving rehabilitation services increasingly come from diverse cultures and ethnic backgrounds or because of chronic disease, advanced age, and/or disabilities, are dependent on others. Fifth, opposing cultural beliefs often cause conflicts between patients' beliefs and values about what it means to be an individual and how these beliefs and values should be

expressed in rehabilitation settings. Finally, these significant changes in the cultural mix of patients and increasing numbers of people who, because of advanced age or disabling conditions, do not match the Western ideal of independence-at-all costs, expose rehabilitation practitioners to new and challenging beliefs and values. In the following sections I identify individualistic and communitarian views of the self and autonomy and how these can collide with the patient's belief about the self and autonomy.

✧ INDIVIDUALISTIC AND COLLECTIVIST VIEWS OF THE SELF

Cultural notions of the self, or of personal identity, range from those that express the self as essentially an object or substance, to those that view the self as essentially a process. The extremes of this range are often associated with Eastern and Western ways of thinking. As Hall states, these ways of thinking are not mutually exclusive. However, although Eastern and Western cultures are similar in some ways, there are "significant cultural differences based upon the *process orientation of much of the former* and the *substance orientation of almost all of the latter* [author's italics]."[3] For example, Descartes' supposition, "cogito ergo sum," establishes a dualism of subject and object, mind and body, time and infinity, and thus the notion of self (the "I" as a person in a body) is understood in relation to "other" persons in bodies. At the other extreme might be an essentially process-oriented Buddhist notion of self, which "is that finite, self-creative, world-inclusive experience which, for a given individual, occurs in the present."[4]

I have chosen from the plethora of possible definitions of the self, a simplified version of Schrag's postulation that humans are self-aware, praxis-oriented, selves who are imbedded in "culture-spheres of science, morality, art, and religion ..."[5] In this concept, the self is "oriented toward an understanding of itself in its discourse, its actions, its being with others, and its experience of transcendence."[5] I use this concept of the self because, as Fleming suggests, from a therapist's perspective, "enabling function [and in the rehabilitation setting, enabling the reconstruction of one's life] would have to address problems of the person's sense of self and future, the physical body, and meanings and social and cultural contexts—contexts in which actions are taken and meanings are made."[6]

A Western Perspective of Self and Autonomy

Broadly speaking, and from a Western perspective, the notion of an individual person as something unique and valued can be traced back to Mills' *On Liberty* in which he asserts that in developing individuality, one becomes more valuable to one's self and to others. He goes on to say of individuality: "for what more or better can be said of any condition of human affairs, than that it brings human beings themselves nearer to the best thing they can be? or what worse can be said of any obstruction to good, than that it prevents this?"[7] This notion of enthusiastic, unbridled development of individual personality,[8] along with the idea of personal freedom, compose perhaps the two most formative influences on the dominant Western culture. Virtually everyone raised in the dominant Western culture assumes their right to personal fulfillment or to realize their individual potential. According to Taylor, this draw to personal fulfillment virtually defines Western liberal societies.[9]

Addelson[10] characterized the practical implications of this notion of (self) individuality as the basic unit for ethics. For example, he maintains that "It is the decisions, actions, and motives of individuals that are important; individuals are judged, rewarded, and punished. Individuals have rights, duties, obligations, and entitlements."[10] Furthermore, he asserted that individuality, at least in the United States, has become the institutionalized way our lives are managed. For example, in the world of work and professions, we organize our thinking about promotions, wages, honors, and reputations around the individual.

There seems to be a very strong, direct line between this philosophical notion of individuality and autonomy and the current bioethical notion of autonomy. Dworkin maintains that

autonomy, a concept that combines individualism and personal freedom, "has emerged as the central notion in the area of applied moral philosophy, particularly in the [Western] biomedical context."[11] According to Jennings, Callahan, and Caplan, noted medical ethicists, the autonomy paradigm assumes that the individual's self-interests and autonomy precede the need for medical help and are independent of the process of receiving that medical intervention.[12] In other words, the individual is first an autonomous person who, because of enlightened self-interest, chooses to use medical services when needed.

Furthermore, Boyd[13] maintains that the "ideal of personhood is linked inextricably to reason." She maintains that persons make reasoned choices about what to do or not do according to their values, moral beliefs, goals, and the like. Rationally and freely acting "according to the will then becomes the root of autonomy consistent with a person's moral law."[14] Of particular interest in examining the notion of autonomy in an individualism-communitarian perspective is Boyd's point that individual autonomy is exercised in a social context (a health care setting, family, or community). She maintains that autonomy is an expression of one's will based on beliefs, goals, values derived from experiences within that context and through which one comes to understand oneself and the world. Given a person has the capacity to make choices as a rational agent, individual autonomy can only flourish in a beneficent context that acknowledges humans are social beings who seek and gain benefit from members of the health care team, family, and community.

A Communitarian Perspective of Self and Autonomy

Within the broad notion of communitarianism, compared to the individualistic perspective, the role and responsibilities of the individual take on very different characteristics. What Bell calls modern-day communitarianism is mostly a Western phenomenon that included a reaction of academicians to Rawls' 1971 book *A Theory of Justice*. Western thinkers like Alasdair MacIntyre, Michael Sandel, and

Charles Taylor challenged Rawls' assumptions about government's duty to "secure and distribute fairly the liberties and economic resources individuals need to lead freely chosen lives."[14] Initially, this particular Western phenomenon largely ignored the fact that for more than 3000 years vast numbers of people in the Middle East, East Asia, Africa, not to speak of Native American and other cultures, have held communitarian beliefs and values about the individual's roles and responsibilities.

It is important to acknowledge that communitarianism is not a monolithic concept, but a complex concept that varies within the many ethnic groups and cultures yet can be considered communitarian in nature. I use the term communitarian to characterize the idea of individuals who keep the group needs and goals, not the individual's, foremost in their minds.[15] Thus, in the broad sense of the word, when a conflict arises between the individual and group, within the communitarian environment, the individual is expected to give up her or his needs or interests in favor of the group, whether the group is based on kinship, tribal affiliation, etc.

Despite much diversity among communitarian cultures and groups, there appears to be one core characteristic that crosses all groups, namely, the notion that the self is defined or constituted by ties to the family or community or to a religious belief.[14] In such a context, individual roles and responsibilities reflect the values and beliefs of the group. The concepts of self-fulfillment and realization of individual potential is not considered or is subservient to fulfillment of the family or community.

Autonomy as the Core of Self

There are many constructs and conceptions of autonomy. In this chapter I focus on the notion of autonomy as self-governance— making choices and decisions about one's behavior in light of one's preferences, rights, and responsibilities. The autonomous person, free of controlling influences and with the capacity for intentional action, acts freely in accordance with his or her self-chosen goals. These can be called first-order preferences, desires, wishes, and the like.[11] On many occa-

sions, these decisions might not reflect a person's autonomy because they are influenced by pressure to conform to another's decision, by the high cost in time and effort to acquire relevant information, and the like. However, a person acting on what Dworkin considers second-order preferences would be a true "test" for autonomy. As he has stated: "Autonomy is conceived of as a second-order capacity of persons to reflect critically upon their first-order preferences, desires, wishes, and so forth and the capacity to accept or attempt to change these in light of higher-order preferences and values. By exercising such a capacity, persons define their nature, give meaning and coherence to their lives, and take responsibility for the kind of person they are."[11]

To cite one example, a college freshman may hope to become a member of a certain fraternity and thereby become accepted by a group he has admired from afar. However, during the pledging process he discovers that fraternity members are prejudiced against homosexuals. Despite his disappointment in learning about the group's prejudice, and the discomfort in doing so, he decides to withdraw his application from the fraternity. He exercised autonomy in that he reflected critically on his first-order desires to become part of a particular fraternity, and exercised his second-order capacity to make decisions based on his higher-order values. In so doing this young man is shaping and giving meaning to his life.

In a second example, one of three daughters of Mexican immigrants may have chosen to live at home and not marry until her parents die. Although she may have met men who she felt she could marry, her second-order preferences for meeting her obligations to her parents outweigh her first-order desires to become married.

Within any given day, many people make first-order decisions and manage their lives successfully even in the presence of a life-threatening disease or in the presence of a severely disabling condition. Take the 85-year-old woman who, after having a CVA (cerebrovascular accident) that left her with right side weakness and trunk instability, has a "fender bender" automobile accident, and decides to give up her automobile driver's license. This was a difficult decision for her because of the convenience of being able to drive to wherever she wanted to go. However, she was able to reflect critically on her first-order preferences for convenience and make a difficult decision based on her higher-order preferences to not harm others. Even in circumstances in which one's autonomy is limited, such as a traumatic head injury or dementia, a person can decide what shirt to wear just before being declared incompetent to drive an automobile, and in the days following that declaration, continue to make decisions about with whom to converse, where to read the newspaper, and all of the other little, seemingly unimportant, decisions in a person's life.

✧ GOVERNANCE

In this chapter I use the term governance broadly to describe a number of models of governing authority, or ways of making decisions and controlling people's behavior, recognizing that these forms of governance are motivated by paternalistic beliefs about doing good for patients. Two familiar models include democracy and autocracy. Democracy denotes the idea that authority and decision making are shared among virtually all of the individuals within that system. In the ideal democracy individuals have the authority and power to represent themselves or choose someone to represent them, and to make critical and even frivolous decisions. In a simplistic way, democracy can be summed up in the phrase: One person; one vote. Autocracy, on the other hand, shares authority, decision making, and ways of controlling behavior with fewer people. Depending on the form of autocracy, one person can have complete authority and control over all within that system. Although these definitions seem extreme and perhaps out of date in the current health care arena, it was not so many years ago when physicians had autocratic power over most, if not all, health care decisions.[15] These forms of governance apply to large hospitals, small hospitals, outpatient clinics, and nursing homes in formalized ways (standard operating procedures, and the like), but also express themselves in the relationships between thera-

pists, nurses, and other professionals through their expectations about patients' following "the rules" implied in treatment plans.

According to Hayle, Michels, and Kari, "An organization's governing structure shapes the processes by which it makes decisions, disseminates information, generates and allocates resources and handles power relationships among its members."[16] In analyzing models of governance in nursing homes, Hale and her colleagues identified two most often used models: the medical model or the therapeutic service model. Both short-term acute care and long-term care settings typically have forms of governance that place all of the authority over what happens during the patient's stay in the hands of the staff. Although these forms of governance may be in the best interest of persons who in days will return to their normal life, for the resident of a long-term care setting, an autocratic model of governance limits the opportunity for people to make choices and express their individuality, for typically, long-term care settings are the residents' *home* (a place connected to family and the larger community, a place where one can "be themselves"). This form of governance creates an atmosphere of powerlessness, impotence, and at the extreme, despair. In the following section I will briefly explore these models and extend them into other settings in which occupational and physical therapists provide their services.

Medical and Service Models of Governance

The medical model of governance typically focuses on disease and disability and looks at problem solving as a process of marshalling resources to cure the disease or of improving function to minimize disability. Knowledge about patients' problems comes from medical and technical experts, with those at the top of the hierarchy, typically physicians, having the greatest amount of power and authority to make decisions about treatment, and depending on the setting, to make decisions about how often and when a resident or patient bathes—decisions that not always have to do with therapy or cure. According to Hayle and colleagues this model fosters dependency down the hierarchy. The patients or residents have few opportunities to express their individual wishes or to make choices and depend on the direct-care workers for self care and other functions, and the direct-care workers depend on the nursing staff for decisions about what to do and when.[16]

The therapeutic service model is very similar to the medical model of governance. It handles power relationships among its members in similar ways: using specialized language, making staff responsible for important decisions, fostering dependence on the staff, etc. This model also offers few, if any, opportunities for patients to make first-order or second-order decisions. This model, however, departs from the medical model in the ways the service model generates and allocates resources.[16] For example, resources (the various disciplines from physical therapy to the spiritual counseling of priests or rabbis) are applied programmatically, and therefore are fragmented into spiritual, physical, social, and other services.

These models seem to dominate health care institutions, yet as Kane, Caplan, Freeman, Aroskar, and Urv-Wong note, "It is not clear by what authority we have the right to so circumscribe a nursing home resident's life and to turn each decision into a health care decision."[17] They go on to say, "We can and ought to arrange nursing home care and other residential care for the elderly in a way that is much more respectful of the personal autonomy of the residents."[17] Jennings, Callahan, and Caplan have asserted that chronic care, much of which occurs in nursing home as well as other residential settings and often includes rehabilitation services, "must restore the fabric of community and a web of mutual support and interdependence, beginning with the cooperative … ties between patients and providers."[12] It seems clear that certain forms of governance would be better at giving individuals opportunities to experience themselves through their discourse with others, their actions, and being with others.

✦ THE SELF UNDER SIEGE

Expanding ethnic and cultural diversity of the United States and growing numbers of older adults and people with significant disabling conditions have created a curious ethical conundrum. Jennings makes the observation, correctly, that in addition to improving function, ethical rehabilitation is oriented to helping the individual patient redesign, reshape, or restore his or her self within the social and cultural context of what gives that person's life meaning and purpose.[2] In extreme cases, rehabilitation patients must recreate a self in light of a massive assault on their sense of self and significant changes in the way they perform and participate in their daily lives. This personal, subjective, rehabilitation process assumes that the patient is an autonomous person, free of controlling influences, with the capacity for intentional action, who acts freely in accordance with his or her self-chosen goals. Rehabilitation practitioners guide, support, and nourish this process. Despite this self-evident need for the patient's active, autonomous participation in the rehabilitation process, we expect those patients to obediently follow our rules and regulations while in therapy, and in the case of rehabilitation in long-term settings, to follow our rules and regulations for life. Furthermore, despite increasing numbers of people from different cultures who have different beliefs about what it means to be an individual, we hold to the belief that independence and the pursuit of self fulfillment is the rehabilitation gold standard.

To the extent that it makes sense to conceive of our patients as autonomous selves who come to understand their uniqueness and individuality through their discourse, actions, and involvement with family and community,[5] it makes sense to construct interventions and treatments that offer patients opportunities to exercise their first- and second-order preferences, wants, and desires in contexts that afford discourse, goal-directed action, and involvement in community.

Hayle and colleagues offer such an alternative model for institutions that promises to offer opportunities for those who have the capacity for autonomous action. This is a participatory civic model of governance based on "the belief that people are capable of contribution and have both a responsibility to make a contribution and a right to be given opportunities for growth in that capacity."[16] This model focuses on individuals' capacities to act and abilities to contribute to the governance of the community. This model assumes that all members of the community have valuable information and knowledge that can contribute to decision making. Rather than a hierarchical approach to relationships, this model encourages interdependency among all members, focuses on contribution and reciprocity among staff and residents, and holds all accountable.

What might residents of a nursing home, hospice, or other residential setting contribute to their community, let alone to the community at large? According to this model, civic responsibility is a process of engagement that starts with the definition of a problem within the setting and culminates in public action and the institutionalized civic action in the broader community. The object of community in this model includes participation in problem solving that first focuses on internal needs of the community. One example from the Lazarus Project will help to explicate this process: The call light story in which tension grew between residents who used call lights and staff whose job it was to respond to call lights. In this setting a Resident Council existed that addressed this issue. After a year of interviewing residents and staff, convening public meetings on the issue, and discussions during ongoing council meetings to define the problem, the Resident Council "decided to provide new residents with a resident-produced list of guidelines about the use, misuse, purpose, and format for call light procedures." Through this community action, residents learned about the uses and purposes of call lights in medical settings and the "staff learned that residents have deeper issues than just quality service and can contribute to problem solving."[16]

✧ CONCLUSION

Rehabilitation professionals are experiencing fast-moving changes in the cultural and ethnic mix of rehabilitation patients as well as increasing numbers of people who, because of chronic disease, advanced age, and/or disabilities, may be dependent on others for some things, but despite this dependence are able to make informed decisions and lead fulfilled, vigorous lives. These changes have put the mainstream Western notions of individual autonomy and appropriate governance on a collision course with communitarian notions of what it means to be an autonomous person and on the notion that people, even though they live in health care–related institutions, have the right to express their mundane, commonplace individuality. Such collisions between ideal individualism and communitarian values and beliefs, mainstream assumptions about autonomy and independence, and beliefs about appropriate governance create for educators the need to develop and teach an ethic that addresses these competing beliefs.

References

1. Johnston P: Bioethics, wisdom, and expertise. In Elliott C (ed): Slow Cures and Bad Philosophers: Essays on Wittgenstein, Medicine, and Bioethics. Duke University Press, Durham, NC, 2001, pp 149–160.
2. Jennings B: Healing the self. Am J Med Rehab January/February(suppl):S25–S28, 1995.
3. Hall DL: The width of civilized experience. In Inada KK, and Jacobson NP (eds): Buddhism and American Thinkers. State University of New York Press, Albany, 1984, pp 14–35.
4. McDaniel J: Mahayana enlightenment in process perspective. In Inada KK, and Jacobson NP (eds): Buddhism and American Thinkers. State University of New York Press, Albany, 1984, pp 51–69.
5. Schrag CO: The Self After Postmodernity. Yale University Press, New Haven, CT, 1997.
6. Fleming MH: The therapist with the three-track mind. Am J Occup Ther 45:1007–1014, 1991.
7. Mills JS: On Liberty. In Elliot CW (ed): The Harvard Classics. PF Collier & Son Co, New York, 1909, pp 203–325.
8. Bronowski J, and Mazlish B: The Western Intellectual Tradition. Harper & Row Publishers, New York, 1960.
9. Taylor C: The Ethics of Authenticity. Harvard University Press, Cambridge, MA, 1991.
10. Addelson KP: Mortal Passages: Toward a Collectivist Moral Theory. Routledge, New York, 1994.
11. Dworkin G: The Theory and Practice of Autonomy. Cambridge University Press, Cambridge, MA, 1988.
12. Jennings B, Callahan D, and Caplan AL: Ethical challenges of chronic illness. Hastings Cent Rep February/March(18):1–16, 1988.
13. Boyd AL: Anagogy of Autonomy. Eubios J Asian and Int Bioethics 10:113–119, 2000.
14. Bell D: Communitarianism. In Zalta EN (ed):. The Stanford Encyclopedia of Philosophy. Winter 2001 ed. 2004.

15. Center for Biomedical Ethics: Rethinking Medical Morality: The Ethical Implications of Changes in Health Care Organization, Delivery, and Financing. University of Minnesota, Minneapolis, 1989.

16. Hayle P, Michels P, and Kari N: The Lazarus Project: Creating a Civic Model for Long-Term Care Governance. The Lazarus Project, Minneapolis, 1995.

17. Kane RA, et al: Avenues to appropriate autonomy: What next? In Kane RA, and Caplan AL (eds): Everyday Ethics: Resolving Dilemmas in Nursing Home Life. Springer Publishing Co Inc, New York, 1990.

6

Creating Community: An Essay on the Social Responsibility of Health Professionals

CHARLES CHRISTIANSEN, EDD, OTR, OT(C), FAOTA

Abstract

Communities are essential structures for the well-being of humankind. The health of communities depends on the trust and goodwill that result when people work together, share in community maintenance, and respect their obligations to the group. The foundation for a strong community also rests on the civil and ethical behaviors of its members. Civility and trustworthiness become part of the social expectations of communities when community leaders model them.

Since social groups traditionally accord professionals special privileges because they are educated and deemed to be trustworthy, this essay asserts that the professional status accorded health professionals confers community obligations on them. It openly contends that the faculty of professional schools should explicitly identify and emphasize these civic responsibilities as obligations of its graduates, and it suggests that curricula should be designed to actively foster social involvement by professional students before they graduate.

Learning activities that foster professional responsibility are identified based on social theory. It is recommended that such content should emphasize the importance of communities and the activities that build social capital. Students should also understand the social obligations of membership in the professions. Through service learning, curricula can assist young professionals to better understand the importance of communities and how they can appropriately fulfill their special obligations to serve as role models for civic responsibility.

"It is in the shelter of each other that people live."—Irish proverb

Universities have often included in their mission statements a commitment to serving society and the communities of which they are a part. This reflects a tacit acknowledgment of the virtues of civic-mindedness and the social obligations of educational institutions to help develop and sustain community well-being. But why are communities important? And what are the virtues of civic-mindedness? Beyond the contribution of educated citizens who perform productive roles, what obligations do universities and professional schools have to contribute to community well-being?

In this chapter, I review the concept of social capital, a term first applied to urban life in 1961 by social critic Jane Jacobs, examine how the concept evolved, and explain why it is important for communities. I then consider how it can be fostered through universities, particularly in professional schools. I suggest that the term *professionalism* implies the presence of behaviors, such as service and altruism, that contribute to social well-being. I conclude with specific recommendations for curriculum content and strategies, such as service learning through volunteerism, that are consistent with the idea that professional schools can be catalysts for the creation of social capital.

✧ WHAT IS SOCIAL CAPITAL?

In this chapter, the term *social capital* is used to describe the extent to which a community or society cooperates, collaborates, and embraces norms and values to create trust and achieve mutual benefits. I acknowledge that the present use reflects the traditional sociological interpretation of Durkheim and that there are other definitions and concepts associated with the term.[1] Robert Putnam, in his popular best-seller *Bowling Alone*, described the collapse and revival of the American community.[2] He noted that the term "social capital," which embodies the broader concepts inherent in the more common term "community," implies a sense of trust, of reciprocal responsibility, and social connectedness. Putnam points out that social capital is a tangible good that benefits both individuals and groups.

For example, when a lawyer provides pro bono legal counsel, for example, her act benefits the broader community by making services available to people who otherwise could not afford it. At the same time, this act benefits the lawyer herself, by creating beneficial social contacts, and helping to establish her reputation as an unselfish, community-minded professional person. The positive consequences of social capital include cooperation, mutual support, trust, and institutional effectiveness.[3]

As a sociological concept, social capital has evolved out of the creation of interdependent communities.[4] Although Americans take great pride in the ideas of self-reliance and independence, it is well known that societies, communities, and organizations exist not as a consequence of independence and individual autonomy, but rather as the result of the efficiency and effectiveness resulting from people working together to achieve mutual benefits. Cooperative behavior represents more than a nice social tradition that evolved from chance activities that produced beneficial results. Rather, it likely represents a genetically encoded adaptation of social animals that contributes to their individual survival, and the evolution of their species.[5] This point is worth exploring in more detail.

✧ ALTRUISM AND COOPERATION FROM THE PERSPECTIVE OF EVOLUTIONARY BIOLOGY

Humans came to live in groups specifically because we are social and occupational beings who are genetically predisposed to exist and act together.[6] Mutuality and reciprocity appear to be an evolutionary necessity.[7] Although the biological basis for humans living in groups is a complex topic, the field of neuroscience has provided some useful theories regarding why and how group living occurred. A key event that coincided with the evolution of group living was the incredible increase in human brain size over thousands of years. Brain size has been closely related to the development of language.[8] These observations suggest that language was important to the development of group living.

One theory proposes that language evolved in early humans as a functional necessity for living in groups.[9] Interestingly, this theory directly relates language development to group activities. Language development correlates with the greater amount of time higher order animals, such as primates, spend in social grooming. From observation of primates, it has been found that social grooming, a basic occupation of personal care and care of others, fosters the development of social relationships. Social grooming requires individuals to be in close, physical proximity to each other for purposes other than sexual reproduction. It is theorized that, in early humans, this closeness enabled the development of social relationships, which were initially important for purposes of mutual support. In turn, mutual support was necessary to protect one's standing in the larger social group.

In early humans, as social groups developed, social grooming extended to other shared occupations or activities, such as food gathering and play within groups, and posturing or fighting with other social groups. In other words, the interaction of shared occupations required language, and language fostered more shared activities.[10]

A more widely accepted theory suggests that language was a consequence of group hunting or protection, which required that individuals be able to direct others to the location of threats or prey. Pinker and Bloom[8] suggest that language evolved in humans for two reasons. First, early humans cooperated in their endeavors, especially those related to protection and support. Second, they had a need to share knowledge about the local environment and ways of doing things with their family and group members in order to sustain the group over time. As humans evolved beyond hunting and gathering to the development of agricultural communities, they learned that there was great benefit to dividing labor.[11] For example, cooperation in the division of labor enabled such innovations as the construction of irrigation systems and the planning and harvesting of crops.

Communities gain stability and a sense of belonging over time by transmitting customs, rules, and beliefs from one generation to the next.[12] This requires the use of language, which evolved to a point during the history of humankind where written symbols could be used to provide an enduring record.[13]

Theories from evolutionary biology propose that cooperation and reciprocal altruism, which were genetically influenced species-survival strategies for homo sapiens and other group-living animals, had a large influence on the evolution of language as well as the evolution of communities.[14,15] The success of some communities through the ages (and not others), led to the development of the idea of social capital, where environments and community goodwill create a sense of security and engender a culture of altruistic behavior.[1,4] Unfortunately, in the United States during recent decades, the social capital of communities has been deemed to be declining, based on organizational membership, volunteerism, and other indicators of altruism.[16,17] If these assertions are true, what implications might this decline have for the future of communities, and what can be done about it?

✦ THE DEMISE OF CIVILITY: A SYMPTOM OF SOCIAL BANKRUPTCY?

Ask nearly anyone these days if they view their world as a kinder, friendlier place to be and chances are good that they will reply in the negative. National polls have indicated that Americans view the public-at-large as less polite, less trustworthy, and less dependable than ever before.[18] In addition to that, road rage, or the use of automobiles as weapons, is also increasing at an alarming rate.[19] These characteristics, which encompass deviations from the human virtues of civility and ethics, would seem to operate together in communities to make them less habitable and less desirable places to live.

In addition, statistics from economic reports, polls, and surveys also indicate that fewer people are volunteering service, membership of service-oriented societies and organizations has declined, and philanthropy has also been on a downswing.[16] Religious involvement, perhaps another indicator of social capital, has also diminished in the past 25 year. In the jargon of sociology, these statistics collectively reflect an erosion of social capital and may help to explain why people generally perceive their communities to be less hospitable living environments.

The causes of this reduction in social capital are several. Consumerism, television, population diversity, autonomy, distrust of government, de-professionalization, and social tolerance for intolerance (or apathy) are among those reasons frequently cited.[20,21] See Figure 6.1.

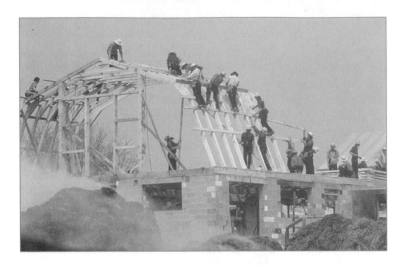

Figure 6.1   ✧   Barn raising. Social capital is created through community cooperation and interdependence. This is exemplified in collective efforts to build physical structures—either for the community at-large or for individuals—as shown in this photo of a barn-raising. Clearly, social capital is created in rural as well as urban communities through such collective efforts.

✦ HOW COMMUNITIES CREATE SOCIAL CAPITAL

The creation of social capital comes directly from acts of civility and kindness sponsored not by governments, but by individuals within informal social networks within neighborhoods, communities, and organizations. Thus, reversing the current downturn in social capital is a process that can occur from the inside out.[22] Advocates for change have argued that it results from perceived trust, civic-mindedness, and generosity, and that this begins with individuals within their communities.[23]

Amatai Etzioni has advocated what he refers to as *communitarian practices*.[24] Similar to other communitarian advocates, Etzioni proposes that we more carefully balance individual rights with a community member's responsibilities to the greater good. Communities develop a sense of commitment and emotional support in times of need as members generate shared beliefs, traditions, and goals through communal activities. Feeling safe and supported by a group engenders feelings of loyalty and attachment. McMillan and Chavis describe four ways in which members generate a "psychological sense of community": this occurs by creating a sense of belonging, through fulfillment of member needs, by providing influence, and by offering shared connections.[25]

These kinds of community-enhancing activities seem more likely to occur if a general climate of trust, friendliness, and goodwill is perceived to exist. The conditions necessary for this environment to occur involve ethical and civil behaviors, ranging from common courtesies to voluntary efforts in community projects. Common courtesies are often overlooked in today's world because what is common sense is not common practice. Common sense is a lay term for what sociologists refer to as normative or expected modes of behavior. As social capital erodes, people spend less time together in shared, mutually beneficial activities. The result is that, too often, group expectations (common sense) does not get communicated.

In recognition of this, The Johns Hopkins Civility Project worked to identify behaviors associated with considerate conduct.[26] As a result, 25 social rules of civility were listed (Table 6.1). These range from using social manners and acknowledging the presence and opinions of others to respecting the environment and giving constructive criticism. Forni asserts that the broader appreciation and application of these rules of considerate conduct create the conditions that make the community and workplace more enjoyable, productive, and healthy environments.[26]

If these changes in conduct of civility are to occur, who among us will provide the motivation and impetus for change? Who will be the role models for turning the tide toward a kinder, more hospitable and trust-inducing social environment? To paraphrase the great French sociologist Emile Durkheim, civility and the

Table 6.1 ✧ **Twenty-five Rules of Considerate Conduct**

Pay attention

Acknowledge others

Think the best

Listen

Be inclusive

Speak kindly

Don't speak ill

Accept and give praise

Respect even a subtle "No"

Respect others' opinions

Mind your body

Be agreeable

Respect other people's time

Respect other people's space

Apologize earnestly and thoughtfully

Assert yourself

Avoid personal questions

Care for your guests

Be a considerate guest

Think twice before asking for favors

Refrain from idle complaints

Give constructive criticism

Respect the environment and be gentle to animals

Keep it down (and rediscover silence)

Don't shift responsibility and blame

Source: From Forni PM: Choosing Civility.
St. Martin's Press, New York, 2002.

actions necessary to create social capital cannot be legislated; they must become a part of the social expectations of communities through the actions of individuals.[27] In the following section, I identify professionals (and students in the professions) as appropriate individuals to lead by example, as an expression of their societal status and "noblesse oblige."

✧ SERVICE: A SOCIAL OBLIGATION OF PROFESSIONALS

Does being professional imply being civic-minded or having a sense of community respon-sibility? If the answer to these queries is yes, then other questions become apparent. For example: What roles do professionals have in modeling civility and ethics? Does professional responsibility implicitly require civic-minded-ness and a commitment to serve others collec-tively? To attempt to answer these questions, it is useful to reflect on the characteristics that constitute a profession and the roles and responsibilities of its members. By virtue of their nature, professions themselves form com-munities of their own.

Goode identified eight characteristics that justify defining the professions as communi-ties.[28] These include: (1) A profession's mem-bers are bound by a sense of identity. (2) Once in a profession, few leave, so that it represents a lifelong commitment or continuing status of membership. (3) A profession's members share values in common. (4) A profession's role defi-nitions are agreed upon and are the same for all members within the group. (5) Within the areas of communal action, there is a common lan-guage, which is understood only partially by the general public. (6) The profession has power over its members. (7) A profession's limits are reasonably clear, though they are not physical and geographical, but social. (8) Although it does not produce the next generation biologi-cally, it does so socially through its control over the selection of professional trainees, and through its training processes as it sends new recruits through an adult socialization process.[28]

In recognizing professions and according them privileges, the members of society support the creation of a community within a commu-nity because members of a profession are, by virtue of their training and commitment to serve, felt to be worthy of special treatment. These privileges include, in addition to a high degree of autonomy, a high level of social respect, and the ability to self-regulate. These privileges accrue as a consequence of the trust extended by the larger society based on its expectation that the profession will adhere to a code of ethics and maintain behavior that is worthy of such privileges. Codes of profession-al ethics generally identify principles of behav-ior that call for altruism, a commitment to service, and behaviors (such as confidentiality, competence, and respect) that ordinarily engender the trust of others.

Through the ages, and to varying degrees, societies have accorded these privileges to four "professions": medicine, law, teaching, and leaders of organized religion. Societies representing these groups have developed codes of ethical behavior, either formally and/or informally. It is not unusual for these formal or informal codes to include statements of responsibility toward the larger society. Consider the renewed call in medical education for honoring the social contract between medicine and the larger society through service and leadership.[29] This expectation of service and leadership is typical of other professional groups as well.

In recent years, sociologists have described an erosion of the respect and autonomy given to traditional professions within society. A term given to this process is *deprofessionalization*. Although there are many reasons given for this trend, one frequently cited is that professions have not lived up to their codes of behavior and have not provided the commitment to service, ethical behavior, and societal leadership expected of them. Although it is not known if the erosion of social capital described earlier is a cause or consequence of the deprofessionalization process, it is likely that a call to renewed commitment to exemplify the ideals of professionalism could contribute to a rebuilding of community through the leadership and professional service commonly expected of professionals.

✧ SERVICE AND SOCIAL CAPITAL

If these codes of behavior are meant to help define professionalism, then actions that reflect courtesy, respect for all, and integrity must be viewed as pertinent to professional demeanors and thus appropriate behaviors to emphasize in the professional education and socialization processes. I argue that health professionals may form a special case wherein the importance of social virtues may be stronger and the imperative greater than it is with other professionals. Many would agree that ethical responsibility is more important among those charged to care for others than in ordinary members of society because human suffering and life itself are at stake. As a result, compassion, trustworthiness, and competence are expected behaviors if health professionals are to deal effectively with the pain, suffering, and grief that accompany disease and injury. It is for these reasons, after all, that Hippocrates deemed it important to include an oath of service as part of the right of passage into the healing arts and sciences.

Moreover, the ethical codes of many health professions imply societal responsibilities in various principles related to beneficence, respect, and integrity. Some even confer responsibility toward society at large. For example, the Code of Ethics of the American Medical Association states in Principle VII that: "A physician shall recognize a responsibility to participate in activities contributing to the improvement of the community and the betterment of public health."[30] Similarly, Principle X of the Code of Ethics of the American Physical Therapy Association also recognizes community responsibility: "A physical therapist shall endeavor to address the health needs of society."[31] The ethical codes of nursing, occupational therapy, and speech-language pathology organizations in the United States similarly allude to obligations to foster the betterment of society.[32–34]

If we accept the premise underlying these behavioral expectations, the next issue is one of determining how best to engender these attitudes and behaviors during the formal education of health providers? In addressing this question, we consider the challenging task of teaching the ethics of social responsibility.

✧ TEACHING THE ETHICS OF SOCIAL RESPONSIBILITY

This writer believes that social responsibility and leadership by example are reasonable expectations for professionals and certainly deserving of attention in the educational process. One approach that has been widely supported as a means for creating the skills and habits of social responsibility is through service-learning. Service-learning is a form of experiential learning where students apply academic knowledge and critical thinking skills to address genuine community needs.[35] Studies have shown that service-learning works effectively to accomplish a number of desirable goals.[36] For example, in grades K-12, service-learning increases social and emotional learning and has positive benefits for academic performance.[37] Other studies have found students with service-learning experience had a greater acceptance of cultural differences and were committed to service now and later in life.[38] In addition to involving the skills necessary to identify and serve community needs, effective service-learning also includes reflection and dialogue, which help a student interpret and solidify values related to community and the larger society.

Social Responsibility: Legislative Support

In recognition of the broad and lasting benefits of service-learning, the U.S. Congress passed legislation in the 1990s called The National and Community Service Trust Act of 1993. This law expanded earlier legislation and established the Corporation for National and Community Service (CNCS), which is responsible for administering all program grants that support the integration of service in the curriculum from primary grades to higher education. Congress passed the legislation with the intent of meeting community needs and renewing the ethic of civic responsibility and the spirit of community throughout the United States. After nearly a decade of activity, the CNCS continues its efforts and its existence has accompanied a resurgence of interest in ways to foster civic responsibility in communities and schools throughout the United States.

Social Responsibility: Curricular Efforts

Happily, recognition of the virtues of service-learning in the health professions has also emerged. The Center for Health Professions at the University of California, San Francisco, has sponsored an initiative called Campus Community Partnerships for Health (CCPH). This program provides expertise and development resources to encourage community-based and service-learning in health professions education. CCPH recognizes the importance of inculcating a respect for the importance of civic responsibility within health profession education.[39]

Fortunately, examples of effective service learning activities in health profession programs are not difficult to find. The author knows of several such programs involving students in nursing, medicine, and the allied health professions. The following example is illustrative of the value of these activities in inculcating an appreciation for community service and an ethic of professional responsibility that embraces the principle of putting the needs of others before self.

Students from all disciplines (including physician assistant studies, occupational therapy, physical therapy, respiratory care, and clinical laboratory sciences) in the School of Allied Health Sciences at the University of Texas Medical Branch participate in a required interdisciplinary course emphasizing core competencies and team learning.[10] This TEAM IDEAL course encourages and provides credit for students who participate in any one of several organized community-service activities, ranging from tutoring local elementary school students from underprivileged families to participation in meals-on-wheels programs and the provision of free health screenings. Students may volunteer for crews that provide house painting and repair for persons with disabilities who reside in the Galveston community. Student participants in these activities consistently report that the experiences help them appreciate cultural and economic situations that may be different than their own and help them realize the importance of such programs to strengthening ties between the university and its surrounding neighborhoods. These activities are discussed in mentored interdisciplinary groups where students can reflect on their experiences and learn the importance of contributing to community well-being. Although programs such as these are enhancing health profession education, they are not nearly widespread enough.

Leaders of academic health centers and local medical and health profession societies may need to place greater emphasis on the importance of such initiatives. Where there are rewards for service-learning innovations, there will be increased efforts. With this in mind, the decision of *U.S. News & World Report* to consider service-learning opportunities as a criterion for ranking institutions of higher education is particularly encouraging. Specialized accrediting agencies would do well to attend to the efforts of educational programs to address civic responsibility in their curricula and to encourage and recognize the use of service-learning strategies.

✧ CONCLUSIONS AND SUMMARY

In this essay, the importance of community to human well-being has been addressed in the context of the individual's responsibility to contribute to it. It has been suggested that health professionals have a special responsibility to provide leadership in this activity as an acknowledgment of their commitments to serve and the privileges accorded to them within society. The obligation of health professions educators to recognize the importance of this agenda toward building social capital and sustaining viable communities has been emphasized. This leads to a recommendation that service-learning strategies can go a long way toward weaving the social fabric that supports strong communities. With concerted effort, the health providers of tomorrow can play an important role in building such communities, even before they officially begin performing their professional roles. But if this is to occur, professional schools must teach them that such responsibilities are attached to the privileges they will enjoy.

References

1. Woolcock M: Social capital and economic development: Towards a theoretical synthesis and policy framework. Theory and Society 27:151–208, 1998.
2. Putnam R: Bowling Alone. Simon and Schuster, New York, 2000.
3. Brehm J, and Rahn W: Individual-level evidence for the causes and consequences of social capital. Am J Poli Sci 41(3):999–1024, 1997.
4. Coleman JS: Social capital in the creation of human capital. Am J Sociol 94:95–120, 1988.
5. Rilling JK, et al: A neural basis for social cooperation. Neuron 35:395–405, 2002.
6. Christiansen CH, and Townsend EA: The occupational nature of communities. In Christiansen CH, and Townsend EA (eds): Introduction to Occupation: The Art and Science of Living. Prentice-Hall, Upper Saddle River, NJ, 2004.
7. Kropotkin P: Mutual Aid: A Factor in Evolution. Black Rose Books, Montreal, P.Q., Canada, 1989.
8. Pinker S, and Bloom P: Natural language and natural selection. Behav Brain Sci 13:707–784, 1990.
9. Calvin WH: The River that Flows Uphill: A Journey from the Big Bang to the Big Brain. Sierra Club Books, San Francisco, 1986.
10. Newmeyer FJ: Functional explanations in linguistics and the origin of language. Lang Commun 11:1–28, 1991.
11. Ofek H: Second Nature: Economic Origins of Human Evolution. Cambridge University Press, Cambridge, MA, 2001.
12. Hauser MD: The Evolution of Communication. MIT Press, Cambridge, MA, 1996.
13. Bloom P: Some issues in the evolution of language and thought. In Cummins D, and Allen C (eds): Evolution of the Mind. Oxford University Press, Oxford, 1998.
14. Trivers RL: The evolution of reciprocal altruism. Q Rev Biol 46:35–57, 1971.
15. Dawkins R: The Selfish Gene, ed 2. Oxford University Press, Oxford, 1989.
16. Putnam RD: Bowling alone: America's declining social capital. J Democracy 6:65–78, 1995.
17. Lemann N: Kicking in groups. Atlantic Mon April:23–26, 1996.
18. Marks J: The American Uncivil Wars. US News World Rep April 22:66–72, 1966.
19. Connell D, and Joint M: Driver aggression in aggressive driving: Three studies by the AAA Foundation for traffic safety. Washington, D.C.: AAA Foundation for Traffic Safety, Washington DC, November, 1996.
20. Carter S: Civility: Manners, Morals and the Etiquette of Democracy. Harper Collins, New York, 1998.
21. Smith TW: Factors relating to misanthropy in contemporary American Society. Soc Sci Res 26(2):176–197, 1997.
22. Rubin I: Function and structure of community: Conceptual and theoretical analysis. In Warren RL, and Lyon L (eds): New Perspectives on the American Community. Dorsey Press, Homewood, IL, 1983, pp 54–61.
23. Youniss J, McLellan IA, and Yates M: What we know about engendering civic identity. Am Behav Sci 40:620–631, 1997.
24. Etzioni A: The Spirit of Community: Rights, Responsibilities and the Communitarian Agenda. Crown, New York, 1993.
25. McMillan DW, and Chavis DM: Sense of community: A definition and theory. J Commun Psychol 14(1):6–23, 1986.
26. Forni PM: Choosing Civility (The Twenty-five Rules of Considerate Conduct). St. Martin's Press, New York, 2002.
27. Thompson K: Emile Durkheim. Tavistock Publications, London, 1982.

28. Goode WJ: Community within a community: The professions. Am Sociolog Rev 20:194–200, 1957.
29. Faulkner LR, and McCurdy RL. Teaching medical students social responsibility: The right thing to do. Acad Med 75:34–42, 2000.
30. American Medical Association: Principles of Medical Ethics. American Medical Association, Chicago, 2001.
31. American Physical Therapy Association: Code of Ethics. American Physical Therapy Association, Washington, DC, 2000.
32. American Nurses Association: Code of Ethics for Nurses. American Nurses Association, Washington, DC, 2001.
33. American Occupational Therapy Association: Occupational Therapy Code of Ethics. American Occupational Therapy Association, Bethesda, MD, 2000.
34. American Speech-Language-Hearing Association: Code of ethics (revised). ASHA Suppl 23:13–15, 2001.
35. Toole J, and Toole P: Key definitions: commonly used terms in the youth service field. National Youth Leadership Council, Roseville, MN, 1992.
36. Morgan W, and Streb M: How Quality Service-Learning Develops Civic Values. Indiana University, Bloomington, IN, 1999.
37. Berkas T: Strategic Review of the W.K. Kellogg Foundation's Service Learning Projects, 1990–1996. W.K. Kellogg Foundation, Battle Creek, MI, 1997.
38. Melchior A: Summary Report: National Evaluation of Learn and Serve America. Center for Human Resources, Brandeis University, Waltham, MA, 1999.
39. Connors K, and Seifer SD: Overcoming a century of town-gown relations: Redefining relationships between communities and academic health centers through community-campus partnerships, 1997.
40. Stephenson K, et al: Changing educational paradigms to prepare allied health professionals for the 21st century. Ed Health: Change Learn Prac 15(1):37–50, 2002.

7

Stigma and Personal Responsibility: Moral Dimensions of a Chronic Illness

PATRICIA BENNER, PHD, RN, FAAN

Abstract

This chapter argues that stigma and responsibility get practically related as moral dimensions of a chronic illness. Persons who are unable to prevent or control their illness are irrationally attributed more responsibility in causing and managing their chronic illness than they have. This informal moral equation is built into the Cartesian view of the "responsibility" of the mind to manage the inert mechanical Cartesian body. Blaming the victim, associated with overestimating the individual's capability and responsibility, is an extreme "mind over matter position." Social and environmental influences for illness are underestimated in a contractual society where moral responsibility rests with autonomous individuals.

Skill acquisition related to managing a chronic illness by patients and by nurses is compared. It turns out that there are commonalities shared by nurses and chronically ill patients at different levels of skill acquisition—from novice to expert. Both must engage in reasoning across time about the particular and both are dependent upon experiential learning despite whatever scientific and technical knowledge they gain about the illness. In both cases, care of a chronic illness is guided by notions of the good and by concerns. An ethic of care is explored, both for the caregiver and care recipient.

✧ MORAL DIMENSIONS OF A CHRONIC ILLNESS

The person facing the diagnosis of cancer in this culture faces stigma, and a set of subtle, unwarranted prejudices that the individual is ultimately responsible for having caused the disease. This stance is common with any illness in Western cultures that stress autonomy and individualism, but seems to be even more prevalent in an illness such as cancer in which the causes and cures are so unclear.[1,2] The following is a research interview with a young woman newly diagnosed with Hodgkin's disease who poignantly depicts the additional burden of self-blame or recrimination that many cancer patients face at some point or another:

I've always taken good care of myself and my body, especially health wise. You know, I've been a vegetarian for over 10 years, but a careful one. And I've been very health conscious—no cigarette smoke, no coffee, caffeine, soda anything. … Cancer is something I am just starting to identify with because that's a difficult word, because I guess it's associated with like toxins, and I just never did any of those carcinogenic things. ...

I'm kind of angry at the stuff that I read where people say that it was your fault that you got it. You know, I wonder, and I've thought about it, but you know could it be because I was under stress or unhappy or depressed or had a difficult year, and it could be, but I would rather think that it is not. Because I look around at my friends, and they're all having struggles and they're under stress from school, and I just don't think that it was my fault. So that's how I'm choosing to look at it right now.[2a]

This study participant describes the searching and pain caused by thinking that one has full responsibility for all actions, thoughts, and feelings and that wrong actions, thoughts, and feelings can "cause" illness. This is an alienated view that the person possesses and controls feelings much like raw material or resources to be managed.[2] Ultimately such an understanding results in a blindness to the limits of personal control. Blaming the victim, associated with overestimating the individual's capability and responsibility, is an extreme "mind over matter position" that is particularly rampant in an extremely individualistic society in which it is believed that the individual has ultimate control and responsibility for any personal event. Social and environmental forces, such as air pollution, pervasive food additives, and early introduction to cigarette smoking, are overlooked or underestimated.[3]

The patient may discover causal links between exposure to toxic wastes at work or in the environment and feel betrayed and victimized. In the case of the patient who may have had known carcinogenic habits (e.g., smoking and heavy alcohol use, or exposure to known carcinogens), acknowledging possible responsibility for cancer may cause great remorse or may bring some clarity and explanation in an otherwise unexplainable capricious event. The patient may prefer having a sense of known linkage to having the uncertainty and lack of control that accompany an unexplained cause. Caretakers, professional or lay, are not immune to these cultural meanings and may inflict more blame and social burden on the person with cancer because the caretaker may link a moral

entitlement to care based on the individual's personal responsibility to prevent illness.

✧ THE CARETAKER'S RESPONSE

Patients' coping may be strongly influenced by the caretaker's own coping with the threat of cancer. Others around the patient (including health care workers) may seek to assign personal responsibility to the cancer patient as a way of warding off the threat of possibly contracting cancer themselves. The young woman quoted below had a very troubling disagreement with her mother because her mother believed that the person defined as patient had to accept responsibility for developing the disease:

My mother feels that it is somehow my fault, so that's kind of strange because it is very important for me not to feel that way. She doesn't feel that I am to blame necessarily, but she is of a different belief than I am right now. And it is hard because I did kind of come from that belief, that somehow, if you got sick, you have to take some sort of responsibility for that. ... (One of the difficult things this week) has been when I was arguing with my mother about the two different ways that we saw why I am sick.[1]

Finding the source of the responsibility within the person who is ill may give an illusion of control or an illusion that the world is just, predictable, and completely interpretable (in social psychology, this fallacy is called the "just world hypothesis"). Blaming the victim may give a sense of immunity to the "disease-free," while evoking a range of feelings, such as helplessness, guilt, loss of control, or victimization, for the patient. Because of the potential for blaming the victim, and placing moral entitlement on receiving care (e.g., one must have lived a healthy lifestyle in order to merit care), nurses, family members, and other health care workers need to be mindful of their own coping with the threat of disease. A consumer warning label must be placed on a "stress management" approach that inadvertently makes the person feel that he or she must manage all distress and be totally "in control" of feelings. The goal of being responsible for a "fighting spirit" or a positive attitude as a prerequisite for health and recovery can place an insurmountable burden on the patient during some of the more distressing times of the illness. Thus any stress-management approach that unwittingly requires that the person step outside of his or her history may only increase the sense of alienation and distress. Eventually the goal is not to step outside one's own history but rather to come to terms with it.

The young woman quoted below describes working through an acceptance of feelings:

I started thinking that because I was depressed that I really got caught up in being depressed ... but now I'm starting to pull back a little bit and realize that I don't have to find out all the answers, that everybody else also thinks about these things. Just because I'm sick, doesn't mean I'm the only one that gets depressed or the only one that thinks about these things. That took the focus off of me, that I can be like that sometimes and not be like that, just as other people are in their wellness."[1]

As this young woman describes, it is easy to lose a sense of legitimacy for feelings. Trying to "manage" all feelings can intensify rather than dampen them. Ascribing a life-threatening or a healing role to emotions can further confuse the everyday issues of living, and make it difficult to feel well, whole, or normal.

A goal of further self-development in the context of dying can be excessively demanding for the patient, and may take away what comfort may be left in the mystery, finiteness, and kinship of the human experience of death. Patients and families may be ill prepared to face the uncontrollable aspects of a terminal illness, unprepared for the possible delirium and loss of bodily control as a part of dying. It is unclear what the expert might reasonably prescribe for a "healthy" death and under what circumstances such prescriptions would provide comfort and help for the dying because meanings and expectations around death and dying vary, as does the actual experience of dying. What the nurse can promise is astute comfort care and pain management along with coaching, presencing (being present and attuned), and assisting patients to maintain their concerns and relationships.

Family Coping and Coping with Caregiving

Families (family is used broadly here to include any significant others) of cancer patients are confronted with a world-changing threat or loss and may experience equal or even more distress than the person with cancer. Glaser and Strauss[4] point out that the patient may be fully absorbed in the situation, and may have adapted to the decreased capacity and well-being whereas it may be difficult for the one standing alongside to see the patient in any terms but the comparative loss. This is not to say that caretakers do not constrict their expectations and understanding of the patient, just that the process may proceed at a different pace than the patient's because they do not share the same physical reality.

One of the most enabling coping capacities is the human capacity to respond to the possibilities inherent in the actual lived situation.[5] Thus a patient and family may come to have expectations around a pain-free hour or around planning a feasible, pleasurable experience. Nurses learn from patients and families over time a range of "situated possibilities" within the bounds of an illness experience and may be effective coaches to patients and families in expanding their sense of situated possibility.[6]

Caregivers, whether professional or family members, can be overextended, and experience fatigue, irritability, resentment, and impatience. Supportive care structures must be provided for family members early, so that respite and rest can sustain the caregiver. Weisman notes that the caretaker who is overwhelmed and extremely fatigued may show signs of abhorrence and avoidance.[7] This is a signal for respite rather than guilt and further demands. Well-timed coaching about the signs of burnout and exhaustion can help the family member be receptive to seeking support when needed. Timing is crucial because family members' concerns and fears are often best alleviated by being present and involved in the care of the loved one, and many warnings of self protection can actually undermine family coping and meanings.

In order to fully understand what the dynamic between caregivers and patients/families entails, we must take into account what the caregiver does to receive and interpret the various kinds of information required to understand the situation. This involves both mind and body. We have two major public discourses on the mind and body and an unsatisfactory array of theories about the relationship between the two. The mind is conceptualized as representational and is measured by beliefs, attitudes, and preferences. It is this view of the mind that we imagine controls the relatively passive body. Our theoretical understandings of the body are typically physiological and biochemical.[8] Both of these scientific and theoretical discourses have much to teach us; however, they cover over what Merleau-Ponty[9] has called the "middle terms." He suggested that our perennial mind-body problems could be resolved if we had shorter conceptual distances between the representing cognitive mind, and the biochemical, physiological body. In between these two understandings lie middle terms that describe the social sentient, skillful body[6] This is the body that has the capacity to dwell in meanings.[10] Examples of middle terms are skills, habits, social practices, common meanings, human concerns, and relationships—the lived social-cultural world. A less objectified view of the body and a fuller appreciation of embodied intelligence have major implications for how we understand treating and caring for our bodies.[6]

A Nursing Perspective on Symptoms

A major influence on how we approach this problem is the Western notion of mind-body dualism developed by the Cartesian model. Under the Cartesian model, the mind is the receiver and interpreter of impressions from the body, and so a symptom is viewed as the mind's subjective interpretation of the body's real disease. Nowhere is Cartesian dualism more entrenched, and nowhere are the limitations of that dualism more obvious, than in the realm of symptomatology. The health care worker's task is to determine what is "really" going on physiologically from the patient's account of symptoms. Furthermore, the separate and nonphysical mind may go astray in its subjective

appraisal and even create bodily symptoms that may or may not be "real." This means that the health care worker must dismiss symptoms that are "merely" psychosomatic and fail to point to underlying disease pathology. This separation and discernment is essential for knowing when to order more diagnostic tests and when to treat, but its language and logic overlook the embodied experiences of suffering and well-being. An alternative vision commonly held by practicing nurses is a consideration of Merleau-Ponty's[9] "middle terms" aspects of the body, described above. For example, nurses assess and manage the effectiveness of technology by "following the body's lead," i.e., understanding embodied patterns.[11] When embodiment is considered as a way of knowing and as a point of engagement with the world, we can consider the body as the ground for a sense of well-being and symptom perception, meanings, and responses.[6]

Symptoms are experienced and appraised differently by the patient and appraised differently by a health care worker depending on the context and history of the symptom.[5] For example, in the case of an acute or a new illness, symptoms may function as an empirical guide for understanding underlying pathology for patient and health care worker. In chronic illness, symptoms function as a familiar signals for an understood, persistent problem. Even before the experience of explicit or nameable "symptoms," one's sense of well-being is experienced. The naming and objectification of "symptoms" is guided by one's self-understanding. Messages from the body, unlike propositions or mechanisms, are partial and imperfectly communicated. The body's strength and adaptive capacities spring from this very ambiguity or indeterminacy. As Merleau-Ponty[9] phrases it, the body enables an emotional connection to the world that allows for attunement, fuzzy recognition of problems, and for moving in skillful, agentic, embodied ways. The social sentient body has the capacity to dwell, to gear into the world, to be in a relationship, to exercise skillful comportment, to seek familiar existential grounds, and more.

As the nursing perspective is concerned with illness as well as disease and human response, and not just as a means to diagnose pathology, in both senses of well-being, distress and the experience of *any* "symptoms" (whether the symptom is considered related to pathology or not) can be heard and attended to in their own right. A nursing approach to symptoms includes symptom perception, response, prevention, and management. Furthermore the management of symptoms includes home remedies, comfort measures, help seeking and receiving, and self care patterns, such as adopting a sick role and seeking respite as well as the use of medical treatments.

Managing a chronic illness does not fit well into a cure-oriented medical system. Those with chronic or terminal illnesses do not fit the cultural paradigm for scientific and technical cures. Caring for the incurable lacks public space, language, and understanding in its own terms. I would not really want the science of medicine to abandon the quest for cures because curative medicine spawns research and a progressive willingness to search for and try new treatments in practice. I too, would like my chronic illnesses cured rather than "managed." However, the power and money flow that accompanies a medico-centric cure approach to disease care causes the human issues associated with experiential learning, craft, or practical wisdom in managing a chronic illness to be overlooked. An emphasis on cure covers the vulnerabilities associated with teaching, coaching, and ongoing management of a chronic illness.

By changing our point of emphasis we can begin to provide the everyday support and attentive care that manage the chronic illness, so that low technology or sustainable technology replaces highly technical cures. For example, treating leg ulcers and foot sores can prevent a large percentage of amputations but this requires attentive care. Likewise, prevention of heart disease could prevent much of the current heart surgery. However, preventive and cardiac rehabilitation require attentive care.

Nurses play unique roles in helping patients manage chronic illness. Learning good technical and scientific management of a disease occurs in the context of learning to cope with the personal, social, and practical implications created by the illness. Like other Western cultures, but perhaps in a more zealous, adoles-

cent way, we have believed in the enlightenment promise of disemburdenment and scientific triumph over darkness, pain, and suffering. We prefer to think positively, citing the latest scientific breakthrough or the one just around the corner, and are prone to assign responsibility or blame the one whose life does match our cultural illusions and promises of control.[2,12] We protect ourselves by pretending that those who suffer must be masochistic or must not have controlled their bodies with their mind, "chosen" healthy lifestyles, or in some other way have earned their suffering.[2] Such folk theories stem from naive theories about a just world and form the moral dimensions of living with a chronic illness, defining what is considered "helpful." The cultural context shapes experiential learning both for nurses and persons with chronic illness. I will use the research on skill acquisition in nursing to think about nurse and patient learning.

✧ FROM ADVANCED BEGINNER TO EXPERT

Do we want medicine to become "life world" specialists? Or do we want to retain the Cartesian vision as a partial but incomplete and, in the end, unsustainable technical vision? Or are there more reasonable positions between these two extremes?

New graduate nurses (advanced beginners) are concerned with mastering the task world, detecting and reporting significant patient changes, coping with the intrusive painful procedures, managing ethical and interpersonal skills as well as the technical skills, making convincing and accurate reports, and communicating with the various levels of health care team members.[13–15] The advanced beginner's day is structured by the assigned reporting tasks, and required patient assessments and procedures. They are caught up with translating their textbook knowledge into relevant patterns of recognition and action. They typically have difficulty recognizing when something is a significant deviation from normal, or whether it can fall within the normal range. They typically "delegate up" their observations of patient conditions, reporting all their observations and asking a more experienced clinician to offer a perspective on the observations they have made. This cannot be otherwise since they have not yet seen a large number of comparison situations. Their practice is guided by general principles and guidelines.

Advanced beginners recognize that they are not operating in the situation with the ease and flow that they see in more experienced nurses. In terms of working with the chronically ill, beginning nurses, like beginning physicians often assume that we already know *what* people with asthma, diabetes, hypertension, cardiovascular disease, cancer, and AIDS have to learn, i.e., that we have the technical-scientific knowledge to teach to patients, and all the patients have to do is to learn the prepackaged skills and techniques of controlling the disease. But as Gadamar notes, and Florence Nightingale before him, this is a fallacy that medical science is building something new rather than restoring an equilibrium already granted by nature.[16] As a beginner, I remember entering with hopes of heroic cures, and omnipotent helping powers, but patients and families in extreme circumstances of suffering taught me that I was one among them and that I only had to discover their stories, their hopes, and have the courage to offer what was possible in the situation. We dare not underestimate what patients can teach nurses about living with a chronic illness.

Situated Possibility—A Non-Normative Notion

Novice patients need to have the task broken down until they can begin to see the bigger picture. Nurses learn firsthand the difficulties associated with adjusting to a chronic illness as an interview on teaching persons newly diagnosed with diabetes conducted by Dr. Harue Masake illustrates:

First, I will say, let's get used to the injection. That is her major fear, and then I will take everything away from you that you have to deal with until you are ready. Then, it is like getting dressed, first the injection, and then start filling the syringes. Next week I think she can do that by herself. Then the next

time we'll do the blood testing and then more into the food. For right now we just focus on not missing meals. Later it will be on how much to eat, what to watch. So we do it in layers. … This is another way of developing trust. Once she feels comfortable enough that she can do this and that she can come back quickly for any kind of help, then we'll move to the next step."[16a]

This is a painfully obvious account to nurses, yet our system of reimbursement and planning for services focuses on the diagnosis and prescription for the disease and overlooks the painstaking work of building a relationship, coaching, empowerment, and bearing witness that is involved in helping people learn to manage their chronic illness. This practice sounds much simpler than it is. Clearly this nurse understands what it is like to work with a novice patient, one who has little or no background experience managing a new chronic illness. This process of coaching changes as new knowledge develops, and as the illness changes.

Competence

The competent nurse (who in this study has at least 2 years of clinical experience) begins to shift his/her attention to the particular in relation to the general. These nurses realize that they must choose a perspective and that the perspective they choose makes a difference. They have a keen new awareness of the limits of the formal knowledge as well as the limits of the knowledge of their colleagues. They are in a position to make more sophisticated judgments of the actions of their colleagues. They talk about noticing patients and families in new ways, now that their skill level allows them to take in more of the situation. They may be aware that the complexity and variety of the situation call for new approaches, namely, pattern recognition and comparison of whole cases, but if they remain committed to analysis rather than synthesis they may not recognize patterns, see trends, or compare this situation with other past situations. They are actively working on modifying their skills of interpersonal involvements for nursing practice. They talk about managing the pain of getting too involved, and the problem of too much distance and disengagement.

In contrast to the advanced beginner, the experienced competent nurse can more effectively use past clinical experience to guide present clinical learning. The focus of the narrative is now more on clinical issues, the clinical condition and management of the patient, and issues of timing and organization of work. The leap in organizational skills is evident upon observation. The performance is more fluid and coordinated and a result of forecasting and developing plans.

There were many reflections on being better able to handle busy complex situations than in the past but organizing work was not a theme compelling enough to talk about unless the organizational and coordination demands were novel or extraordinary.

The competent nurse actively thinks about the future in order to plan the present care. This is a conscious attempt to anticipate what is likely to occur in the future. The future is reflected upon in order to provide guidelines for the present. This is not an integrated grasp of the present situation in terms of the future, which is a characteristic for the expert. Thinking about the future offers an analytical tool for the competent level nurse, whereas for the expert typical futures are incorporated in understanding the present situation.

A major form of clinical learning for nursing and medical students is that of recognizing what constitutes a sign and symptom in real life. This meshing of clinical (practical) knowledge with formal theoretical knowledge is evident in the beginner but becomes more nuanced and sophisticated in the competent nurse and, for the first time, the competent nurse becomes a repository of firsthand perceptual knowledge:

N. I have a tendency to go to more experienced nurses and say this is what I found, is there something I missed? Is there something that's not quite making sense? Or, I haven't seen it quite this way before. It's really nice now to find people coming to you sometimes, not too often.

I. How do you know when to go to a more experienced nurse when things don't fit together so well?

N. I know I don't feel as comfortable with head traumas. I'm not familiar with some of the signs about herniation or head injury. We have a couple of nurses who are just excellent. You just say, 'I just want to make sure I'm doing this okay. Could you just verify with me what I'm finding?' Also, I don't deal comfortably with cardiac patients because we don't deal with that a lot. We have a lot of healthy hearts.[15]

Formal descriptions do not automatically lead to recognition of the actual signs and recognition of contextual and relational responses; they require time to assimilate and recognize. Clinical expectations can become too esoteric and complex so that the basics are overlooked, as the following nurse reflects after a successful but perhaps avoidable resuscitation: "I think I was looking for more complex things instead of just saying this is basic shock. It was pretty much the basic shock symptoms and I don't know, maybe she would not have coded if everybody would have acted more quickly."[15]

This kind of reflection is crucial for clinical learning and illustrates the experiential distance between the formal signs and symptoms as they are learned in the classroom and the recognition of these in the actual clinical situation.

I suspect that patients, too, have to learn these particular patterns of their symptoms as well as their own impediments to recognizing and responding to symptoms early in an illness cycle. Helping patients discover early warnings and coaching them in reading their own bodily responses can help patients move from competency to proficiency. For example, when giving a person with diabetes a machine to measure blood sugars, it is a good idea to suggest that they guess what their blood sugar is before reading the meter. This way, the use of technology can increase skill in reading the body, instead of de-skilling the patient by decreasing the attentiveness to bodily sensations associated with particular activity and eating patterns.

Proficiency

Increasingly, practice is guided by good outcomes. It is no longer enough to have performed efficiently, or to know the right answers.

The performance must now be connected to good outcomes. For example a nurse responds to the interviewer's question about what makes a good code in the following way: "The guy wakes up and talks to you. That's the only qualification. A code can be messy and horrid, but if he wakes up later and talks to you, it's worth it."[15]

Nurses talk about having a good grasp of a situation, or being comfortable rather than being confused, overwhelmed or lost. Since their anxiety is now generally lower, they can begin to trust their emotional responses to guide their attentiveness and calls for help. Emotional responses offer a "fuzzy" recognition strategy that they now can relate to specific situations. Now nurses cope with their emotional responses to problems, errors, and things that do not go as planned as crucial to clinical learning. That they even sense disappointment in the patient's clinical course grows out of their increasing involvement and agency. Learning skilled know-how requires attentiveness and openness to learning from new situations and from an increased grasp of the complexities:

I. Have you taken care of a person with the same hypotension?

N. Oh, many.

I. What kind of questions go through your mind now that did not go through your mind then?

N. Are they volume depleted? Do they need blood? Are they dilated, do they need a little tone?

I. Do you have a checklist that you go through?

N. Yes.

I. You didn't have a checklist before?

N. You have little bits and pieces but it just doesn't all fit together.

I. Didn't they present the checklist in the heart course?

N. They do present it in the heart course, but still, different things happen with different patients, so it's not exactly as the heart course presents it. Every patient is a little bit different. So, it's not always, as easy as going down the list and saying this other factors. But they did present a list. A sort of understanding the concepts of pre-load and after-load, that doesn't come from—you do not understand that for awhile.

Second Nurse: They gave you a definition and you can spin it back.

N: Right, you can spin out a definition like that, but you cannot picture what is going on in that heart until you have had a few of these hearts and realize what is really going on.[15]

The nurse must learn to see the relationships between therapeutic actions and patient responses in the actual practical situations before the possibility of real agency and responsibility can develop that is relevant to the clinical situation. Also embedded in this narrative is the recognition of the particular in relation to the general and learning the concrete manifestations of the formal categories. This is a critical juncture for recognizing the limits of formal knowledge and an increasing sense of responsibility. In coaching chronically ill patients, timing, recognizing teachable moments, and recognizing the adaptive tasks that the patient/family is struggling with are crucial.

Becoming Situated and Recognizing Changing Relevance

The hallmark of the proficient stage is to recognize when the clinical situation has changed so that things that were not important in the past may now be very important. We call this changing relevance. Gaining a sense of salience means that the clinical situation is meaningful, in that some things stand out as more or less important without reflective thought. Changes in the clinical situation and recognition of these changes loom large in the narratives. Proficient nurses now have an increased ability to recognize changing relevance, which includes both the recognition and the orchestration of skilled responses to the changing situation. For example, a person with asthma may learn to recognize that a combination of heavy exposure to allergens, fatigue, and stress may require more modifications and self-care strategies than would be the case with any one of these factors alone.

Clinical Expertise

The clinical nurse has a different level of sophistication in recognizing the particular in relation to the general. For example, instead of talking about the objective properties of drugs in general, they now talk about how specific patients respond to drugs, as when asking, how does this patient respond to Nipride or dobutamine? Much of the content of their exemplars has to do with developing new knowledge, or with ethical dilemmas. We have found that observations were a key to describing expert practice, because the expert typically talks about new learning, puzzles, or dilemmas in their group interview sessions.

The expert nurse's agency and responsibility is evident in three major areas: (1) negotiating clinical knowledge; (2) keeping track of what's going on with less experienced nurses' patients and augmenting their clinical assessments; and (3) being responsive to and advocating for the patient and family concerns in ways that are close to patient/family actual concerns and needs.

What it means to be a responsible agent acting in a clinical nursing situation is determined by one's perceptual grasp of the situation. Agency for the advanced beginner is accomplishing tasks; for the competent nurse it is setting goals and making plans that are achieved. For the proficient nurse, agency takes on new experientially based possibilities to recognize new issues and changing relevance directly in the clinical situation. For the expert, "reading the situation" is based on expected changing relevance and includes actions based upon the patient/family responses.

Expert nurses are tutored by the situation, and attend to, in particular, the patient's responses. The following example illustrates articulation of the coaching, transformation, and skill required to empower a patient to take up the project of managing her diabetes. As a home care nurse Deena Bunzel received the report that a 75-year-old woman refused to give her own insulin after repeated infections, and staunchly refused to call on family members for help. Bunzel states:

I am blessed with a gift to connect with people, even when they don't want it, and that began the process with Jewell. After two weeks of daily instruction, I was now met with a willing participant, organized with glasses and good lighting to do her fingerstick Fasting Blood Sugar, review her diet choices, critique her snack choices, and enjoy her humor. "Never, will I stick myself!" she said. We explored her ideas: she is too old to learn: "Can't teach old dogs new tricks, you know?"; and she would not need the insulin long, anyway, so why couldn't I just do it. By this time, she was enjoying my daily AM visits. We learned about each other's preconceived ideas: the difference in our idea of "old," and "learning," and "independence." Each step of the way, we both learned to alter our plan, and I changed my teaching strategy more times than I can relate. She required constant reminders of the infections she had endured, which is where this all began. She also needed to know that I thought she could learn, that I believed she could stick herself, and that I knew she could manage her diabetic regime ALONE.

I felt the pressure from my supervisor to limit my home visits because insurance money is running out. I feel the pressure so I "suggest to her" that the following Monday, she may choose to give me a shot, or give herself her own insulin. She responds with a look of incredulous surprise!! I reply: "It's your choice on Monday." I am amazed at Jewell. She is prepared to give her own insulin. She says: "I can't stick you!"

She did a magnificent job, including reiterating all my teaching. We were progressing, and from there we polished off the other dynamics of diabetic education, decreased the visits to 3 times a week, then two times and then weekly. She currently lives independently in the same complex at age 80, and manages her diabetes with blood glucose of 120–180 without any assistance. She continues to keep her physician appointments and all the records as we did initially. She had one infection about two years ago, and immediately called for the Visiting Nurse's to fine tune her regimen.[16b]

This example of teaching persons with diabetes makes the skilled coaching and teaching of expert nurses visible. Change, growth, and empowerment come as the nurse bears witness to the patient's plight, informs, presences herself, understands, instructs, humors, and encourages in a patient, consistent way. The skillful teaching and relational skill of the nurse are essential to good symptom management and for empowering the patient to take up his or her life in ways that are acceptable and possible. Situated possibility is central to the human condition—it is all any of use ever have—and it is often quite enough.

Phronesis and Relationship

The practices of nursing and medicine carry within their tradition moral sources for meeting the other in respect and in solidarity with the human condition of embodiment, finitude, vulnerability, and human possibilities. The helping professional must be schooled in skills of involvement, in meeting the other—in receptive ethics.[17]

Nurses in practice, even in the most bureaucratic settings, struggle with a relational or care ethic. Nursing as a socially organized set of caring practices brings to the discussion of bioethics ethical concerns about how to meet, encourage life courage and growth, how to protect, nurture, and comfort those who are vulnerable and in need of care.[6,17] But nursing, when truest to its tradition, does this with an acknowledgment of the distinctiveness and separateness of the other, and with the understanding that the need for care is universal and helpers share the same human possibilities as those they would help.[6] This stance is distinct from the technical expert who only holds an external relationship to an object of craft or fabrication. Although nursing as a discipline can claim rationality, knowledge, and skillful ethical comportment in its caring practices, it cannot coherently claim a narrow rational technique that guarantees mastery over the outcomes of caring relationships with concrete finite others.

This places nursing as a discipline more firmly in the Aristotelian tradition of phronesis and praxis rather than poiesis or making, the technical rationality of producing outcomes.[5,13–15] A justification of right actions based upon moral principles, while useful for institutional policies and procedures and for justified ethical decision making, especially in dilemma or breakdown cases, is not sufficient for generating or discovering the good in concrete particular caring relationships. This calls for wanting the other to flourish, to be met and recognized—what Iris Murdoch would call finding the good in others with no ulterior motive or point to prove.[18,19] That this art would seek the good in situations of risk and vulnerability requires more than a diagnostic armamentarium for fixing pathologies and deficits—it requires that the good possibilities in actual concrete situations and concrete relationships be acknowledged and nurtured. In meeting the other and in caring practices one finds "situated possibilities" rather than norms or static goals.[6] There can be no guarantees in such a fragile and risky set of caring practices. "Helping" that dominates, takes over, or promises of what is not feasible must be vigilantly resisted.

Norwegian nurse philosopher and ethicist Kari Martinsen[17] has written about the necessity of metaphysics and a critical social ethic for nursing that is life affirming and nurturing: "Ethics, life-philosophy and metaphysics are cornerstones in nursing. ... Caring for others and loving one's neighbor are the most natural and fundamental aspects of our lives. And also so difficult."[17]

Martinsen, influenced by the works of Karl Marx and K.E. Logstrup,[20] critiques the extreme individualism of the modern self-centered and self-assertive individual. In Martinsen's words:

Life with fellow man demands a certain way of living: Not to interfere, control or master the other person. To be open and empathic yet restrained induces an ethics of reception. The attitude towards life is gratitude. In our world of productivity and results, this becomes critical ethics ... The battle between conquering and receiving appears in human relations. In human relations, power can be used to destroy the other, or used to expand the other's life-space by receiving him/her. Hope lies in receiving, not in conquering each other. Receiving the other with confidence is criticism of the violent idea of growth, to which we are expected. It is counterweight to progress and competition which creates loneliness and tension. Receiving the other in confidence is seeing and defending the unqualified human values, in a society which measures them according to qualifications and usefulness. It is seeing what has been given us—seeing the other as creation and irreplaceable. It is seeing the potential in the person who never achieved anything."[17]

Martinsen's work resonates with my work in articulating notions of good in the everyday practice of nurses.[6,13] I am convinced that nurses encounter the fundamental demands that the lives of others be received and responded to as members and participants in a common humanity or, as Logstrup[20] and Martinsen[17] put it, as a response to the fundamental gift of life. First-person experiences, or stories from nursing practice, point to meeting the other in vulnerability, situated possibility, and respect for the life of the other. Nurses have informal narrative dialogues about "knowing the patient and family"[21] whereby their judgment is guided by knowing the particular concerns and clinical trajectory of the patient. Within knowing the patient and family, the nurse is able to make qualitative distinctions about what will be experienced as care and what will be experienced as controlling and dominating.[22] Despite our many theoretical and practical reasons for being skeptical about the human possibilities of a receptive ethic, the discovery of these sovereign life expressions against all odds holds out the distinct possibilities of care and allows us to explore and encounter the sovereignty of the good.[23] Charles Taylor[24] makes the point that our sense of moral obligation is dependent on the broader and more fundamental sense of what it is good to be:

But ethics involves more than what we are obligated to do. It also involves what it is good to be. This is clear when we think of other considerations than those arising from our obligations to others, questions of the good life and human fulfillment. But this other dimension is there even when we are talking about our obligations to others. The sense that such and such is an action we are obligated by justice to perform cannot be separated from a sense that being just is a good way to be. If we had the first without any hint of the second, we would be dealing with a compulsion, like the neurotic necessity to wash one's hands or to remove stones from the road. A moral obligation comes across as moral because it is part of a broader sense which includes the goodness, perhaps the nobility or admirability, of being someone who lives up to it ...."

If we give the full range of ethical meanings their due, we can see that the fullness of ethical life involves not just doing, but also being; and not just these two, but also loving (which is short-hand here for being moved by, being inspired by) what is constitutively good. It is a drastic reduction to think that we can capture the moral by focusing only on obligated action, as though it were of no ethical moment what you are and what you love. These are the essence of the ethical life.[24]

A recent observation of care planning and reporting between hospice nurse and physician Dr. Derek Kerr[25] explained following the notions of good care with all its particularities and contingencies. For example, rescue treatment is not usually applied in managing terminal pneumonias in hospice care. However, Dr. Kerr explained, "In the case of pulmonary infection which is distressingly malodorous, or provokes a troublesome cough, then oral antibiotics would be prescribed." The person's humanity, facing death, and closing down a life in the context of a particular life and disease guide medical and nursing interventions. The ethical concerns related to patients' rights are different from those related to providing as good a death as possible for a particular patient, once the patient's rights related to dying and treatment are settled.

Discernment and risk are ever present as judgments are made about increasing narcotics or providing palliative care that will ease the days and allow persons to face their death as they are able. Notions of good are fragile and come with risks of not doing or being good in a situation.[25a] It is easier to guarantee rights than it is to ensure fidelity to the good in concrete contingent situations. Practical reasoning (phronesis) about facing death and providing comfort and dignity are not reduced to "choice" or "control" though choice and control figure into concerns and discernment as the person finds his or her way toward death. Many more particular life goods are at stake than choice. For example, the moral art of holding open a life so that social death does not occur before physical death, and so that leave-taking rituals and the human task of facing death are possible, are fragile goods that require connection and discernment. They cannot be guaranteed, but they can be nurtured by telling our practice stories where the good is actualized, and by creating work environments that support and encourage caring practices between health care practitioners and patients. Rights are essential and remedial, but not the end of ethical concerns.

❖ SUMMARY

It turns out that there are commonalities shared by nurses and chronically ill patients at different levels of skill acquisition—from novice to expert. Both must engage in reasoning across time about the particular and both are dependent upon experiential learning despite whatever scientific and technical knowledge they gain about the illness. Acute episodes of illness are always situated in the midst of varying circumstances and resources. Neither can predict the future with certainty, but both, with experience, gain experiential wisdom that enables them to engage in informed forethought about the signs and symptoms and consequences inherent in their illness. Both are guided by their situated concerns, though the content of those concerns are quite different. Most concerns are related to the person's notions of good … what they care about … what they consider important. Both expert nurses and expert patients can gain perceptual acuity or intuitive grasp of situations that are similar or notably dissimilar from past experiences; therefore, both must acknowledge the wisdom of this perceptual, tacit, or intuitive understanding that is based upon experience. The patient's and the nurse's quality of engagement with the situation versus level of disengagement or distraction will influence whether they are able to act in an expert manner.

But nurses and patients remain different to each other despite the quality of the relationship. The patient's illness and concerns shape their own life world in ways that caring for the ill person does not influence the nurse's world. This notion of caregiver and one cared for being other, but no wholly other[26] is central to an ethic of care. Boundaries must be respected as well as the limits of control, and notions of good and concerns that guide each person's actions. Experiential learning for the patient depends on observation and reporting of others, and also direct experience of the symptoms, their meanings, and their context … all of which are bodily and embodied. The patient, like the nurse, lives his or her own bodily experience in the context of their life world. This is why a receptive ethic, and ethic of care, is required by both nurse and patient, but also why it remains central for cure, recovery, reha-bilitation, and managing an ongoing chronic illness.

References

1. Leder D: A tale of two bodies: The Cartesian corpse and the lived body. In Welton D (ed): Body and Flesh, A Philosophical Reader. Blackwell Scientific Publications Inc, Oxford, 1998.
2. Benner P, et al: Moral dimensions of living with a chronic illness, autonomy, responsibility, and the limits of control. In Benner P (ed): Interpretive Phenomenology. Sage Publications Inc, Thousand Oaks, CA, 1994, pp 225–254.
2a. Larson P, et al: A clinical ethnography of two cancer trajectories. An unpublished pilot study sponsored by the Oncology Nursing Society, UCSF, 1990.
3. Sontag S: Illness as Metaphor and AIDS and its Metaphors. Picador USA, New York, 1977.
4. Glaser BG, and Strauss AL: Awareness of Dying. Aldine de Gruyter, New York, 1965.
5. Benner P, Hooper-Kyriakidis P, and Stannard D: Clinical Wisdom and Interventions in Critical Care, A Thinking-in-Action Approach. WB Saunders Company, Philadelphia, 1999.
6. Benner P, and Wrubel J: The Primacy of Caring: Stress and Coping in Health and Illness. Addison-Wesley Publishing Co Inc, Menlo Park, CA, 1989.
7. Weisman AD: Coping with Cancer. McGraw-Hill, Inc, New York, 1979.
8. Dreyfus HL: Being-in-the-world, A Commentary on Heidegger's Being and Time, Division I. MIT Press, Cambridge, MA, 1991.
9. Merleau-Ponty M: The Phenomenology of Perception. Translated by C. Smith. Routledge and Kegan Paul, London, 1962.
10. Polanyi M: Personal Knowledge: Towards a Post-Critical Philosophy. University of Chicago Press, Chicago, 1958/1962.
11. Benner P: The role of articulation in understanding practice and experience as sources of knowledge. In Tully J, and Weinstock DM (eds): Philosophy in a Time of Pluralism: Perspectives on the Philosophy of Charles Taylor. Cambridge University Press, Cambridge, 1995, pp 136–155.
12. Lowenberg JS: Caring and Responsibility, the Crossroads Between Holistic Practice and Traditional Medicine. University of Pennsylvania Press, Philadelphia, 1989.
13. Benner P: From Novice to Expert: Excellence and Power in Clinical Nursing Practice. Prentice-Hall, Saddleback, NJ, 2000.
14. Dunne J: Back to the Rough Ground, Practical Judgment and the Lure of Technique. Indiana University Press, Notre Dame, 1993.
15. Benner P, Tanner CA, and Chelsa CA: Expertise in Nursing Practice: Caring, Clinical Judgment and Ethics. Springer Publishing Co Inc, New York, 1996.
16. Gadamer HJ (ed): Truth and Method. Sheed and Ward, London, 1960/1975.
16a. Masake, H: Unpublished pilot research data. UCSF, 1995.
16b. Deena Bunzel: Nursing narrative presented at UCSF, 1995.
17. Martinsen K: From Marx to Logstrup. Tano Publishers, Oslo, Norway, 2003.

18. Murdoch I: Metaphysics as a Guide to Morals. The Penguin Press, New York, 1992.

19. Taylor C: Philosophical reflections on caring practices. In Phillips SS, and Benner P (eds): The Crisis of Care: Affirming and Restoring Caring Practices in the Helping Professions; 1996.

20. Logstrup KE: The Ethical Demand. Notre Dame: University of Notre Dame Press, 1997.

21. Tanner CA, et al: The phenomenology of knowing a patient. Image 25(4):273–280, 1993.

22. Rubin J: Impediments to the development of expert clinical knowledge and ethical judgment in critical care nursing. In Benner P, Tanner CA, and Chelsa CA (eds): Expertise in Nursing Practice: Caring, Clinical Judgment and Ethics. Springer Publishing Co Inc, New York, 1996, pp 170–192.

23. Murdoch I: The Sovereignty of the Good. Routledge and Kegan Paul, London, 1970.

24. Taylor C: Iris Murdoch and moral philosophy. In Antonaccio M, and Schweiker W (eds): Iris Murdoch and the Search for Human Goodness. University of Chicago Press, Chicago, 1996, pp 3–28.

25. Conversation with Derek Kerr, M.D., Hospice Physician, La Guna Honda Hospital, San Francisco, CA, 2000.

25a. Nussbaum M: The Fragility of Goodness: Luck and Ethics in Greek Philosophy. Cambridge University Press, Cambridge, UK, 1986.

26. Levinas E: Alterity and Transcendence. (M.B. Smith, transl.) Columbia University Press, New York, 1999.

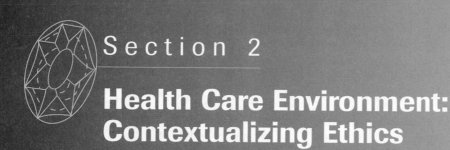

Section 2

Health Care Environment: Contextualizing Ethics

8

The Ephemeral Ethics of Evidence-Based Practice

CHARLOTTE BRASIC ROYEEN, PHD, OTR/L, FAOTA

Abstract

"[H]ow to intervene with wisdom and courage [?]. Let us trust ourselves to be guided by our own values"[1]

This chapter explores the ephemeral ethics of evidence-based practice as a mandated mantra within occupational therapy and physical therapy. First, a view of evidence-based practice as a medical import from England will be presented and the current status reviewed. Second, the ephemeral ethics of evidence-based practice will be introduced. Third, selected research and scholarship will be presented, including insight into what occupational therapists and physical therapists think about evidence-based practice. Fourth, the TRIO model of ethics for practice in occupational therapy and physical therapy will be presented and explained, including (a) habits of the mind, (b) habits of the heart, and (c) habits of the art. Fifth, best practice in occupational therapy and physical therapy will be hypothesized to emanate from integration of habits of the mind with habits of the heart and habits of the art. Sixth, a simple mnemonic device provides a framework for guiding such integrated practice and encapsulates the factors a therapist might consider when striving for best practice: ETHICS (E, evidence-based; T, theory driven; H, humanistic; I, individualized; C, client centered and culturally sensitive; and S, spiritual and therapeutic use of self). Finally, a summary and conclusions about the utility of the TRIO model of ethics and the ETHICS framework for guiding best practice will be presented.

I find it a bit of a paradox that I—not formally trained in ethics—am contributing a chapter to this book about ethics in occupational therapy and physical therapy. Admittedly, however, lack of expertise rarely limits my opining upon a topic. (Consider that an artifact of a strong "J" personality variable—rendering judgments is just part of this type of personality.) In addition, I submit that my informal training in ethics, ranging from parental expectations, a decade and a half of receiving and teaching Presbyterian Sunday School, socialization into the profession of occupational therapy, and the osmotic effect of long-term exposure to Jesuit ideals and culture has sensitized me to need to reflect upon the moral dimensions of life in general and occupational therapy and physical therapy practice specifically. Why else would I be sitting here on a weekend grappling with profound issues dealing with how therapists think about and execute their practice in service to society? Thus, I submit that my early life experiences and "on the job" education, combined with repeated exposure to those actually educated and expert in ethics,[1a] has inspired me to consider how ethics relates to best practice in our fields. And, I consider this perspective particularly as coupled with the powerful, externally initiated movement of "evidence-based practice" (EBP) permeating our professions. A view of how evidence-based practice, as a mantra, came to be, follows.

✦ A VIEW OF EVIDENCE-BASED PRACTICE

With an eye to the humorous, evidence-based practice in medicine has been contrasted with other practices in medicine, such as eminence-based medicine, vehemence-based medicine, eloquence-based medicine, diffidence-based medicine, and confidence-based medicine.[2,3] In a serious vein, evidence-based practice appears as nearly a zealot movement in our fields, focusing our practice primarily and directly on what research and science reveals about how to intervene. Occupational therapy and physical therapy did not invent evidence-based practice. Rather, it is a long trail from point of origin—evidence-based medicine[4]—to our fields that delineates how it came to be paramount in our worldview. Arrival of evidence-based medicine as a "movement" from England has been likened to the import of the music of the Beatles—rapid, pervasive, and dominant. Evidence-based practice appears to be a politically correct, preeminent strategy in occupational therapy[5,6] and physical therapy.[7,8]

I argue that just as the imported music of the Beatles has an important and long-lasting role in the blends and genre of music we appreciate (classical, country, jazz, etc.), so too imported strategies for evidence-based practice should have a role in how and what we practice as therapists, but not an exclusionary role—perhaps not even a dominant role. For just as a musical diet restricted to the Beatles would be dulling without other types of music, adherence to evidence-based practice as a primary guide to practice is, in my mind, beyond dulling, moving into bad practice. Predominant or exclusive use of evidence-based practice as a guide for intervention leaves out other critically important parts of what we should do and how we should do it, part of the ethics of practice alluded to by Purtilo.[9]

Herein lays the essence of the ephemeral ethics of evidence-based practice. At first blush, it sounds like a fine idea and the right thing to do. But, after reflection, the truth of evidence-based practice dissipates, and one realizes that there is so much more that goes into working with humans than a one-dimensional view using only research evidence. Primary use of evidence without considering all the other variables that are just as important—such as clinical reasoning,[10] caring,[11] cultural context,[12] socioeconomic status, life history, as well as personal values and goals, is likely the wrong thing to do. Thus, the ethics of using research evidence and doing right is ethereal—good at a glance but it just doesn't hold up and dissipates when considering the multitude of other factors going into human health and engagement in occupation.[12a] For example, Friedman argues that evidence-based practice has limitations especially when applied to a single patient with multiple diseases.[13]

At the same time the United States experienced increased accountability for health care costs,[14] evidence-based medicine arrived from England. A coincidence, you say? Perhaps. Evidence-based medicine has been widely accepted as the way for medical professionals and professions related to medicine [occupational therapy and physical therapy] to be more accountable in the interventions they provide.[15] Thus, in some ways evidence-based medicine serves as an effective constraint on what and how services may be offered to individuals. Medicine was the first profession to define and advocate an evidence-based approach to practice,[14] in response to the findings that numerous studies revealed, namely, that practitioners tend to rely on experiential knowledge to guide practice rather than appraising the research evidence.[15] In the larger sense, evidence-based practice can be viewed as the process of understanding evolving from sources of knowledge, clinical experience, professional and scientific literature, and professional peers as well as the client.[16] In the best sense, evidence-based practice involves integrating clinical experience with the best available evidence derived from systematic research[17] and the integration of information into the management of patient care.[18] Too often, however, it appears that evidence-based practice has been functionally and practically reduced to reliance upon data from large-scale controlled clinical trials to justify and fund intervention. A current standard of acceptance of levels of evidence-based practice is presented in Table 8.1.

I am not original in labeling evidence-based practice a mantra. Typically, in evidence-based medicine the gold standard for knowledge and truth is randomized controlled trials.[15,19] Indeed, a hierarchy of knowledge of evidence is commonly based upon Sackett.[20] As a norm, evidence ranges from the "best" being randomized controlled trials to the "worst" or "weakest" being qualitative research. A hierarchy of evidence was similarly attempted in English law centuries ago. It didn't work then, and it might not work now. Accordingly, English law evolved into a more flexible system such that "weight given to each bit of evidence should be determined by detailed appraisal of the characteristics of that evidence."[21] And, indeed, we see an evolution of the standards of evidence for practice in different fields. For example, in early intervention Patrick, Mozzoni and Patrick's single-subject design research is considered "good" evidence.[22]

The benefit of evidence-based practice may also be its weakness, e.g., we think we know something. We might know something about generalities based upon populations. But we know nothing about how any given intervention will actually play out in a real-life situation, with the "n of 1." Given the real complexities of real life, we cannot adequately predict. It may be considered the mismatch or dissonance between evidence and what Knottnerus and Dinant refer to as clinical reality.[23]

At first blush, the concept of using research evidence to prescribe action makes sense. And certainly, clients have a right to interventions that are grounded in solid evidence.[14] But upon reflection and consideration, many thorny issues concerning evidence-based practice arise that are ethical in nature. To illustrate, Kerridge[24] identified that evidence-based medicine (and I argue its corollary in our fields' evidence-based practices) is based upon consequentialism or the proposition that the value of an action be measured by its consequence. Yet, a myriad of concerns arise, such as (a) important outcomes may not be readily identifiable, (b) whose needs or objectives are being met by the outcomes, and (c) some supposedly desirable outcomes may not be consistent with values or culture of the participant. Tonelli and Callahan[25] provide a thoughtful discussion of how basic assumptions of what we know and how we know it (epistemology) is fundamental to understanding evidence-based practice and how it is not a match when evaluating complementary and alternative medicine (CAM).

We face the problem that criteria for internal and external validity (that is, clinical applicability) may conflict. Clinical studies are usually performed on a homogeneous study population and exclude clinically complex cases for the sake of internal validity. Such selection may not, however, match the type of patients for whom the studied intervention will

Table 8.1 ✧ Sacket's Method for Grading Research for Evidence-Based Medicine	
LEVEL OF EVIDENCE	CATEGORY OF TYPE OF DATA
I	Large randomized controlled trials
II	Small randomized controlled trials
III	Nonrandomized prospective studies
IV	Nonrandomized historical cohort comparisons
V	Case studies

be considered. Medical practice is often confronted with patients presenting several problems. Older patients and women are underrepresented in clinical trials, and patients with comorbidity, a common phenomenon at older ages, are generally excluded. Evidence from patients selected by referral cannot easily be generalized to patients seen in primary care with less severe or early stage clinical pictures. And some important needs for evidence are missing. For instance, although drug trials usually provide evidence about starting drug treatment, doctors are increasingly confronted by patients taking multiple long-term medications but have no proper data on evidence-based drug cessation. Gregson and Meal identify the incompatibility of the epistemology in quantitative meta-analysis such as used in evidence-based practice and the epistemology and reasoning in expert practice.[26] The incongruence of the differing epistemologies further fuels the ephemeral nature of the ethics of evidence-based practice. Goding and Edwards particularly view this in terms of a dichotomous relationship between reductionism (evidence-based practice) and a holistic approach.[27]

Thus, what at first seems clear (evidence-based practice is good) becomes transient—the ephemeral ethics of evidence-based practice. What was right becomes foggy and perhaps not even right when working with a particular client with a particular problem in a particular situation.

Thus, the rightness or ethical justness of using evidence-based practice is clear for populations, but truly ephemeral when it comes to literal application with a particular person. Gibbs and Gambrill discount two ethically related arguments against evidence-based practice.[28] First, they discount the import ascribed to researchers as authority figures. Second, they discount the equal abilities of all methods in determining truth. But their theoretical discussion of counterarguments for evidence-based practice fail to include discussion of its ephemeral nature as argued in this chapter.

The American Occupational Therapy Association and the American Physical Therapy Association have been active in developing evidence-based clinical guidelines in various areas of their respective practice specialties. An evidence-based approach to assessments is increasingly common in both fields.[18] Yet the real issue may not be just dissemination of information about evidence-based practice. The real issue may be how to change practitioners behavior based upon the "best available evidence," due to the large gap between research findings and routine care.[17,29]

✧ A VIEW OF EVIDENCE-BASED PRACTICE FROM THE FIELD

This section of the chapter describes a sort of "what is" in terms of therapists' understanding of evidence-based practice. It is presented as a grounding for the next section on the TRIO model as an ethical standard for guiding practice. In the fall of 2002, a self-selected group of occupational therapists and physical therapists working in early intervention were queried "What is evidence-based practice?"[29a] providing a "snapshot" assessment into a topical area for a view from a cross section of involved participants. Participants' responses clustered into four main categories are presented in Table 8.2.

Of the four categories of responses, the first includes those responses focusing on evidence-based practice primarily as techniques or protocols that are "proven" and correct, a simple interpretation of evidence-based practice as "the" correct procedure to implement in practice. The second category is the consideration of evidence-based practice as synonymous with the outcomes measurement documenting performance of a client in current intervention for accountability. This category may be interpreted as consideration of evidence-based practice as the collection of data about assessment of client performance. A third category is related to the first, but reflects a somewhat larger view of intervention as more complex than a single procedure, yet still supported by rationale and evidence. The fourth category is practical understanding of evidence of what works. Not listed in these categories is a single, outlier response that illustrates yet another level of meaning for evidence-based practice and one that appears to be at a higher level than the

Table 8.2 ✧ Participants' Responses by Category, Meaning, and Illustrative Sample		
CATEGORY	MEANING	ILLUSTRATIVE SAMPLE
1. Procedures and fact	Learning effective procedures	Learning techniques that have proven to be effective based upon studies.
		Following treatment.
2. Outcomes measurement	Accountability	A way of determining whether your therapy is effective based upon evidence/facts.
		Therapy designed toward use of observable behavioral outcomes as a means toward management improvement.
3. Textbook	Support for interventions	Providing services that are based on a clear rationale and have been validated by some type of research along a continuum.
		Interventions that are directly supported by current research as being effective.
4. Practice	What works	Practice that has been used and shown to work.
		Method of treatment that is based upon proven research.

others, the gestalt or global view of "systematic investigation of phenomena that directly affects how, why, when, etc., of the therapeutic process." The reason this response reflects a higher level is that it explicitly recognizes intervention as a collection of phenomena and does not restrict intervention to just the procedure or what works, which is the risk of evidence-based practice. This preliminary assessment of order of EBP reveals the need to promote a broader view of our interventions not just as evidence of value of procedures. The single outlier response about evidence-based practice suggests a need to acknowledge that best practice is more than just knowing the science. This identified need brings us to the proposed TRIO model of practice for occupational therapy and physical therapy.

✧ TRIO MODEL FOR PRACTICE

In her Mary McMillan Lecture, Purtilo stated that "The tools of ethics are designed for sifting through muddy details of everyday life, examining them for why, to whom, and how we show care and be accountable.[9] In this chapter, two tools of ethics (TRIO model and the framework of ETHICS) are presented to assist in reaching the goal of how we show care in service. The TRIO model of practice is based upon three interacting habits—(1) habits of the mind, (2) habits of the heart, and (3) habits of the art.[30]

Habits of the Mind

Evidence-based practice as the mantra for our professions is focused on the science of what we do. This is directly related to habits of the mind or cognitive-based knowledge and facts about our interventions, procedures, and techniques, henceforth referred to as habits of the mind. Although I would not quibble with the incredible importance of knowing what interventions work with what populations under what conditions such as advocated by Holm for occupational therapy, two other critical phenomena are also part of our practice— habits of the heart and habits of the art. Each will be addressed in turn.

Habits of the Heart

Habits of the heart refer to the emotional components of not just the therapist but also of the client during intervention. Cognition does not operate in a vacuum in humans, but rather in the context of our emotional state at any given time. Indeed, cognition and emotion may be considered as opposite ends of realms of the same construct. Adapted from the concept of metacognition, I have turned the phrase "metaemotion of occupation"[31,32] to promote this reflective process, the conscious and subconscious understanding of how one feels about what one is doing, an essential part of the therapeutic process for any given interaction.[33]

Habits of the heart are what intrinsically draw many of us to a helping profession, such as occupational therapy or physical therapy. Habits of the heart also relate to the intuitive process that many of use in daily life as well as in intervention delivery. The recognition of intuition as a legitimate and powerful component of appropriate human action is a newly rediscovered part of brain theory, and most certainly operates during the intervention process for many therapists.[33]

Habits of the Art

Habits of the art refer to the psychomotor traits of the corporeal body as well as the spiritual self during therapeutic encounters. Therapeutic use of self is an old term from Rogerian psychology that has fallen out of vogue, but is part of the core of what a therapist brings to any therapeutic intervention.[34] Recognition of the importance of habits of the art is most clearly seen when one observes a "master clinician" in action. The master clinician knows how to place his or her hands. The master clinician knows how to say the right thing. The master clinician knows when to say the right thing. The master clinician knows how to elicit motivated behavior through intentional actions. The master clinician knows how and when to disclose in order to facilitate rapport. This skill set is not a result of cognitive processing—though the skills are undoubtedly cognitively related. They are the artist's skills in action, transforming the meeting of two or more beings into a therapeutic encounter.

Students and TRIO Practice

As educators, we all know students who excel at habits of the mind, so to speak. They are the students with high grades, who master content and the science of our professions quite well. But, in the clinical setting, and in competency-based testing, they struggle with the intangible from the realms of heart and art—they cannot practice emotional intelligence well, nor can they perform and master psychomotor and/or therapeutic use of self toward rapport-building strategies well. Such students could and do excel in understanding and articulating evidence-based practice—but they cannot do best practice because their habits of heart and art are not well developed.

In essence, such students typify the ethical dilemma posed by practice viewed only from habits of the mind (such as only considering or primarily considering or exclusively considering evidence-based practice for intervention planning). Best practice, as presented in the TRIO model, is a blend of all three habits. Those expert in procedures and interventions, regardless of evidence-based statistics, are doomed to failure without incorporation of the dimensions of habits of the heart and habits of the art. It is for us to dust off our values, renew our commitment to holistic practice, and well articulate practice grounded not just in science, but also in heart and art.[35]

But how do we do this? Vast resources in the United States as well as elsewhere fully support evidence-based practice or habits of the mind. Who shall support the moral imperative of best practice including habits of the heart and habits of the art? We are they.

✧ *ETHICS* AS A WORKING GUIDE TO BEST PRACTICE

As a humble contribution to the daunting task of renewing our professions' commitment to practice incorporating the TRIO model, an admittedly "cute" device of a mnemonic based upon ethics legitimately evolved. As Glaser noted elsewhere in this book, we all need guides in whatever we do. If we are to practice in accordance with best practice, ethical principles, and the morally just position incorporating habits of the mind, habits of the heart, and habits of the art, then a road map or path of reason might well serve our quest. Hence, ETHICS is one such proposed roadmap. ETHICS is a framework for best practice, encapsulating factors an occupational therapist or physical therapist might consider when striving for best practice using the TRIO model.

E, Evidence-Based

As previously identified, Holm from occupational therapy and others from physical therapy advocate use of a research evidence base for practice.[36] They are correct and we should do so. But, we cannot stop there—best practice requires so much more than knowledge of the research evidence about effects of interventions under specified conditions. And, "the so much more," is, in part, guided by the concepts in the rest of the ETHICS mnemonic.

T, Theory Driven

There will never be sufficient research in any field to address what to do (re: intervention) in all circumstances or conditions. Inevitably, there is a point where there are no facts, and insufficient empirical data to direct actions. At this juncture, the relevance of theory is reaffirmed and reestablished. It is theory that suggests to us possible courses of action when no data reveal what to do. Thus, theory has been and ever shall remain a key factor in practice, since best practice requires use of a complete theory or developing theoretical reference when confronting the unknown.

H, Humanistic

Science alone—such as a restricted focus upon evidence-based practice—without consideration and action based upon respect for humanistic principles of interacting with others, fails to ensure good practice. Several authors in this book emphasize that good practice requires, first and foremost, that we be "good" human beings, and best practice requires that we integrate humanistic principles into how and why we interact with our clients.[37] Our long tradition of caring is embedded within this presumption.[11,38–45]

I, Individualized

For the most part, most of evidence-based practice is predicated upon aggregates or collections of individuals as populations. In such science, the individual does not exist within a contextual framework and individual performance can be predicted only in terms of probabilities of occurrence. In contrast, in best practice we work with individuals first and foremost—unique configurations of wants, needs, desires, and meanings that constitute an individual. Population-based methods can prescribe neither what to do with, nor how to act, with a given individual in a given situation. An individualized approach using science data, coupled with habits of the heart and habits of the art tailored to the unique "n of 1" for a particular encounter, is how best practice is approximated.

C, Client Centered and Culturally Sensitive

This component of the guide to best practice relates to whose need gets met—it should be the clients! Not the third-party payer, not the referral agency, not the protocol, and certainly not a preordained method of a "top down" or "biomechanical" or an "orthopedic" approach to the particular person involved. Rather, a client-focused approach directs therapists' actions to the unique meaning, purpose, and activities, or occupations, engaged in by a person and the functional needs to achieve engagement in occupational processes. Further, culturally sensitive care connotes an approach related to humanistic care—fundamental and profound respect for the unique nature of each person who enters into a therapeutic encounter. It must be viewed as a sacred space.

S, Spiritual Sensitivity and Therapeutic Use of Self

Over 20 years ago I was chastised by Margaret Rood for improperly approaching a patient who had suffered a stroke. I approached him in a rather buoyant, exuberant manner and it did not match nor suit his rather dampened and cognitively compromised situation.

Rood challenged me to emotionally match the situation—to do something that in current time is akin to what Damasio would call a somatic marker.[33] It was a huge lesson in therapeutic use of self—of self as a tool for the therapeutic encounter. And it is through this therapeutic use of self that we allow for or facilitate the therapeutic encounter that can allow for a form of spirituality to emerge within the sacred space.

✧ SUMMARY AND CONCLUSIONS

This chapter has led the reader on a journey though the ephemeral ethics of evidence-based practice, including a review of what is considered to be evidence-based practice and how it came to be in the fields of occupational therapy and physical therapy. It provided an introduction to the issues and a selective review of related research as well as a pertinent assessment of therapists' knowledge. The inevitable clash or schism between a prescribed practice or method of intervention for a given individual based upon aggregate data compared to best practice incorporating the TRIO model of practice—habits of the mind, habits of the heart, and habits of the art—was addressed. Finally, a guide for therapists whose goal is better practice based upon the mnemonic of ETHICS has been delineated as a road map for the continual quest for best practice.

In conclusion, I suggest that use of the TRIO model and the ETHICS guide for better practice can assist us to "intervene with wisdom and courage [by trusting] ourselves to be guided by our own values"[1] rather than being guided by another medical model of practice, such as evidence-based practice, to the exclusion of our own values. The "bottom line," so to speak, is not just that one's practice be evidence-based,[46] but that in addition to such habits of the mind that habits of the heart and habits of the art be included. To achieve this requires not just a focus on evidence-based practice, but a more global and complex strategy incorporating working together, continuing education, expert interactions, and discussion opportunities toward changing therapists' behaviors in the

direction more consistent with best practice standards.[47] Perhaps our self-reflection question is not, "Is my practice evidence-based?" but rather, "Is my practice grounded in ethics?"[46]

I leave you with a final comment for rumination—old scholarship by today's standards of the newest and the latest—but a comment representing the timeless: "The end of art is the beginning of science; for when it is seen what is done, then comes the question of why it is done."[48]

References

1. Piccard-Greffe H: Back to the future—Muriel Drive Memorial Lecture. Can J Occup Ther 61(5):243–249, Dec 1994.
1a. Some of these colleagues are Dr. Beverly Kracher, Associate Professor of Business Ethics of Creighton University; Dr. Gail Jensen, Associate Dean of the School of Pharmacy and Health Professions of Creighton University Medical Center; and Dr. Ruth Purtilo, Director of the Center for Ethics and Health Policy, also of Creighton University Medical Center.
2. Isaacs D, and Fitzgerald D: Seven alternatives to evidence based medicine. Br Med J 319:18–25, 1999.
3. Isaacs D, and Fitzgerald D: Seven alternatives to evidence-based medicine. Oncologist 6:390–391, 2001.
4. Dobouloz C, et al: Occupational therapists perceptions of evidence-based practice. Am J Occup Ther 53(5):445–453, 1999.
5. Taylor MC: Evidence-based Practice for Occupational Therapists. Blackwell Science, Oxford, 2000.
6. Luebben AJ: Ethical concerns; human occupation. In Kramer P, Hinojasa J, and Royeen CB (eds): Perspectives in Human Occupation. Lippincott Williams & Wilkins, Philadelphia, 2003, pp 297–311.
7. Turner P, and Mjolne I: Journal provision and the prevalence of journal clubs: A survey of physiotherapy departments in England and Australia. Physiother Res Int 6(3):157–169, 2001.
8. Law M: Strategies for implementing evidence-based practice in early intervention. Infants Young Child 13(2):32–40, 2000.
9. Purtilo RB: Thirty-First Mary McMillan Lecture: A time to harvest, a time to sow: Ethics for a shifting landscape. Phys Ther 80:1112–1119, 2000.
10. Mattingly C, and Fleming MH: Clinical Reasoning: Forms of Inquiry in a Therapeutic Practice. FA Davis Co, Philadelphia, PA, 1994.
11. Benner P, and Wrubel J: The Primacy of Caring: Stress and Coping in Health and Illness. Addison-Wesley Publishing Co Inc, Menlo Park, CA, 1989.
12. Iwama M: Toward culturally relevant epistemologies. Am J Occup Ther 57(5):582–588, 2003.
12a. The reader is referred to N. Pollock and S. Rochon, "Becoming an evidence-based practitioner" (31–46) for an insightful analysis and discussion of how to try to integrate evidence with these other factors. In

Mary Law (ed): Evidence-Based Rehabilitation: A Guide to Practice. Slack, Thorofare, NJ, 2002, pp 31–46.

13. Friedman N: Evidence-based medicine: The key to guidelines, disease and care management program. Ann Acad Med-Singapore 31(4):446–451, 2002.

14. Hammell KW: Using qualitative research to inform the client-centered evidence-based practice of occupational therapy. Br J Occup Ther 64(5):228–234, 2001.

15. Taylor MC, and Savin-Baden M: Whose evidence are we applying? Br J Occup Ther 65(5):200–213, 2001.

16. Curtin M, and Jaramazovic E: Occupational therapists' views and perceptions of evidence-based practice. Br J Occup Ther 64(5):214–222, 2001.

17. Straus SE, and Sackett DL: Using research findings in clinical practice. Br Med J 317:339–342, 1998.

18. Fritz JM, and Wainner RS: Examining diagnostic tests: An evidence-based perspective. Phys Ther 81(9):1546–1564, 2001.

19. Ballinger C, and Wiles R: A critical look at evidence-based practice. Br J Occup Ther 64(5):253–255, 2001.

20. Butler C, et al: Evaluating research in developmental disabilities: A conceptual framework for reviewing treatment outcomes. Dev Med Child Neurol 41:55–59, 1999.

21. Barton S: Which clinical studies provide the best evidence? [Editorial]. Br Med J 321:255–256, 2000.

22. Patrick PD, Mozzoni M, and Patrick ST: Evidence-based care and the single-subject design. Infants Young Child 13(1):60–73, 2000.

23. Knottnerus A, and Dinant, G.J: Medicine based evidence, a prerequisite for evidence based medicine. Br Med J 315(7116):1109–1110, November 1, 1997.

24. Kerridge I, Lowe M, and Henry D: Ethics and evidence based medicine. Br Med J 316:1151–1153, April 11, 1998.

25. Tonelli MR, and Callahan TC: Why alternative medicine cannot be evidence based. Acad Med 76(12):1213–1220, 2002.

26. Gregson PR, Meal AG, and Avis M: Meta analysis: The glass eye of evidence-based practice. Nurs Inq 9(1):24–30, 2002.

27. Goding L, and Edwards K: Evidence-based practice. Nurs Res 9(4):45–57, 2002.

28. Gibbs L, and Gambrill E: Evidence-based practice: Counter arguments to objections. Res Soc Work. 12(3):452–476, 2002.

29. Chilvers R, et al: Evidence into practice. Application of psychological models of change in evidence-based implementation. [Editorial]. Br J Psychiatry 181:99–101, 2002.

29a. One hundred and fifteen early intervention occupational and physical therapists attended a 2-day conference on "Contemporary Practice in Early Intervention: An Institute for Pediatric Therapists" in Carlisle, Pennsylvania, sponsored by the Child and Family Studies Research Program of Thomas Jefferson University and the Commonwealth of Pennsylvania. Of those therapists attending the session, I presented "Practice Based Evidence and Natural Environments"; 68 shared their written responses to the question, "What is evidence-based practice?" at the beginning of the talk.

30. Royeen CB: The 2003 Eleanor Clarke Slagle Lecture. Chaotic occupational therapy: Collective wisdom for a complex profession. Am J Occup Ther 57(6):609–624, 2003.

31. Royeen CB, and Duncan M: Meta-emotion of occupation: A new twist for mental health. Paper presented at the AOTA Annual Conference, Philadelphia, PA, 2001.

32. Royeen CB, Duncan M, and McCormack G: Reconstruction of the Rood approach for occupation based treatment. In Pedretti S (ed): Occupational Therapy: Practice Skills for Physical Dysfunction. ed 5. Mosby, St. Louis, MO, 2001, pp 576–587.

33. Damasio AR: Emotion, Reason, and the Human Brain. Avon Printing, New York, 1994.

34. Hosking P: Utilizing Roger's theory of self concept in mental health nursing. J Adv Nurs 18(6):980–984, June 1993.

35. Welsch I, and Lyons CM: Evidence based care and the case for intuition and tacit knowledge in clinical assessment and decision making in mental health nursing practice: an empirical contribution to the debate. J. Psychiatr Ment Health Nurs. 8(4):299–305, August 2001.

36. Holm MB: 2000 Eleanor Clarke Slagle lecture. Our mandate for the new millennium: Evidence-based practice. Am J Occup Ther 54(6):575–585, 2000.

37. Goodwin JS: Chaos, and the limits of modern medicine. JAMA 278:1399–1400, 1997.

38. Hightomer-Vandamm MD: Nationally speaking: Caring is the key, it always has been. Am J Occup Ther 34(3):239–240, 1980.

39. Baum CM: 1980 Eleanor Clarke Slagle Lecture. Occupational therapists put care in the health system. Am J Occup Ther 34(8):505–516, 1980.

40. Devereaux EB: Occupational therapy's challenge: The caring relationship. Am J Occup Ther 38(12):791–798, 1984.

41. Gilfoyle EM: Caring: A philosophy for practice. Am J Occup Ther 34(8):517–521, 1980.

42. Cannon N: Eighth Nathalie Barr Lecture: Caring for the patient. J Hand Ther 7(1):1–4, 1994.

43. Dychawy-Rosner I, Eklund M, and Issacsson A: Caring dynamics as perceived by staff supporting daily acceptance for developmentally disabled adults. Scand J Occup Ther 15:123–132, 2001.

44. Hamlin RB: Embracing our past, informing our future: A feminist re-vision of health care. Am J Occup Ther 46(11):1028–1035, 1992.

45. Peloquin SM: Art in practice: When art becomes caring. [Doctoral Dissertation]. Medical Branch at Galveston, University of Texas, Galveston, 1991.

46. Greenhalgh T: "Is my practice evidence-based?" [Editorial]. Br Med J 313:957–958, 1996.

47. Roberts AE, and Barber G: Applying research evidence to practice. Br J Occup Ther 64(5):223–227, 2001.

48. Whewell W: The philosophy of the inductive sciences founded upon their history. Frank Cass Publications, London. The philosophy of the inductive sciences, founded upon by their history. A facsimile of the 2nd edition, London (1847) with a new introduction by John Hervivel, 1847/1967.

9

Examining the Moral Role of Physical Therapists

Herman L. Triezenberg, PhD, PT

A b s t r a c t

A research study that was conducted to learn more about the unique moral role of physical therapists is discussed in this chapter. Participants in the study consisted of a sample of 15 individuals who met specific selection criteria—expertise and knowledge. At the completion of the series of individual semistructured interviews, all participants were invited to attend one of two focus group sessions. This paper discusses the main question posed in the study, "What characterizes the moral role of a physical therapist in today's health care environment?" Based on the responses of the participants in this study, the author suggests that the rehabilitation encounter presents a specific set of moral responsibilities that are part of the professional identity of the rehabilitation professions. The results suggest that the role of rehabilitation professionals has unique characteristics that distinguish it from the roles of other health professionals. I propose a model that divides the moral role of the physical therapist into two categories of interactions: interactions with the patient and interactions with the nonpatient. Based on the responses of the participants, I propose specific characteristics and responsibilities that are part of these relationships. I further suggest that understanding more about the unique characteristics and responsibilities of the moral role of physical therapists will help educators more clearly define their goals in ethics education for students in rehabilitation.

✦ INTRODUCTION

Changes in the health care delivery system over the last 10 years have affected health care practitioners in a variety of ways. Some changes have been positive, although many changes have been considered by health care providers as negative and as a threat to the profession and to patient care. The changes have forced health care providers and professions to reevaluate their role in the delivery of health care.[1–5] A discussion of the positive and negative effects of the shift to managed care is not the focus of this paper, but the turmoil and self-examination that characterized the late 1990s and early 21st century provide the backdrop for the study. Physical therapy and other rehabilitation professions also participated in this period of self-examination. Physical therapists and occupational therapists were forced to look more closely at their role in the care of individuals within the health care system.[5–9] Many began to question the value and cost of the care that was provided by rehabilitation professionals. Rehabilitation professions and clinicians felt under siege by uncontrollable forces. Many segments within the rehabilitation professions began to display the characteristics of an oppressed population as described by Paulo Freire in *The Pedagogy of the Oppressed*.[10]

There were certainly financial concerns and loss of rehabilitation positions during this time, but there also appeared to be a deeper question regarding the values and beliefs at the core of rehabilitation. Prior to and during this period many authors noted that discussion on the specific issues, values, and moral role of the rehabilitation therapist was lacking in the literature of occupational therapy and physical therapy.[11–15] The time appeared right for reflection on the question of the unique moral role of rehabilitation professionals and hence the investigation discussed in this chapter.

✧ METHODOLOGY

The methodology used in the study was a semistructured individual interview technique combined with two follow-up focus group interviews. This technique was chosen as an appropriate tool to use to identify the values and beliefs of a defined group.[16–19] Participants in the study consisted of a sample of 15 individuals who met the following selection criteria: (a) they had practiced physical therapy for more that 5 years, (b) they had received additional training or a degree in a discipline related to social/behavioral aspects of patient care and/or ethics, and (c) they were recognized as contributors to our understanding of the social/ behavioral and/or ethical aspects of physical therapy practice through their history of publications and/or professional presentations. Thus, the investigator selected the participants for their expertise and knowledge. All 15 of the individuals identified and invited to take part in the study agreed to participate. At the completion of the individual interview each participant was invited to attend one of two focus group interviews for further discussion.

The semistructured interview guide used in the study contained six questions. This chapter will focus on the responses obtained from the first question posed, "What do you feel characterizes the moral role of a physical therapist in today's health care environment?" This open-ended question was designed to generate a wide variety of responses. The initial question was followed by a series of clarifying questions relating to the values, moral duties, and responsibilities that were a part of the moral role described in the initial response of the participant. Interviews were recorded and transcribed. The transcriptions of the interviews were evaluated by the investigator, coded for themes, and recurrent themes identified.

✧ FINDINGS AND INTERPRETATIONS

The initial question and follow-up questions prompted a wide range of responses from the participants. In this chapter, I will try to identify and describe the areas where the respondents were in agreement. I will also present some of the thoughts presented by a small number or single individual that provide a new perspective and greater insight.

Areas of Agreement
Moral Component of Rehabilitation

The first area of agreement that emerged from this study was that all of the participants believed that physical therapists are moral agents in their role as rehabilitation professionals. Each participant confirmed and expanded the belief that the role of the physical therapist had a moral dimension. One participant stated,

> As a physical therapist we act as moral agents in almost everything that we do. In almost everything that we do there will be moral or ethical content to it.

All respondents appeared to assume as a starting point that the role of the physical therapist has a moral component. This belief is supported by numerous discussions in the professional literature of the rehabilitation professions.[11–16,20,21]

Primacy of Patient

The second concept of general agreement is that the moral role of the physical therapist is defined primarily by the characteristics of the relationship between the physical therapist and the patient. The participants each began their responses by describing the therapist-patient interaction as the central consideration in the moral role of the therapist. The respondents expressed this belief in a number of ways.

The central role of the physical therapist is to be helpful to the patient that comes to them.

I think that as a fiduciary, the highest duty is always to the patient.

We have to place the patient's needs first, I guess the sort of classic, old-fashioned fiduciary relationship that characterized the profession. That is what we have got to do.

So the moral role then becomes having the courage to do what you know is best for the patient in the face of forces that would encourage you to set other priorities.

I think primarily we have a role to make sure that we're doing the best that we can for our patients.

You really have to stay focused on what is in the best interest of the patient.

The language used in these and other statements by the respondents place the consideration for the needs and welfare of the patient as the starting point for discussion of the moral role of physical therapists.

Moral Obligations to Nonpatient

A third belief that nearly all the informants expressed was that in addition to the patient, physical therapists had relationships with and moral obligations to other individuals and organizations. The respondents identified a variety of groups and individuals they felt they had an obligation to including: self, society, health care colleagues, the profession, employers, and third-party payers. The response of one informant addresses many of the individuals and groups identified by the participants.

We are first of all responsible to the patient. And I think that we are responsible to ourselves, too, to provide quality care. We are responsible to our employers. We are responsible as well to third-party payers. We are responsible to society as a whole.

Another informant expands the list further to families, the profession, and colleagues.

Our primary responsibility is to our patients, ourselves and our patients. And then certainly to their families and then to our employers and to the profession. We also have a responsibility to colleagues. All kinds of colleagues, everybody working in the system, physicians, nurses, etc.

The importance, order, and moral obligations to these different groups or individuals varied greatly among the respondents and there was no specific order of priority identified by the participants.

The responses discussed above describe three areas of agreement among the participants: (1) the role of the physical therapist has a moral component, (2) the relationship of the therapist to the patient is the central consideration in that moral role, and (3) the therapist has additional moral obligations that are derived from relationships with individuals and groups that are not patients. The belief that the role of the physical therapist has a moral component is a basic belief underlying this study and the discussion will focus on defining that moral role.

To begin defining the moral role, the investigator separated the responses of the participants into two categories of individuals with whom physical therapists have interactions. The first category consists of their patients and the second category is the variety of individuals and groups that fall outside the direct therapist-patient relationship or nonpatients. The participants in this study identified specific characteristics associated with the therapist's relationships with these different individuals or groups.

Definition of the Patient

All participants in the study recognized the relationship of physical therapists with their patient as the central consideration in defining the moral role of physical therapists. Their responses also indicated that some differences existed among the participants on who should be included in the definition of the "patient." Two categories of patients emerged from the responses of the participants: (a) direct patients, and (b) extended patients.

Direct Patients

In referring to the "patient," all participants in the study recognized the individual who is being treated by the physical therapist as the patient. Special requirements and consideration are identified by all participants for that individual who comes to the therapist for treatment of a particular problem that falls within the scope of physical therapy practice. Some responses include:

I use patient pretty liberally to mean anyone we are providing services for. ... it is the person who is seeking help from us.

It seems to me that the central role of the physical therapist is to be helpful to the patient that comes to them, and by helpful I mean by attempting to meet whatever needs they express to the physical therapist when they come to them for treatment.

I look at ethical therapy really on that individual therapist and patient level. In that sense, I think it involves responsibility in providing professional medical care to an individual based on her needs within the scope of our practice.

These responses identify the patient as an individual who obtains assistance from a therapist for a specific problem. One of the respondents added the qualification that the problem presented by the patient falls within the scope of physical therapy practice. Maintaining services within a defined scope of practice is an important consideration that was discussed by many of the informants. Scope of practice was further discussed by the participants relating to the therapists' interactions with other health care professionals.

The participants believed that the relationship between the physical therapist and the patient being treated was unique. The patients being treated by the therapist composed the first category of patients. The special relationship that existed with the patient that the therapist is treating was considered by all respondents to be a central component of the moral role of the therapist.

Extended Patients

Many of the participants expanded the definition of "patient" to include not only those patients who are currently being seen by the physical therapist, but also those who need the care offered by a physical therapist, and are unable to access that care. One respondent stated:

One of the issues is that we have these individual responsibilities to the people in front of us, but we have responsibility to all people who need our care.

I think it is crucial that we make our primary accountability to people whose condition falls into our line of work and can benefit from our intervention.

Some respondents chose to include in their discussion of patients individuals who are potential patients or future patients and even those who the therapist could help avoid the need of physical therapy services. This inclusion greatly expanded the definition of "patient."

If we are a profession, society has granted us the privilege to be a profession and society has licensed us, so I see our responsibility as a societal one, to all those patients that are we are treating, all those patients that need our services, and then all those ... I think we are just getting our teeth into the fact that all those citizens out there that if we were to help them now we could prevent them from needing traditional physical therapy services in the future.

I guess I would say the patient because they are the reason we are here. Only because the patients create the collective society, so they are kind of inherent in society because all of them are potential patients of ours someday.

This group of "extended patients" included: (a) potential patients, (b) future patients, (c) individuals who could benefit from physical therapy services but can't access them, and (d) individuals who could be helped to avoid physical therapy by early intervention and education. Components of this group were described by many of the respondents, but there was no clear consensus on the exact composition of this category of patients. It was also unclear if the moral responsibilities of the therapists to the "extended patient" are the same as the responsibilities the physical therapist has to the "direct patient."

Characteristics of the Physical Therapist/Patient Relationship

Most of the respondents began their response to the initial question by identifying the relationship of the therapist to the patient as the primary relationship. The respondents then discussed what behaviors of the therapist should characterize that interaction. From the responses of the participants, the investigator identified five themes that will be presented as five characteristics of the physical therapist/patient relationship (Table 9.1).

Characteristic 1: Advocacy

The characteristic that was identified most often by the participants to describe the physi-

Table 9.1 ✧ **Characteristics of the Physical Therapist/Patient Relationship**	
Characteristic 1.	The physical therapist serves as an advocate to address the needs of the patient.
Characteristic 2.	The actions of the physical therapist are centered on the patient and are performed in the best interest of the patient.
Characteristic 3.	The physical therapist develops and acts within a collaborative relationship or partnership with the patient.
Characteristic 4.	The physical therapist serves as a bridge to bring the patient to a new place or increase the ability of the patient to function independently.
Characteristic 5.	The physical therapist skillfully applies a specific and unique set of skills to address a patient's particular set of problems.

cal therapist's relationship with the patient was advocacy. The advocacy role for the patient was considered by many of the respondents to be the most important component of the moral role of a physical therapist. Advocacy was described by the respondents as an active role in which the therapist learns about the needs of the patient, understands their constraints, and then assists the patient to achieve the best possible outcomes. One respondent described the importance and responsibility of advocacy in the following way:

The central piece is really advocating for the patient in seeking and having a good understanding of where the patient is coming from in an environment that has a scarcity of resources and reimbursement issues. You really have to stay focused on what is in the best interest of the patient and balancing that with the institution and organization factors. ... To look out for the patient's perspective and to see the world from the patient's perspective and then begin to help the patient negotiate their systems as best as possible.

Another participant described advocacy in a way that presents it as a promise to the patient that the therapist will not abandon the patient. This individual also saw the responsibilities of the role of advocate as being a guide for the actions of the therapist.

And advocacy in terms that you keep at it until you have solved the problem. That is the persistence and responsibility that you assume, that you don't abandon a patient. That you become their guide, as you will. They in a sense become your guide as you walk through this promise you have given.

Another informant considered advocacy the most important concept to consider when teaching ethics to physical therapy students.

I was actually thinking that it feels to me in teaching the ethics course that almost all of it is around advocacy and allocation of resources which aren't the only issues in ethics, but they seem to be the driving ones. That is the role we've got to assume.

The role of advocate was viewed by many of the participants as a role that broadens our responsibilities to the patient from a solely clinical role to a broader patient management role involving new areas of knowledge and skill.

We've been developing a model that advocates nothing new or different, but trying to put that advocacy role in a more prominent place as part of the role of a physical therapist. That is what we need to be doing and it's coming out of viewing the role of physical therapists as more broad than having clinical knowledge and expertise. I think people have not yet recognized what that means to have all of these expectations of these other skills and also the need to know what the administrative practices are and the reimbursement policies, and all of that. ... it has to be part of their function. And if that is there, then this advocacy role has got to become more prominent and what I worry about is that the physical therapist is able to carry out that role.

Characteristic 2: Patient Centering

The respondents in the study identified the responsibility to place the needs of the patient ahead of the needs of the therapist as a major characteristic of the therapist/patient relationship. This perspective was described by some respondents as "other-centered."

So being other-centered is really the value. The value is not me but thee and from that perspective comes the work of the physical therapist.

In the area of self-interest versus other-interest, they [therapists] must always choose other-interest. That is a value I think that we all should subscribe to.

One respondent stated further that the interest of the patient must supersede the interests of more than just the therapist but also other competing interests.

Again it goes back to that issue that we are here primarily to put patients first and how we do that in ways in which we have other decision-makers coming in, reimbursors, making decisions, referring providers, making decisions that we question. Are those in the best interest of the patient?

This same respondent stated that the basis of the obligation to put patients' interests first rests in the position of power that we have over a patient.

The first thing that I think about is the idea that we are in somewhat of a position of power, if you call it that, and that we should see to it that what is done is done in the best interest of the patient, and that it is not done for our benefit but hopefully for the best of the patient.

Other informants add the warning of the consequences of not putting the needs of the patient first.

Self interest is an important issue that may tend to shift priorities to putting one's own financial interests before that of the patient. I think that the giving in to real or perceived demands of government, managed care entities, or third-party payers may compromise the value of the relationship and the morals and ethics of physical therapists.

But under health professional ethics you do have an affirmative duty to put the patient's interests first, even above your own self interest.

Placing the best interest of the patient before that of the therapist was identified by many of the respondents as an important component of the moral role of the therapist.

Characteristic 3: Physical Therapist and Patient Partnership

Many of the respondents characterized the relationship between the therapist and the patient as a partnership involving collaboration in decisions involving the patient. Some of the responses emphasized the need for the therapist to ensure that the patient is an active participant and not a passive recipient in rehabilitation. The term "collaboration" was often used to describe the relationship between the therapist and the patient.

I think it is back to what I think is at the center is that we deliver more to the patients to help them do what is best for themselves. I see the role as therapists to not only do something to the patient, but working with the patient. I think that it is very much collaborative.

Other informants emphasized the importance of the therapist being available to the patient as another responsibility of this partnership. This was described in terms of walking with the patient or standing beside them.

One clear duty is to walk beside the patient and families through the long haul. To walk with them I think is a very strong characterization of the role. I think persistence in terms of finding the many sources and being there with them by their side.

But I think to be a good physical therapist, sometimes you have to be able to walk with the patient for a while. And so it is not a matter of you guiding them all the time and carrying, but somehow you have to walk exactly. You have to talk with them and understand all the dimensions of their life. At the same time I think this introduces a lot of boundary issues. I think that is something that we have not really explored enough. What are those boundary issues and how do we deal with them, because what's being asked of the physical therapist is to be very close to the patient, very close physically and psychologically at times to understand how they can help their lives.

These two responses suggest that there is a responsibility for the therapist to enter the life of patients, to be available to them, to walk beside them, and to be with them for the long haul. The last quote also addresses the need to examine the boundaries of the close relationship between the therapist and the patient.

Other respondents emphasize the collaboration and reciprocity that characterize the partner relationship. In these responses the participants point out the importance of respect for the patients and their choices.

There is a heart to physical therapy and the heart of good physical therapy is the celebration of the therapist's and the patient's joint humanness with all the problems and all the potentials. So, I'm going to make mistakes and they're going to make a mistake. But together we will go through it.

A lot of collaborative activity is finding common ground and then being able to proceed with collaboration. And I suppose that a value that goes along with that is respect and ultimately respecting the patient's wish, even if it is injurious or harmful, and to understand that it is the patient's choice. And while you would like to bring them to another point, you may be unsuccessful. That each person is responsible for their own life in this world and you do

what you can to walk beside them and bring them to paths that are perhaps healthier or more satisfying, but in the end you must respect their rights and their issues.

Characteristic 4: Bridge to Function

A number of respondents saw that an important characteristic of the therapist's relationship with the patient was to be a bridge to a role or functional ability. The emphasis on the return to function was considered a unique component of the therapist's relationship with her or his patient. One respondent stated:

We have a whole language that supports that we are a bridge back to a social role. We are bridges back to society in a more dramatic sense than a lot of other health professionals.

Other informants emphasized the importance of functional improvements and the necessity of progress toward greater independence as a result of the therapist's interactions with patients. Physical therapists help patients to help themselves.

Our job is to help the patient to help themselves, and I've come to realize that in that regard physical therapists are different from most other health professionals. So in terms of our moral role, we enter the profession wanting to help others and we learn that our helpfulness or our doing good is to help them to help themselves.

If one has respect, mutual respect, that also includes knowing where the patient is coming from. If you start from that place, you are starting from a good position and other things will follow. I see that as a fundamental to rehabilitation because we are there to assist or facilitate, and help them do for themselves.

Well, I think that all of us in rehabilitation have the same goal and that is to work toward the highest or deepest level of independent function with the patient as possible.

These responses link the therapist/patient interaction in rehabilitation to the attainment of functional skills. The therapist has a moral responsibility to help the patient increase in functional ability. The respondents also emphasized the importance of helping their patients help themselves and progress toward greater functional independence.

Characteristic 5: Provide Unique Benefit

Many of the respondents stated that the relationship of the therapist and patient is dependent on the therapist having a unique set of skills that is of value to the patient. These skills are specific to the role of the physical therapist and help the patient address a problem or improve function. The respondents described the importance of the physical therapist providing the patient with a unique service or set of skills that helps to address a problem. They saw the role of physical therapist as unique.

All the morality of the profession has been legitimated around the idea that we can relieve a certain condition and suffering that nobody else can do.

The nature of physical therapy is that we are involved with people from birth until the moment of death in trying to help them with movement disorders that interfere with function and best quality of life.

Many respondents considered the intensity of the relationship and the length of involvement with the patient as a unique part of the role of the therapist. A number of the respondents also emphasized that in their interactions with their patients physical therapists were responsible to limit the scope of their practice to their areas of skill and responsibility. In relation to limiting the scope of practice one informant discussed the responsibility of the therapist to exercise "due care."

So if one is a moral agent as a physical therapist, first I think the profession's duty would be kind of professional duties of due care, of trying to limit one's scope to those areas that most fully respect a combination of what a client/patient brings as his/her ends or would like to accomplish, and what health care professions generally put as their limitation. So scope, if you want to think about it as a character trait like humility or judiciousness or would like to think of it as the duty of due care. I think the moral dimension of physical therapy has to take into account its scope, its appropriate scope. So dispositionally and in terms of actual behaviors we aren't all things to all people or

even all things, we're not health professionals who can do anything to be of help.

Many of the participants identified the importance of the therapist providing a unique service for the patient that is within a defined scope of practice.

Interactions with Nonpatients

All respondents in this study recognized that physical therapists have interactions and relationships with groups and individuals who are not patients. The other interactions described by the respondents also created moral requirements on the actions of the physical therapists. The participants also considered these relationships to be a component of the moral role of the physical therapist.

Definition of Others

The respondents identified a variety of individuals and organizations that were part of this category. The one common characteristic that they possessed was that they had some interaction or relationship with physical therapists or the profession of physical therapy and are affected by the actions of physical therapists. They were, however, not involved in a patient/therapist interaction. This included health care colleagues, peers, professional organizations, third-party payers, health care administrators, social service agencies, insurance companies, governmental agencies, institutions of higher education, and the society as a whole. It is a wide and diverse group that spans a number of different types of relationships and interactions.

To begin the analysis of the responses by the participants of this diverse group, the investigator divided the group into three categories based on the amount of contact the therapist has with the individual or group and on the direct influence the actions of the therapist would have on the entity. The first category consists of physical therapy colleagues and physical therapy professional organizations. The second category is composed of all the other health care colleagues that physical therapists interact with and the organizations and agencies involved in the provision of health care services. The third category includes society at large, social services organizations, governmental agencies, and other interest groups. This division was not proposed by the participants in the study, but was developed by the investigator as a useful tool for organizing the responses.

Category 1 of Nonpatients: Physical Therapy Peers and Professional Organizations

There was a sense among many of the participants that for physical therapists their relationship with the profession of physical therapy and other physical therapists was an important area of moral responsibility. One respondent described this responsibility as maintaining a "good thing."

I put our profession second because one of my personal values is that I think we provide a good, we do a good thing. And if we want to continue to recognize that and allow us the opportunity to do that good thing, then we have a responsibility to make sure the profession survives. And that is a good thing because of the patients, that's not necessarily because we need the work, but because society will be better off.

Another respondent stated that communicating to others about the values of the services that the profession of physical therapy has to offer is an important part of a physical therapist's responsibility to their profession.

I think we have an obligation to the profession in terms of helping patients understand what physical therapy has to offer. Sometimes it can get short shrift because it can look like self-interest, but I think the profession of physical therapy when it is performing in the area that we would like to think that it is promoting physical therapy as a benefit, as a good for patients, something that will enhance their lives, their function. I see the professional role there and that we as physical therapists should be acting in a way that is supportive of those things.

Another respondent also identified the responsibility of physical therapists to define their area of expertise and make it clear what they do to help the patient.

I think our responsibility is to continue to identify our area of expertise. I don't think we have finished doing that. I believe we are on to something that is really unique and going with your function, neuromuscular physiology. The language that we've developed and that lies behind it is something that nobody else is doing.

There was also a feeling by a number of the respondents that as a member of a profession, physical therapists had a moral responsibility to the profession to comply with the Physical Therapy Code of Ethics and Guide to Professional Conduct.

The duties are multifaceted. Certainly compliance with the Ethical Code of Conduct as enunciated by the professional association, that being the Guide for Professional Conduct. That's the rule's utilitarian component of the ethical mix.

Some respondents identified the responsibility of the physical therapist to help ensure that all members of the profession act ethically.

If you know that somebody is doing something that is not particularly ethical or legal or sort of borderline, you have a responsibility to do something about it, to confront them or do something. I think that is really hard for us.

Category 2 of Nonpatients: Health Care Colleagues

The respondents recognized that physical therapists have relationships and interactions with a variety of individuals from other health care professions. An important characteristic of these relationships should be to optimize the care of the patient.

I think certainly the issue of who we as physical therapists are as members of the whole health care delivery team. And that would encompass everything from the issue of primary care provision, certainly multidisciplinary and interdisciplinary approaches to patient care and how we work with others in delivering health care to optimize the patient outcome as opposed to the outcome for us as a physical therapy profession.

Other respondents emphasized the need to stand with colleagues and work together.

We also have the responsibility of fidelity to colleagues, all kinds of colleagues, everyone working in the system. We have to stand together and make decisions together. Stand up for each other. It is wrong I think to criticize or bad-mouth the decisions that are made by colleagues in front of patients. It weakens the whole system.

Another informant identified our responsibility to interpret for other health care professionals the language that we have developed to describe rehabilitation.

I think we have the duty of interpretation for some areas of health care that aren't necessarily within our narrow screen of language and ends. I'll say medicine and nursing. I remember struggling with how one would talk about a benefit when it was maintenance. Medicare and Medicaid had requirements that we were having to justify and we always had to keep showing benefit and improvement. And we didn't have a good language for that. So we had to develop a language and interpret it backwards.

The "duty of interpretation" as described by the participant involves a responsibility to provide and explain the meaning of terms that can be used as a tool to communicate more clearly the needs and progress of patients receiving rehabilitation services.

Category 3 of Nonpatients: Social Agencies and Society at Large

This category of society includes all the interactions physical therapists have with other groups and agencies that do not have an active role in the provision of health care services. This would include governmental agencies, much of the business community, many of the social agencies, and the society at large. Many of the respondents identified a general responsibility to society and the various groups that compose it. Some of the respondents stated the need for physical therapists to focus on the needs of society.

I think that we have got to focus on what society needs from us and that goes from individual patients to also include the community. It is a broader view. I don't think that physical therapists have a broad view.

Another responsibility that was identified by the participants was that physical therapists need to look at our place in the delivery of health services and to evaluate how we are contributing to the cost of health care. The concern for stewardship of resources was one that was voiced by many of the respondents.

I think that with the changes in health care we're having, we need to look at our position in society as well as how we are contributing to costs as well as cost conservation. So more social awareness is necessary.

So we have to have some responsibility to ourselves as a profession, but we also have responsibility to the people who are paying, the insurance company. Especially if they are going to trust us to make decisions about what the patient really needs.

A number of the respondents also emphasized the need for physical therapists to participate in creating changes in social policies that affect individuals in our scope of responsibilities.

I think that the profession as a whole tends to overlook their larger responsibility that is to effect the best outcome for a single patient or client may indeed be to participate in change policy.

✧ DISCUSSION

In this chapter the investigator identified two primary categories of relationships: relationships with patients and with nonpatients. The responsibilities that physical therapists have within these different relationships have their origins in different moral obligations. The relationship that therapists have with patients is based on a fiduciary relationship that includes direct responsibility to the individual patient and patient-centered behaviors. The relationships that physical therapists have with individuals or groups of nonpatients are not based on a fiduciary relationship, but appear to come from a social contract that defines the role of the physical therapist in the context of its usefulness in addressing a defined social need. The interaction patterns in these latter relationships are more collaborative and complementary. They appear to be based on good citizenship, value to society, and fairness. See Figure 9.1.

Physical Therapists as Moral Agents

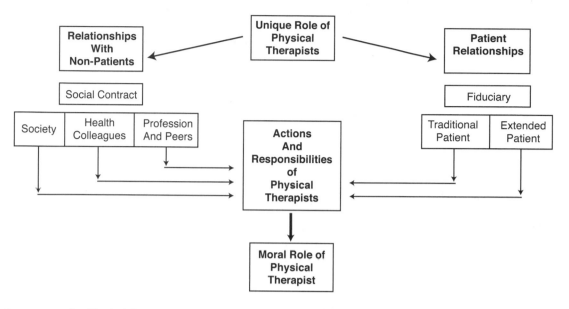

Figure 9.1 ✧ Physical therapists as moral agents.

Defining the Central Responsibilities of the Moral Role of the Physical Therapist

The responses of the participants indicated that the center of the moral role of a physical therapist was their individual interaction with their direct patients. This interaction was often presented as a very personal and intimate relationship. It was described as walking with the patient, entering the life of a patient, and putting the patient's needs ahead of their own needs. This personal relationship also presented moral requirements for behavior that reflect this personal role.

The relationships that physical therapists have with nonpatients were identified as an important component of the moral role of physical therapists, but did not receive the central position given the therapist's relationship with their patient. The responsibilities therapists had to nonpatients were usually discussed as additions to the primary moral role of the therapist and were often mentioned as responsibilities that therapists often forget to consider. The focus of the responsibilities that therapists have

to nonpatients was directed toward promoting better organization of society through collaboration, fairness, and abiding by social agreements and rules. These responsibilities were less personal and more directed toward interactions with groups and organizations, and toward affecting policies.

The two different types of relationships present different responsibilities for inclusion as components in the moral role of the therapist. The responses of the participants indicated that therapist-patient interactions are the central and most important component of the moral role of the physical therapist. The responsibilities and behaviors that are described as a part of the therapist-patient relationship are therefore at the core of the moral role of the physical therapist.

The relationships and interactions that physical therapists have with nonpatients create other moral responsibilities that need to be included in the moral role of the therapist. These responsibilities and relationships have a major impact on the patient-therapist relationship through organizational policies, codes, laws, and professional interactions that set the social context within which the therapist-patient interaction takes place.

Uniqueness and Value of Rehabilitation

A unique component of the role of physical therapists identified by many of the discussants was the relationship that the therapist has with the patients. The respondents described the role of therapist as being centered on the promises and commitment that therapists make to their patients. The therapist promises to come to the patient with the knowledge, skill, and motivation to help the patient reach a better place in her or his life. The therapist also promises to serve as an advocate for their patients to help them achieve their goals. These promises involve standing besides the patient, working as partners with the patient to achieve goals, staying with them through the long haul, being a guide, and putting the needs of the patient ahead of the needs of the therapist.

The respondents in this study also identified a set of responsibilities that arise from the therapist's relationships and promises made to society. Therapists have agreed to abide by the laws that govern practice. They have agreed to provide a service that benefits the citizens. They have agreed to stay within a defined scope of practice. They have also agreed to follow employment contracts and institutional policies. The relationships and promises made to different groups create the responsibilities outlined in Table 9.2.

Some of the responsibilities that are included in that table are that the therapists define clearly their skills, communicate effectively the needs of rehabilitation patients, collaborate with other health professionals to provide best patient care, work to achieve the best care for the segment of the population entrusted to their care, and work toward meeting the health care needs of society.

The responsibilities that physical therapists have to their patients and the responsibilities to nonpatients are often complementary. Promoting the best interest of individual patients should also be in the interest of the larger society. Communicating clearly and collaborating with other health care professionals

Table 9.2 ✧ **Responsibilities of Physical Therapists' Interactions with Nonpatients**

Profession and Peers:

1. To act in ways that strengthen the profession.
2. To define the skills and expertise associated with the profession.
3. To inform others regarding the value of the services offered by physical therapy.
4. To maintain the standards of behavior that are described by the profession in the APTA Guide to Professional Conduct and Code of Ethics.

Colleagues:

1. To work with other health professionals in a collaborative way that maximizes the outcomes achieved by the patient.
2. To communicate clearly and effectively with other health professionals.
3. To define and interpret the language of rehabilitation to health professionals who may not be familiar with the terminology used to describe patient care and progress.
4. To respect the skill and opinions of other health care professions in their interactions with patients.

Society:

1. To help address the health care needs of society.
2. To provide expected services to members of society within a define scope of practice.
3. To be good stewards of the health care resources allocated for physical therapy services.
4. To provide oversight of organizational and governmental policies and work to ensure policies that are in the best interest of the segment of society that falls within the scope of rehabilitation care.

should be in the best interest of the patient as well.

There also appears to be potential for stress and conflict between the different responsibilities. Examples of these conflicts are numerous. Many of the conflicts involve agreements made with employers and organizational policies that threaten the promises made by the therapist to the patient. The respondents in this study identified managed care and reimbursement issues most often as the practice issues that threaten the moral role of the therapist. Most of the threats that were identified by the respondents involved nonpatient relationships putting restraints on or conflicting with the therapist-patient relationship.

✦ SUMMARY AND FUTURE RESEARCH

The results of this study point to the need for physical therapists to be attentive to the responsibilities of both the relationships therapists have with their patients and the relationships with nonpatients. Although the core of the therapist's moral role is the relationship with the patient, the social context and the relationships that therapists negotiate with nonpatients will greatly affect the ability of therapists to fulfill their responsibilities to patients. This study suggests that it is the rehabilitation professional's responsibility to bring these two areas of responsibility into harmony.

This study has additional implications for the education of rehabilitation professionals. To teach applied ethics to students in a professional education program, it is helpful for the educator to have a clear understanding of what constitutes the moral role of that profession. In both physical therapy and occupational therapy there have been a number of articles written relating to the teaching of ethics in the professional curriculums of these professions.[22-27] Most of this literature has been directed toward descriptions of current practice and pedagogy. The current study was conducted to provide a better understanding of responsibilities and behaviors that are associated with the moral role of the physical therapist. The study could be replicated in occupational therapy.

References

1. Gold MR, et al: Cost-Effectiveness in Health and Medicine. Oxford University Press, New York, 1996.
2. Morreim EH: Balancing Act: The New Medical Ethics of Medicine's New Economics. Georgetown University Press, Washington, DC, 1995.
3. Emanual EJ: Justice and managed care: Four principles for the just allocation of health care resources. Hastings Cent Rep 30(3):8–16, 2000.
4. Kronick P, et al: The marketplace in healthcare reform: The demographic limitations of managed competition. N Engl J Med 148:52, 1993.
5. Thomasma DC: The ethics of managed care: Challenges to the principle of relationship-centered care. J Allied Health 25:233–246, 1996.
6. Lopopolo RB: Hospital restructuring and the changing nature of the physical therapist's role. Phys Ther 5(1):38–44, 1999.
7. Blan R, et al: The experience of providing physical therapy in a changing health care environment. Phys Ther 82:648–657, 2002.
8. Purtilo R: Managed care: Ethical issues for the rehabilitation professions. Trends Health Care Law Ethics 10(1–2):105–118, Winter/Spring 1995.
9. Miller PA, and Solomon P: The influence of a move to program management on the practice of physical therapy. Phys Ther 82:449–458, 2002.
10. Friere P: Pedagogy of the Oppressed. Seabury, New York, 1970.
11. Purtilo RB: Understanding ethical issues: The physical therapist as ethicist. Phys Ther 54:239–242, 1974.
12. Guccione AA: Ethical issues in physical therapy practice: A survey of physical therapists in N Engl Phys Ther 60:1264–1272, 1980.
13. Sim J: Ethical considerations in physiotherapy. Physiotherapy 69:19–120, 1983.
14. Triezenberg HL: The identification of ethical issues in physical therapy practice. Phys Ther 76:1097–1107, 1996.
15. Barnitt R: Ethical dilemmas in occupational and physical therapy: A survey of practitioners in the UK National Health Service. J Med Ethics 24:193–199, 1998.
16. Swisher LL: A retrospective analysis of ethics knowledge in physical therapy (1970–2000). Phys Ther 82(7):692–706, 2002.
17. Fontana A, and Frey JH: Interviewing: The art of science. In Denzin NK, and Lincoln YS (eds): Handbook of Qualitative Research. Sage Publications Inc, Thousand Oaks, CA, 1994, pp 361–392.
18. Seidman I: Interviewing as Qualitative Research, ed 2. Teacher's College Press, New York, 1998.
19. Mishler EG: Research Interviewing: Context and Narrative. Harvard University Press, Cambridge, MA, 1986.
20. Barnitt R: What gives you sleepless nights? Ethical practice in occupational therapy. Br J Occup Ther 56(6):201–212, 1993.
21. Clawson AL: The relationship between clinical decision making and ethical decision making. Physiotherapy 80:10–14, 1994.
22. Barnitt RE: 'Deeply troubling questions': The teaching of ethics in undergraduate courses. Br J Occup Ther 56:75–110, 1993.
23. Haddad A: Teaching ethical analysis in occupational therapy. Am J Occup Ther 42(5):300–3304, 1998.
24. Triezenberg HL: Teaching ethics in physical therapy education: A Delphi study. J Phys Ther Educ 11:16–22, 1997.
25. Pinnington L, and Bagshaw A: The requirement for ethical reasoning in occupational therapy education. Br J Occup Ther 55(1):419–422, 1992.
26. Purtilo RB: The structure of ethics teaching in physical therapy: A survey. Phys Ther 59:1102–1106, 1979.
27. Triezenberg HL, and Davis CM: Beyond the code of ethics: Educating physical therapists for their role as moral agents. J Phys Ther Educ 14(3):48–58, 2001.

10

The Impact of Advances in Medical Technology on Rehabilitative Care

REGINA F. DOHERTY MS, OTR/L

Abstract

Occupational therapists and physical therapists have a moral obligation to be knowledgeable and competent in technology to best address the needs of our patients. Awareness is the key to technology, without it we are left behind, as practical application is limited if we do not truly understand technology functionality. New technologies have advanced the abilities of health care and the use of these technologies present important ethical considerations. As rehabilitation practitioners, we bring "function" to medicine and technology. We must develop and refine skills of ethical reasoning and moral agency to advance our clinical practice. Rehabilitation practitioners have a valuable contribution to make to our clients and the technology field by developing and communicating a language of function. In order to best do that, we must take risks and answer difficult questions from patients and the interdisciplinary team with ease. Ethics education and mentoring is key to developing and advancing this skill in clinicians. It is our duty to observe the ethical components of our practice and serve as legitimate stakeholders in the care of the patient.

✧ INTRODUCTION

In the 17th century, conquering surgical pain was a challenge that faced many physicians and patients. Surgery was often referred to as barbaric and was avoided at all costs. Accounts of horrid yelling and screaming from both children and adults plagued surgeons for years. Imagine the dilemmas that presented to our practicing predecessors when decisions were riddled with such events. If only they could save life without having to induce pain and suffering. Then a group of Boston dentists and physicians discovered ether as a means to conquer pain during surgery. On October 16, 1846, William T. Morton and John Collins Warren went down in history as making medicine's greatest discovery. Their patient, Gilbert Abbott, underwent the successful administration of ether for resection of a vascular tumor. Gilbert informed curious onlookers when he awoke that he had experienced no pain during this process. Warren turned to the observant crowd and stated "Gentlemen—this is no humbug." From that point on a new era of medicine began.[1]

Today anesthesia is a standard of care for all patients undergoing surgical treatment. Medical discoveries in the 21st century continue to advance the abilities of medicine and science. Just as Morton and Warren strove to make health care better a long time ago, so too do providers today. New discoveries and medical technologies have allowed for great advances in the care of patients, and in turn have advanced the practice of medicine and the humanities. How do these advances influence health care professionals? How does the public view medical advances? What value do we as a society place on medical innovation, and how does the use of technology have an impact on how individuals function in their day-to-day lives?

In this paper I will explore the delicate balance that occurs between technological advances and the everyday lives of those assisted by them. I will begin to reflect upon how occupational therapy (OT) and physical therapy (PT) practitioners can be best prepared to work with patients who are assisted by advanced technologies and how they can best use critical reasoning skills to balance the clinical and ethical needs of these patients. I will then look toward the future of rehabilitative science and its collaboration with medical science, exploring the role of occupational and physical therapists in evaluating the impact of technology on function, and bringing to the forefront of technology issues related to quality of life.

✦ TECHNOLOGY IN CLINICAL PRACTICE

In order to begin thinking about how rehabilitative practice and technology intersect, let us look at the following cases and reflect on some of the ethical concerns and considerations that they present.

The case of Phil raises several ethical considerations. To effectively treat Phil and maintain good moral standing, his occupational and physical therapists must achieve technical competence in treatment of Phil given his combined diagnosis of CVA and cardiac disease with LVAD dependency. They must learn the ins and outs of the LVAD machine to accurately predict how this, combined with his hemiplegia, will alter his daily activities. The occupational therapist and physical therapist must balance their obligation of caring for Phil, while maintaining objectivity in the face of mounting pressure from the medical team. They must have the courage to face the difficult questions that Phil will ask them, and have moral courage to best advocate for Phil to the surgical team when/if lack of progress is encountered. They must be prepared for difficult questions from Phil such as, "If I can't go home, can't they take this LVAD out and let me die?" The occupational therapist and physical therapist must also carefully consider the question of how aggressively to treat Phil, and how to prioritize Phil's treatment with other patients in times of high volume or staff shortages.

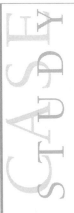

Phil is a 55-year-old firefighter who presents to the emergency room with 10 out of 10 chest pain. Cardiac catheterization revealed 80% to 90% blockage in all coronary arteries, severe pump dysfunction, and severe myocardial ischemia. He is taken urgently for coronary artery bypass grafting and a left ventricular assist device (LVAD) is placed to pump for his heart as a bridge to transplantation. Over the next 24 hours he is watched closely in the ICU (intensive care unit). The medical team begins to note a sudden facial droop and decreased muscle tone in his right arm. Diagnostics are run and an additional diagnosis is confirmed—Phil has had a left middle cerebral artery CVA (cerebrovascular accident). Rehabilitation services are consulted to help Phil become "as functional as possible" so that he can eventually be considered a transplant candidate. His therapists can count on the fingers of one hand the number of stroke patients that they have worked with who were on an LVAD. Phil's LVAD is pneumatic, not electric, and he can never leave the hospital while using it. This technology is keeping Phil alive. It replaces the pumping action of his heart and will sustain his cardiac output. Since this technology requires intense nursing and medical care, no free-standing rehabilitation hospital will accept him. He will need to receive all his rehabilitation services in the acute care setting. His progress is slow. He is depressed and has had many additional medical set backs. Phil starts refusing occupational and physical therapy with increasing frequency. Many months pass and the chances of him being considered a candidate for the transplant list are slim. His surgical team does not want him to "lose hope." His occupational and physical therapists often ask Phil what his goal is, to which he replies—to feel better and go home. They struggle with the reality that this will never happen.

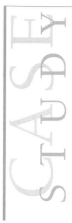

Lucy is a 20-month-old child with cerebral palsy secondary to an anoxic injury sustained during birth trauma. She spent the first six months of her life in the acute hospital and rehabilitation setting, and has had five subsequent hospital admissions since then. On the most recent hospital admission, which was for a g-tube revision, the mother was informed by one of the senior residents that they were doing a study (phase one trial) on the benefits of hyperbaric oxygenation treatment (HBO_2) for children in Lucy's condition. He told her she should consider the benefits of enrolling Lucy in that trial. The next day you arrive to see Lucy for treatment. The mother tells you that she has signed up Lucy for "a great treatment that will help Lucy's brain heal." She says, "right now it is experimental, but soon everyone will be doing it. That's why they need kids like Lucy to sign up." You ask her if there are any risks to the experiment and she says that there are none of which she is aware. You know from your past experience in treating children with carbon monoxide poisoning that HBO_2 can cause complications including barotraumatic lesions (e.g., ear pain, rupture of tympanic membrane, lesions in sinuses) and ocular effects (such as myopia and cataract growth) as well as seizures.

Communication is a moral imperative in the case of Lucy. The rehabilitation practitioner must obtain the facts of the case. They must consider how the hope and belief of "healing" can be strong motivators for family. They must also consider the greater likelihood of therapeutic misconception in the rehabilitation medicine population, knowing that many of these research participants and families may associate the word research with treatment or cure.[2] The practitioner must advocate for the patient by openly communicating with the researcher to explore the process of informed consent, knowing that a phase one trial is one that is used to test drug/treatment safety, not dosage of effectiveness. Consent is a process of shared decision making, which includes both informed consent and informed refusal. Again there is a need for the practitioner to balance the moral obligation to the patient with the moral obligation to the greater good of future children through research.

Rick's case highlights pharmaceutical and medical technology combined for a positive outcome. Rick is a technology success story with improved rehabilitative potential as a

Rick is a 40-year-old male admitted to the hospital status post sudden onset of right-sided weakness and slurred speech. It was Friday and Rick had taken the day off to work in the garden. He had a lot to do to get the yard ready for his daughter's high school graduation party, which was scheduled for that Sunday. His wife joked with him before she left for work that the place had better be in "ship shape" when she got home. While beginning the day his symptoms suddenly appeared. He called his wife at work around 11:00, who immediately called 911. Emergency medical services arrived and noted that Rick had a significant weakness (0/5 in the right arm and hand, 2/5 in the right leg). Their preliminary diagnosis was CVA. Rick was brought to the hospital where an MRI (magnetic resonance imaging) of his brain was immediately performed. This revealed a clot in his right middle cerebral artery, obstructing flow to the surrounding brain tissue. Because his wife was with him earlier in the day and was able to confirm that he was doing well, the time frame of his symptom onset was known by the medical team to be less than 8 hours. Rick was then deemed a candidate for tissue plasminogen activator (tPA). Administration of this clot-breaking drug is seen as a lifesaver for some stroke victims. It can break up the clot, restoring normal blood flow to the brain, but in doing so, there is risk that the broken up clot may cause residual damage. Rick, with the assistance of his wife, decides to consent to the treatment. tPA is administered and over the next 24 hours Rick's clinical presentation is much improved. He is able to use his right arm and leg functionally. His strength is returned to 4/5 in the arm, 3/5 in the hand, and 4/5 in the leg. He meets his occupational and physical therapists the next morning, his neurological prognosis is very optimistic.

result. His case reminds us of our moral obligation as professionals to educate society on stroke symptoms, increasing public awareness and potentially improving our clients' outcomes.

These three cases (Phil, Lucy, and Rick) highlight the use of technology with varied outcomes. Technology allows our patients to heal after surgery and survive through crises. Technology can be a lifesaver, a bridge, and it can be the difference between poor quality of life versus good quality of life. Technology brings with it a balance of benefits and burdens, a balance that occupational therapy and physical therapy practitioners must be prepared to understand.

Technology—"High" versus "Low"

The practice of occupational and physical therapy would clearly not be where it is today if not for the many technologies that medical science has provided. There are varying types and ranges of technology. There is "low tech and high tech," ordinary and extraordinary, and for each type there is an individual client consideration. The following are a few examples of the ranges of technology seen in clinical practice:

✦ Use of supplemental oxygen (low tech) to full respiratory support via intubation and mechanical ventilation (high tech)

✦ Use of a Glucometer (low tech) to continuous venous-to-venous hemodialysis (CVVH) (high tech)

✦ Use of a puff-activated call bell switch (low tech) to use of a fully established environmental control unit (high tech)

Technology—Its Power

Although this chapter will mainly address extraordinary "high" technology, such as life-sustaining treatments, it is important to remember that all technology is individualized in that it is as advanced as its user (the patient and or family) view it to be.

Our patients are living longer and fuller lives. Disabilities are being prevented and in some cases impairment minimized through the use of medical and technological advances. Technology allows the person who has lost a voice the ability to communicate, the person who has lost the strength to walk the ability to be mobile, and the person whose heart has lost the ability to pump to beat. These are our clients. These are the patients who inspire us as they resume life and rehabilitate. Technology also brings with it difficult decisions. It possesses such great benefits, that it becomes difficult to imagine living without it. Just as it can save lives, it also may increase pain and suffering, and in turn burden those it can no longer save.

But technology has power. It is spotlighted on the pages of our newspapers, is talked about among social circles, and it is broadcast on American television in dramatic fictional and nonfiction forms. Its benefits are so well boasted, that society has become accustomed to expecting it. Technology today has an intrinsic and extrinsic value medically and socially.[3]

✧ CORE PROFESSIONAL VALUES AND TECHNOLOGY

In order to better understand the value of technology, we as rehabilitation professionals must explore our own values. What are the values that are inherent to the professions of occupational therapy and physical therapy? What standards help guide us in applying our science and practice? If we look at the professional codes of ethics of these professions we see many guiding principles and standards that assist us in interpreting ethical principles professionally, but we still need to reflect further. We need to reflect upon what makes us unique.

Function as a Core Value

As a professional group, occupational and physical therapists highly value function: it is inherent in our practice. It is a value that we try to instill in our patients, our colleagues, and our students. Function first, maximizing functional potential, prognosticating functional outcome, however it is phrased, it is a core of the occupational and physical therapy professions. Despite impairment, disability, or handicap the patient's function and ability to engage in roles is valued first. Second to this is the technology. An expert occupational therapist or physical therapist can walk into a hospital room that is riddled with technology—a patient attached to a ventilator, multiple IV lines, artificial skin, a heart pacing wire—and still see only function. They turn to the distraught wife and begin to talk about who this person is. One of the first questions they ask is, "What did he like?" or "Tell me about your husband," already acknowledging his important life roles. This is what makes us different than others. We bring function to medicine. This is a driver of our professions. It is an intrinsic value that we hold true, no matter what practice setting we are in.

Advocacy as a Core Value

Advocacy is another core value held by the rehabilitation practitioner. Occupational therapists and physical therapists have always served as strong advocates for the patients they treat. The concept of advocacy as it specifically relates to technology will be discussed further in this paper.

So how can we better prepare to address the intersection of technology and our professions? How do we best mentor our newer colleagues and students to gain a broader understanding of the benefits and burdens of technology? First, we need to ensure a greater awareness of technology. Part of this awareness should be an understanding of the technology itself, as well as its functional strengths and limitations. We must embrace educational opportunities that appear medically oriented and bring forth the questions that we have regarding the "technicalities" of technological devices so that we may understand them as well as or better than other members of the health care team. Only then can we help educate our patients and families on how the technology will affect their lives. Take the case of Phil, the 55-year-old firefighter on the LVAD. His therapists needed to have a thorough understanding of the operations of the LVAD; everything from the shelf life of the battery to the way the valve exited the skin at the abdomen. Only then could

they be aware of how to educate Phil on how to bathe and dress himself and how to become portable and walk out of his room to socialize with others. They also had to gain an understanding of what Phil needed to be responsible for in terms of maintenance of this device. This was a new role for him. He was a health care consumer. Some of these responsibilities were simple, such as performing a battery check (pushing one button to get a read-out). Others are more complex and require having the cognitive processes, endurance, and strength, for example, to hand pump his device in the event of a power failure.

✧ TECHNOLOGY FUNCTIONALITY

Awareness is the key to technology. Without it we are left behind, as we can no longer apply function if we do not truly understand technology functionality. Some practitioners will contend that they do not practice in a technologically based setting, so they do not need such a thorough understanding of this technology. (To this point I would argue, learn now or be left behind.) Technology will continue to advance and practitioners in all settings will be affected by it. Upon the writing of this chapter, the Centers for Medicare and Medicaid Services issued a decision memorandum approving the use of the LVAD as destination therapy for beneficiaries with Class IV chronic end stage heart failure.[4] These patients must meet certain conditions, however; this is just one example of a broadening technology application from research to clinical trial to hospital use to home application. It will affect rehabilitation services in many ways. There will be many ethical questions that will need careful consideration. For example, how do we best advocate for this population should we find them demonstrating new cognitive deficits at home? What about the client who functions independently at home with the LVAD who is now newly diagnosed with cancer requiring surgical treatment? How does the LVAD have an impact on decisions related to cancer care given that the context of life with the LVAD has now changed? Whether a technology is in current use, or is part of a patient's past medical history, understanding of the technology will only advance the therapeutic relationship that is developed between clinician and client.

Many of our patients are survivors. They come to us with impairments and limitations as a result of a physical or psychological trauma. For some this is an obvious trauma, such as a motor vehicle accident, for others it is the life-altering event of being diagnosed with cancer or kidney failure. To understand and better treat our patients we must be aware that many of them are survivors of health care crises. As a result they have particular learning needs of which to be aware. Loss and control are two important themes that drive patient learning needs. Health care practitioners have reported encountering difficulty dealing with the physical and mental complications of the survivor and their continuing illness, yet few identified coping strategies to manage these problems.[5] The formal processing of difficult ethical issues is an effective strategy for practitioners to use in order to better care for survivors (and themselves).

✧ ETHICS EDUCATION AND MENTORING

Early ethics educational and socialization activities should be a staple in the physical therapy and occupational therapy curricula and integrated into mentorship during clinical practice. Ethics must be taken seriously early in the educational process and cases must be discussed early in the careers of future practitioners so that practitioners can problem-solve how they feel and begin development of moral decision making as it will relate to their professional roles. Socialization must also be integrated, i.e., not only having a client with a spinal cord injury or other disability come into the classroom as a well model, but also having students go into the sick model and observe patients on life support where team meetings are conducted regarding difficult decisions. The well population and the population of individuals who are sick or disabled must spend time together to better understand each other.

This valuable time will broaden the perspective of physical therapy and occupational therapy clinicians when we are asked to evaluate an individual's quality of life. It is a big job; we should be academically, clinically, and morally prepared to do so. Experiential and academic training in moral human reasoning is an important component of clinical reasoning development. It is also part of character development to instill the values of the profession.

Mentorship opportunities that focus on ethical questions and dilemmas must also be made available to practicing clinicians. Clinicians skilled in ethical reasoning should support those who are newly developing this skill so that their practice and clinical reasoning can appropriately advance. Novice clinicians need guidance to actualize the emotional components of difficult cases and professional support to impart moral courage to their actions. Advanced clinicians with skills in ethics consultation and assessment can effectively provide this support. They can assist the practicing clinician in distinguishing the ethical dimensions of the case from the other overlapping dimensions (such as legal dimensions) and assist them in identifying morally acceptable options. Participation in multidisciplinary institution-based ethics committees is also an important role for the rehabilitation practitioner.

Some practitioners will have practical wisdom. We know that practical wisdom and ethical discussions are closely related.[6] When we teach critical thinking, we ask students to think, reason, and choose alternatives. We should teach ethics in a similar model, integrating personal decisions and socialization experiences to help practitioners develop their own moral character. This will lead us to a greater reflection on ethical issues and more sophisticated ethical discussion can then occur.

✧ ADVOCACY SKILLS AND TECHNOLOGY

The third way to ensure a successful interplay between technology and the occupational therapy and physical therapy professions is to encourage clinicians to be strong patient advocates and resources for functional application of technology. As stated previously, awareness of the technology, and understanding of the individual as a whole makes us a natural advocate for patients who are impacted by technology. We must overcome hierarchical barriers and be confident that our contribution to the care of these patients is essential. Society will value the input that physical and occupational therapists can have on how to help patients live quality lives with technology; for example, helping our patient's family members understand the functional implications of a devastating diagnosis, such as permanent vegetative state, to help decide whether or not to continue the use of ventilator support. Use of strategies inherent to the profession, such as roles clarification and values assessment, are of key assistance to the team and the family for the most effective proxy decision making process. If we are comfortable with the moral challenges these discussions bring, we can help our colleagues in the medicine and other health care fields with the broader application of technological advances. We must advocate for the patient who has no voice. We must help our colleagues understand disability, its limitations and its abilities. As an example, we know from the research that patients with tetraplegia and those with neuromuscular disease report life satisfaction and a good quality of life despite the need for ventilator assistance,[7,8] yet how many times have we heard ICU nurses say, "Well, he already has multiple sclerosis, why would we expect he would want to live on the ventilator too?" We must share our professional knowledge with our physician and nursing colleagues and be ever-present in discussions regarding care planning for clients with both new and preexisting conditions. We also need to be prepared to engage in future decisions related to genetic conditions. The field of genetics is rapidly expanding, with prenatal (cystic fibrosis gene) and presymptom (breast cancer gene) diagnostics being offered. This advanced knowledge will change the future of health care for populations of well people as well as people who are disabled.

Some of the barriers to strong advocacy are obvious. Technology can be frightening. If we don't understand it, it is easier to defer to our physician colleagues in explaining its impact on a patient's life. We also must acknowledge that these are difficult discussions to have. We must develop a comfort in addressing the "elephant in the room"[9] and, in the case of the use of technology at end of life, develop the skills to initiate, broach, and continue the discussion. Dying is a part of living. When we talk about care planning and quality of life with a cancer patient, we must be comfortable addressing questions that they have about living well through the dying process. The social culture of America is, at times, a barrier to this process, as death is not as openly talked about in this culture as it is in others. Paradoxically, technology is more openly discussed, maybe because it is viewed as a way to avoid eventual death. Socially, the information age will continue to grow, allowing patients greater control over their own health care. This, in combination with the advanced directive/advanced life planning movement, may help raise consumer awareness regarding technology and for this we must also be prepared.

✧ TECHNOLOGY ASSESSMENT AS A TOOL

When we look to the future of medical and rehabilitative science, we must consider how the occupational therapy and physical therapy professions will be affected, both from a traditional clinical and an emerging practice perspective. Health technology assessment is a growing need in the United States. As technology advances and the consumer's need for outcome-specific data increases, the field of health technology assessment will likely broaden. Health technology assessment is the careful evaluation of a medical technology for evidence of its safety, efficacy, cost, and cost-effectiveness, and its ethical and legal implications.[10] An important objective of technology assessment is to facilitate positive effects of technology and assist in the development of health care policy and the practical decision-making that is associated with the use of medical technology.[11] Research on technology has generally been focused on biomedical aspects rather than functional application and ethical aspects. Occupational therapy and physical therapy practitioners have much to contribute in this area. Rehabilitation practitioners are skilled in assisting patients and families with goal setting and goals clarification. We can use our skills in activity analysis and functional prognosticating to have meaningful discussions with patients regarding how technology will interplay with their lives, and how it can (or cannot) best match/meet their life goals and role performance. Technology brings with it many consequential moral questions concerning its introduction and application.[11] Occupational therapy and physical therapy practitioners who are well trained in ethical analysis add the life-cycle perspective and are able to provide valuable insights into the use of technology.

There are many social and political barriers to health technology assessment. It has experienced varied attention and prioritization on the national level. The private and public sector responsibilities related to technology assessment fall under many national agencies and institutes (National Institutes of Health, Agency for Health Care Policy Research, Food and Drug Administration); however, priorities are separately coordinated and a broader evaluation of outcomes is difficult to actualize. Despite this fact, consumers demand the services that they have seen or read about, and coverage decisions must be made regarding emerging technologies.

Technology may solve a medical problem, but it takes a rehabilitative practitioner to best apply it to solve a functional problem. Technology is an intervention. To best evaluate this intervention we must look critically at outcomes. Technology outcomes must include not only those related to morbidity, mortality, and client satisfaction, but also outcomes such as occupational performance, role competence, adaptation, health and wellness, and quality of life. These too must be emphasized as a priority in the evaluation and application of emerging technology, both at the clinical and national levels. Occupational therapists and physical therapists must participate in and be strong advocates for this type of technology evalua-

tion. Only then can technology's true effect on health, well-being, and life satisfaction be better known.

✦ CONCLUSION

The field of rehabilitation will continue to change through advances in medical technology, as will the field of medical technology through the expertise of rehabilitation practitioners. Integration of formal ethics training in both the academic and clinical setting is an essential component of clinical and moral reasoning development for rehabilitation practitioners. We must be both ethically sensitive and skilled in the language of ethics. As medicine and technology continue to advance, so too will the social and ethical implications of caring for our patients.

References

1. Fenster JM: Ether Day: The Strange Tale of America's Greatest Medical Discovery and the Haunted Men Who Made it. Harper Perennial Library; 2002.
2. Blackmer J: The unique ethical challenges of conducting research in the rehabilitation medicine population. BMC Med Ethics 4(1):E2, 2003.
3. Callahan D: Living and dying with medical technology. Crit Care Med 31(5):Suppl, 2003.
4. Phurruough SE, Farrell J, Ulrich M, Long K, on behalf of Centers for Medicare and Medicaid Services. CAG 00119N. Coverage Decision Memorandum for Ventricular Assist Devices as Destination Therapy. Available at: http://www.cms.gov/ncdr/memo.
5. Marguart SM, and Sauls J: Survivorship. Living through a life altering event. Crit Care Nurs Clin North Am Sep 13(3), 349–355, 2001.
6. Devettere R: Practical Decision Making in Health Care Ethics—Cases and Concepts. ed 2. Georgetown University Press, Georgetown, 2003.
7. Bach JR, and Barnett V: Ethical considerations in the management of individuals with severe neuromuscular disorders. Am J Phys Med Rehab 74(1):S34–S40, 1995.
8. Bach JR, and Tilton MC: Life satisfaction and well being measures in ventilator assisted individuals with traumatic tetraplegia. Arch Phys Med Rehab 75:626–632, 1994.
9. Quill TE: Initiating end-of-life discussions with seriously ill patients. Addressing the "elephant in the room." JAMA 284(19):2502–2507, 2000.
10. Perry S, and Eliastam M. The national center for health care technology. JAMA 245:2510–2511, 1981.
11. ten Have, H: Medical technology assessment and ethics: Ambivalent relations. Hastings Cent Rep September/October, 1995.

11

Professional Responsibility and Advocacy for Access to Rehabilitation Services: A Case Study in Lymphedema Services in Vermont

LEE NELSON, PT, DPT, MS

A b s t r a c t

Lymphedema is a swelling of soft tissues as a result of an accumulation of protein-rich fluid in the extracellular spaces from disruption of lymphatic transport. In Europe and many other parts of the world, the identification, diagnosis, and treatment of this medical entity is made by physicians and health care professionals well versed in the lymphatic system. In the United States, however, lymphedema is frequently referred to as an "orphan" disorder or "step-child" due to a dearth of medical specialists, and specially trained therapists able to effectively identify and treat it. It is, therefore, frequently underidentified and, at times, neglected or ignored. Individuals who have received treatment for cancer, primarily breast cancer, comprise the largest population of individuals in the United States with lymphedema. People with this condition may experience discomfort or pain, emotional distress, sadness and depression as well as impairments in mobility, strength, and function. The current preferred treatment involves a protocol of education, massage, compression bandaging, and exercise. This chapter addresses ethical issues that arise when the medical sequelae from a chronic condition, such as lymphedema, are not well known or researched and are not well recognized by the medical or health community. In the past few years, as this medical condition has gained better recognition within the health community in the United States, issues with acceptance of this treatment by physicians and insurers alike, given a sparse research base upon which the treatment is predicated, have also arisen. This chapter focuses on the development of education, clinical practice, advocacy, and research initiatives for this underrecognized medical entity. The issues of scarce resources and justice for chronic conditions requiring rehabilitation services are discussed. Issues of professional responsibility for advocating for improved access, contributing evidence for a specific new practice while continually monitoring the results of intervention are also addressed.

For the more commonly known, well-recognized physical impairments, disorders, and disabilities, such as those resulting from stroke, spinal and head injuries, amputations, etc., the rehabilitation process can be lengthy and complex, but usually one for which protocols and plans of care have been identified and agreed upon by members of rehabilitation teams. The process frequently is characterized by periods of progress, regression, and inevitably, plateaus, but rarely is cure the outcome. Thus the primary role of the rehabilitation professional in this process is to assist individuals in regaining functions required to accomplish activities of daily living. Ultimately the goal is to foster a high quality of life through interventions designed to maximize a person's level of physical, psychological, vocational, and social functioning given the limitations imposed by the condition.[1]

The purpose of this chapter is to show serious ethical issues that arise if the patient's quality of life is being seriously compromised by the sequelae of medical or surgical care when those sequelae are chronic conditions not well known, well researched or well recognized by the medical or health community. I will use the case of secondary lymphedema to illustrate the basic ethical problem and describe the experience of the Vermont Lymphedema Network to show how one group of therapists exercised their professional responsibility to become advocates for access to needed care. At the heart of the problem is lack of access to rehabilitation services, a situation shared to some extent by many types of patients requiring rehabilitative services. My hope is that the lessons and themes addressed here will be instructive to faculty and students alike as they consider such basic ethical aspects of rehabilitation practice as beneficence, justice related to access, and the strategies therapists can employ to address ethical issues when they arise.

✦ REHABILITATION AND COST CONCERNS

In the past few decades in the United States, the more traditional focus of the rehabilitation professional's primary role has, at times, collided with cost-containment initiatives. As the costs of attempting to support various dimensions of a person's functioning have escalated, health professionals increasingly have been given a message that this level of support is prohibitive financially. Not surprisingly, ethical questions regarding rehabilitation have been called into play, requiring rehabilitation professionals to examine their moral obligations, not only first and foremost that they have to their patients, but also to society. What is it about the rehabilitation process and the individuals in need of rehabilitation that currently has caused society to become so focused on the costs of rehabilitation? According to Caplan, much of it has to do with societal views of individuals needing rehabilitative care:[2]

Those most often in need of rehabilitative services are those already undervalued by the society. Many are elderly. Some have congenital disabilities. A large proportion are unable to work. In a society that places great value on youth, vigor and industriousness, and manifests an ongoing trust in the power of science and medicine to reverse the effects of disease and disability, there are powerful stigmas and little prestige associated with patients who lack both highly valued characteristics and the capacity for cure.[2]

Caplan highlights that ours continues to be a society that saves and salvages people through the use of advanced technology and other life-saving measures; however, the social supports and financial assistance needed to help them truly carry on with an acceptable "quality of life" oftentimes is missing. Because rehabilitation focuses on this "quality" of individuals' lives, it is often given "the short shrift in the distribution of health care resources."[3] Health professionals, recognizing the scant resources, have to look to new ground for ways to reconcile their role as professionals and their duty of beneficence with their insufficient resources to do what is best for the individual patient. In short, even in cases of "commonly known, well recognized" impairments or disabilities, ethical challenges arise around the rehabilitation process.

✦ REHABILITATION CARE AND LYMPHEDEMA

Lymphedema is a condition of swelling in various body parts sometimes occurring after treatment for cancer. For many years it has been considered to be more of a "cosmesis" than a medical issue. According to the Vodder School definition:[4]

Lymphedema is a swelling of a body part, most often an extremity, resulting from an accumulation of fluids, in such proportions to be palpable and visible. Lymphedema occurs when the lymph vascular system is not able to fill its function of reabsorption and transport of the protein and lymph load. Lymphedema occurs whenever lymphatic vessels are absent, underdeveloped or obstructed. The condition most often causes a feeling of embarrassment and causes decreased mobility, discomfort and often repeated episodes of infection, cellulitis and lymphangitis. This can lead to general depression and a general worsening of the patient's life and health. Fungal infections can be very frequent and these place a greater load on the lymphatics. Severe cases are associated with thickening of the skin, hardening of the limb (fibrosis), leakage of lymph and massive swelling (elephantiasis).[4]

As the above definition describes, much more than the typical "cosmetic problem" is involved. In addition to the swelling, people with this condition may experience discomfort, pain, emotional distress, sadness, and depression as well as recurrent bouts of cellulitis. Cellulitis itself can be an emergent situation, requiring immediate medical care and administration of antibiotics in order to minimize more serious systemic effects. Psycho-social issues involving body image, pain, impairments/disability, and altered vocational capabilities can be overwhelming for many individuals. People survive the cancer diagnosis but then live on to develop this chronic condition of lymphedema, and for many, this becomes a much more difficult, long-term, troublesome challenge. As Benner indicates: "Cure of a disease or medically controlling a chronic illness are not the same as recovery from an illness and regaining a livable embodied relationship to world and others."[5]

The impact that lymphedema can have on a person in terms of cosmetic deformity, risk for infections, discomfort, and potential disability can be profound. In addition, physicians, in pursuit of ruling out the possibility of cancer recurrence, may trivialize these symptoms because they are not of a life and death nature, and add to the person's distress.

✧ LYMPHEDEMA: TYPES AND TREATMENT

There are different types and causes of lymphedema; however, for the purpose of this chapter, I will limit discussion to secondary lymphedema, i.e., where a cause is known. The reasons for this are that (a) the number one cause of lymphedema in developing countries is due to treatment for cancer; and (b) the most frequent type of cancer for which lymphedema is treated in the United States is breast cancer with resulting arm and trunk lymphedema. In order to better understand the ethical issues stemming from attempts at identifying and treating this disorder, some background information about lymphedema may be helpful.

An estimated 266,000 new cases of breast cancer are expected to occur among women in the United States in 2003.[6] In Vermont, that estimate is tagged at 500 new cases, with 100 women dying of the disease. Because there is not a national lymphedema registry, the actual number of individuals living with lymphedema secondary to any type of cancer treatment in the United States overall or the state of Vermont is not specifically known. However, with regard to lymphedema caused by breast cancer treatment (the most studied of all cancers and lymphedema), reports of the incidence of lymphedema vary widely and are dependent on a number of factors, including willingness/access to report, extent of axillary treatment, methods used to define/measure lymphedema, and length and completeness of follow-up. The incidence ranges from 6% to 30%.[7,8] However, physicians and health care professionals involved with breast cancer care generally feel that approximately 15% to 30% of individuals with breast cancer develop lymphedema following treatment. This means that of more than 2 million breast cancer survivors in the United States, there may be approximately 400,000 coping with the swelling, discomfort and, at times, disability resulting from lymphedema.[9]

Given this high number of cases in the United States, why hasn't lymphedema received the recognition in the United States that it has for the past three or four decades in Europe, Asia, and Australia? The answer is not easily found or understood. Little is written by way of research or anecdotally; therefore, much is left to supposition. According to Weissleder, general ignorance and lack of training at the university level is partially the reason, coupled with the fact that lymphedema care is time consuming to both diagnose and treat. He also feels that treatment results in the United States have not been as convincing as in Europe, due to lack of quality training and education of the therapists performing the treatment.[10]

As can be gleaned from the definition of lymphedema, this chronic condition can seriously compromise health status. According to an international consensus document drafted by the International Society of Lymphology, the preferred treatment for lymphedema is called combined physical therapy (CPT), also known as Complete or Complex Decongestive Therapy (CDT) or Complex Decongestive Physiotherapy (CDP).[11] Currently, CDT appears to be the preferred nomenclature. This treatment is gentle, safe, effective, and noninvasive. The treatment consists of: (a) education in skin care and tailored exercises, (b) manual lymph drainage (sometimes referred to as manual lymph massage), and (c) application of multilayered compression bandaging and garments. The first phase is quite intensive and generally lasts from 1 to 4 weeks until the edema reduction and improvement in skin integrity have plateaued. Treatment occurs about 5 times per week. The second, a maintenance phase, involves treatment aimed at maximizing and preserving the gains achieved in phase one. CDT should be performed by skilled therapists who have received advanced education and training in this area. And, although this treatment approach appears more effective than other options in minimizing the effects of lymphedema, the availability of quality treatment centers and qualified, skilled therapists is limited. There are currently 149 programs listed with the National Lymphedema Network as Lymphedema Treatment Centers, although there are only 2 listed as Treatment/Diagnostic Centers and only 1 as a Diagnostic Center. This shows an increase in numbers in the past few years as contrasted with approximately 99 facilities being listed as treatment centers in 1998, and only 1 listed as a diagnostic center, but is still limited.[12] Therefore, even with better methods of identifying and managing lymphedema, access to care may still be problematic.

✧ GEOGRAPHIC DIFFERENCES IN CARE

Lymphedema has been referred to as an "orphan disease" in the United States due to the fact that it has largely been ignored by the medical community.[13] Foldi refers to lymphology, or the study of the lymph system, as the "stepchild of medicine" due to the omission of the requisite knowledge base in medical and postgraduate education in Europe also.[14] So it may be a matter of degree regarding the differences in the detection and treatment of lymphedema in the United States compared with Europe and other continents. The challenge of properly identifying and treating lymphedema appears to be common in many countries. However, this geographical difference historically is considerable and has had a negative impact on people in the United States who have survived cancer but find themselves living with the chronicity of lymphedema.*

Based on the social and medical backdrop, it is easy to see that the standard of care has been quite different among continents. Up until the 1990s in this country, the concept of "therapeutic nihilism"(i.e., no treatment at all) was

---

* It is difficult to trace this difference as little is written about this. However, it is estimated that up until the past 5 to 10 years, there were approximately 15,000 therapists certified to treat lymphedema in Europe whereas the whole of North America had only about 450. In addition, there were medical specialists called lymphologists who could primarily treat this condition or serve as consultants to primary physicians. Women in Austria and Germany were offered care in a "spa" setting where treatment, meals, and residence were offered for the better part of a month until the lymphedema improved and they could resume their home life and activities of daily living. Given the social medicine backdrop of these countries in paying for this extensive type of care, payment was generally not as much of an issue or barrier as it has been most recently in the United States.

prevalent and the most common response to a woman concerned that she might have lymphedema, or that she would like to have it treated, was that she needed to "learn to live with it" or that she "should be thankful to be alive."[9] One woman in Vermont who had endured the severe consequences of lymphedema for nearly 25 years after surviving 2 bouts of breast cancer, with a grossly lymphedematous arm, was finally sent to an orthopedist in New York City at her own urging and insistence, hoping to finally find someone who knew something about lymphedema. She was appalled, dismayed, and angered when the professional recommendation she received was to have her arm amputated because there was no other treatment that could be offered. Imagine this being an acceptable alternative when this woman, had she lived in Europe, would have received intensive conservative treatment with close follow-up, and likely very favorable results.

✧ ONE COMMUNITY'S EFFORT TO ADDRESS THE ETHICAL ISSUES

Assessing what has been described, numerous ethical issues emerge, e.g., issues of professional responsibility, distributive justice, advocacy, access to care for chronic conditions, and concerns around evidence-based medicine. Recognizing the depth of problems surrounding lymphedema identification and management, a group of therapists trained in lymphedema care formed a state-wide network, called the Vermont Lymphedema Network, in 1999. The members work together to address these issues. Our initiatives and activities are described throughout the rest of this chapter.

✧ OVERVIEW OF THE SITUATION

Given the magnitude of what needed to be done, a long-term plan of education, treatment, and research in our state community was charted to raise the consciousness of the various aspects of lymphedema; concurrently, specific initiatives for action also were drawn up. The major problems were:

◆ Insufficient knowledge on the part of physicians, nurses, physical therapists, and occupational therapists about identification and preferred treatment of lymphedema. In addition, there were anecdotal stories of therapists making lymphedema worse by using traditional therapeutic techniques, such as deep tissue massage, vigorous exercise, and compression pumps with excessive pressure. Therapists were not trained in lymphedema care of what *not* to do, nor could they identify lymphedema so that patients could be referred to trained lymphedema therapists for further examination and possible treatment.

◆ Insufficient knowledge on the part of insurers about the medical underpinnings of lymphedema. Patients (many of whom found care through self advocacy and assertiveness, i.e., telling their physicians that they knew care was available and insisting on a referral) presented for treatment only to find out that their insurance company would not recognize lymphedema as a medical entity. A frequent response was that it was something that could be "lived with," and until there was evidence that there was a medical issue as a result of having lymphedema and/or double blind research studies could be produced about treatment effectiveness, that reimbursement for care would not be forthcoming.

◆ Lack of sufficient and quality research on the identification, diagnosis, measurement, and treatment of lymphedema. Much of the literature originated in Europe, some of which is still in untranslated German, and none had a strong research base. There was very little in the way of intervention studies, and the existing ones suffered from lack of uniformity of methods and measurement. There has been and continues to be criticism of the National Lymphedema Network's 18 Steps to Prevention, as none of the recommendations were based in research findings.

✦ Insufficient numbers of qualified, trained health professionals to treat lymphedema in our geographic area. Within a few months of initiating a practice in lymphedema care, 50 to 60 people were on a waiting list, some of whom lived 2 to 3 hours away and were willing to make the daily commute for several weeks just to get care. There was only one other therapist in my community trained in lymphedema care at that time. The scenario is a commonly heard one once the awareness of lymphedema improves in a community.

✧ ISSUES OF PROFESSIONAL RESPONSIBILITY

Having a deeply rooted sense of professional responsibility is essential for every health care professional. But, knowing how to act on it in this situation to effect change and influence policies and practices required a stretch in every direction. The dual identity underlying the definition of professional responsibility, i.e., accountability and responsiveness, was a primary consideration in drawing up a plan to address the challenging situation that presented itself.[15] Central to our mission was how to execute the duties of beneficence, nonmaleficence, and fidelity while developing meaningful ways to advocate for the needs of individuals with lymphedema collectively with the very specific goal of decreasing the barriers to access, quality of care, and payment issues.

As health professionals, my colleagues and I found ourselves in a conundrum in several ways. In thinking through the guiding principles that would offer some structure and support, we placed our focus on professional responsibilities. To whom were we accountable? It was difficult to navigate the physician, insurer, and consumer waters with so little evidence to go on, but we felt that empirically we had sufficient evidence that the treatment was effective and therefore we needed to start somewhere with building our case. Glaser's three realms of ethics, described in Chapter 16, highlights that our problem had personal, organizational, and societal dimensions.[16] Although there were

anecdotal and collective stories about the success of the preferred treatment method of combined decongestive physiotherapy, we lacked a strong body of literature to specifically support this treatment.

How could our personal/professional ethic of care be shaped to move ahead with this initiative? Physical therapists have multiple accountabilities and encounter many difficulties and challenges when attempting to do the right thing for the patient while remaining ever-cognizant of reimbursement interests as well as defending skilled care.[17] The same is true for occupational therapists. Pellegrino talks about the inherent responsibilities of a professional in saying:[18]

To be a professional is to make a promise to help, to keep that promise, and to do so in the best interests of the patient. It is to accept the trust the patient must place in us as a moral imperative, one that the ethos of the marketplace or competition does not expect us in our society to honor. The special nature of the helping and healing professions is rooted in the fact that people become ill and need to trust others to help them restore health.[18]

As Hack describes the use of the word "fiduciary" in the health care arena, we recognized that we did have a fiduciary responsibility, i.e., a responsibility to put patients' trust in my abilities to advocate and do what was prudent for them first.[19]

In 1997 I became certified in a European method of lymphedema care. I was fortunate to be friends and work with a physician who several years previously had been diagnosed with breast cancer and subsequently developed lymphedema a few months later. Her inability to find a health professional in our community actually caused me to undertake studies in lymphedema. Upon finishing my coursework, I decided to start a private practice on a part-time basis specializing in the treatment of individuals with lymphedema. At that time, most insurance companies did not know what it was and therefore, were not willing to reimburse for it. And, because manual lymphatic drainage is sometimes called manual lymph massage, a number of insurance companies declared that they don't pay for "massage," their assumption being that it was done for relaxation purposes and not for therapeutic reasons. Currently there is a CPT code for manual therapy that actually names manual lymphatic drainage as part of a bundled code. However, at the time I started my practice there was no such code, so charging for care became an issue, as it couldn't be done in an accurate, forthright manner.

The issue of how to charge became an exercise in ethics as there was truly no way to legitimately charge for the care I had rendered. I typically ended up receiving prior approval and asking each insurance company how I should bill for services, so as not to appear fraudulent, by using a code that did not match the service. And then, I would document exactly what had happened. In addition, several insurance companies indicated that they might be willing to reimburse for services, but needed evidence from "double blind studies" showing the effectiveness and efficacy of complex decongestive physiotherapy. There were none. The research base for lymphedema is sparse. When we asked if there was compelling evidence for their choice to cover compression pumps, the answer was consistently no, but because it was a long-standing practice, no one chose to challenge it.

But, there were other staggering and important issues that emerged upon attempting to provide care for people with or at risk for lymphedema. One of the biggest hurdles that needed attention had to do with physicians and other health care professionals having any knowledge that treatment for lymphedema was available. Another had to do with their skill level, as well as their willingness to identify and diagnose lymphedema, and subsequently refer appropriately. Although edema/swelling can result for a number of reasons, it seemed that diuretics were prescribed for all swelling without specific knowledge of the etiology. Diuretics typically don't have much effect on lymphedema due to the size of the protein molecules left sitting in the interstitial fluid, and their propensity for drawing in more fluid. But when physicians and/or patients were asked if the diuretics helped and they responded in the negative, they also indicated that it was all that they knew to do for it, so they just kept doing it in light of negative results.

Using the principles elucidated in my profession, I used the APTA Code of Ethics and Guide for Professional Conduct as a springboard for thinking through related actions.[20] Subsequently, I have found several parallel ideas in the AOTA Code of Ethics.[21] In the actual situation I referred solely to the APTA documents; the reader will be introduced to the various principles in the order that I used them. In several key areas I have added items from the occupational therapy documents to show their similarities. The following bear particular relevance to the situation at hand:

APTA Principle 2.1 A—Patient/Physical Therapist Relationship:[20]

... Patient/clients often come to the physical therapist in a vulnerable state and normally will rely on the physical therapist's advice, which they perceive to be based on superior knowledge, skill and experience. The trustworthy physical therapist acts to ameliorate the patient's/client's vulnerability, not exploit it.

These patients were all extremely vulnerable. And, although I had a sound experience in general physical therapy, in the beginning, I did not have depth in the treatment of lymphedema. Beyond that, the "superior knowledge" was based on advanced training in this area and the well-founded hope that treatment would be effective; but, this was not based on extensive research and this proved to be an uncomfortable spot to be in.

APTA Principle 3.2—Just Laws and Regulations:[20]

A physical therapist shall advocate the adoption of laws, regulations and policies by providers, employers, third-party payers, legislatures, and regulatory agencies to provide and improve access to necessary health care services for all individuals.

Principle 3.3—Unjust Laws and Regulations:[20]

A physical therapist shall endeavor to change unjust laws, regulations, and policies that govern the practice of physical therapy.

Principle 1 of the AOTA Code of Ethics also addresses this:[21]

Occupational therapy personnel shall demonstrate a concern for the well-being of the recipients of their services (beneficence).

Principle 1C of this same code specifically identifies advocacy as a role of occupational therapy personnel:[21]

Occupational therapy personnel shall make every effort to advocate for recipients to obtain needed services through available means.

With levels of awareness and knowledge about lymphedema low among medical and health professionals, it was very difficult to advocate for improved management of it. However, given that lymphedema services were only being reimbursed by a few insurers in the state of Vermont, we knew we had to initiate something. We devised a blueprint for educating and lobbying the major insurers of the state. We set and carried out well-constructed agendas for meetings with medical directors and case managers over 1or 2 years through presentations of case studies, research studies, and anecdotal results. These attempts initially were met with across the board denials, but eventually evolved into invitations to submit requests for prior authorization, and reviews by medical reviewers/case managers. We saw the door begin to open to a professional dialogue that would initially influence and eventually change the reimbursement for this chronic condition. In my opinion, the cornerstone of this change had to do with promoting the acceptance that treatment for lymphedema fell into the therapeutic category and was medically necessary due to the high risk of developing cellulitis. Providing a cost analysis of treatment versus multiday intravenous or oral antibiotics was helpful in viewing combined decongestive physiotherapy in a different light.

APTA Principle 7—A physical therapist shall seek only such remuneration as is deserved and reasonable for physical therapy services:[20]

7.1.C A physical therapist shall recognize that third-party payer contracts may limit, in one form or another, the provision of physical therapy services. Third-party limitations do not absolve the physical therapist from making sound professional judgments that are in the patient's best interest. A physical therapist shall avoid underutilization of physical therapy services.

This principle resonated strongly for the entire network of practitioners dealing with this issue on a daily basis. The final area for consideration of professional responsibility is found in Principle 10—A physical therapist shall endeavor to address the health needs of society:[20]

10.1 A physical therapist shall render pro bono publico (reduced or no fee) services to patients lacking the ability to pay for services, as each physical therapist's practice permits.

Given that Vermont Blue Cross/Blue Shield was the first insurer, except for Medicare, to begin reimbursing for lymphedema services (and this didn't fully occur until November 1998), therapists providing care prior to that were essentially offering some care on a pro bono basis if they were accurate/honest in submitting charges based on services rendered. It was quite difficult to examine a patient and professionally know that she or he could benefit from treatment, and not go ahead and provide the needed services due to the patient's lack of resources. We wrote and were successful in obtaining grants (primarily from the Susan Komen Foundation) that provided partial funding for women who were uninsured or underinsured to obtain the necessary treatment and related supplies or garments that were needed.

APTA Principle 10.2 regarding community health:[20]

A physical therapist shall endeavor to support activities that benefit the health status of the community.

In the broader context of contemplating responsibility to society and in relationship to principles 10.1 and 10.2, the issue of cost-effectiveness weighed heavily. When looking at all the health care needs of our society, how should we go about determining if this one condition, i.e., lymphedema, is more or less worthy to be reimbursed than another? What evidence is there for effective treatment? If our national health policy was one of rationing care, where would lymphedema fall? ... near the bottom or top of the list? The moral and ethical justice issues were paramount. Although I had enough experience to know that treatment truly helped. ... did it help enough? Did the beneficial effects last long enough? Would something else help more? I had a sense that focusing in on any one patient, individually, would not yield the results of affecting care for the subpopulation of people with lymphedema and might be perceived as focusing on a much narrower professional interest. Physical and occupational therapy were playing a critical role in advocating to society via the health insurance industry to "care" for and about one small—but not insignificant—clinical entity. We were also asking the medical and other health professions community to trust that the direction we were plotting was not only a good one, but also an efficacious and cost-effective one. As Purtilo stated, a sense of strong professional self-identity in providing services that would meet the health care need, coupled with strategies aimed at going beyond the individual patient and surveying the societal landscape to provide responsible care for a larger population was what was needed.[22] With this in mind, multiple initiatives were begun.

Before describing these initiatives, however, the other critical issues demanding attention and analysis that wove their way throughout this scenario along with professional responsibility were justice and access to health care services, the role of a health professional in advocacy for a cause, as well as the research base for practice

✧ DISTRIBUTIVE JUSTICE/ ACCESS TO CARE

In reviewing the roots of justice in access to health care, several documents bear mentioning for a comprehensive understanding of the issue. Of particular note in the 20th century was the United Nations Universal Declaration of Human Rights, issued in 1948, 3 years after the founding of the United Nations.[23] Article 25 of this declaration states that:

Everyone has the right to a standard of living adequate for the health and well-being of himself and of his family, including food, clothing, housing and medical care and necessary social services, and the right to security in the event of unemployment, sickness, disability, widowhood, old age or other lack of livelihood in circumstances beyond his control.

It is interesting to note that not just sickness or disease was addressed in this declaration; it also included the word "disability" implying sequelae from illness or sickness that could progress to disability. And, of great import was use of the word "right." Shortly thereafter, in 1952, in the United States, the President's Commission on Health Needs of the Nation supported the intent of the U.N. Declaration by declaring that access to health care is a "basic human right."[24] Twenty years later, the President's Commission for the Study of Ethical Problems in Medicine and Biomedical Research issued a statement that did not include health care as a right, but indicated "society has an ethical obligation to ensure equitable access to health care for all."[25] It declined to declare health care as a right and favored the social responsibility language.

And today, this ambivalence between health care as a right versus as an ethical obligation or moral responsibility remains within our society. Some attribute possible reasons for this philosophical shift to the rising health care costs coupled with technological advances that have occurred in the past 30 years.[26] Some find that as costs have spiraled there has been an intertwining of economic and ethical problems, with each needing careful thought and analysis prior to forming health policy. The economic problems have to do with controlling costs while distributing resources, whereas the ethical problem involves the fair distribution of resources while providing equitable access to health care.[27] The United States is one of the few industrialized democracies that has not recognized health care as a basic human right. This decision is against a backdrop of 43.6 million people in the United States, 15.2% of the total population, lacking health care insurance, and an additional 17% who are underinsured.[28] Nearly 15% of our gross national product is spent on health care compared to much lower percentages for many other countries and yet our access levels and our proportions are still not sufficient. When considering the relationship between access to health care and insurance coverage, the data show that the lack of access is associated with both poorer health outcomes as well as underutilization of services.[29]

With specific regard to lymphedema and breast cancer, it appears that the constellation of underrecognition of this condition by physicians combined with the use of the word "massage" in the treatment, as well as a legacy of lack of treatment options being explored in this country, left a void in the ability of individuals to request a reasonable treatment option. As this persisted decade after decade, language identifying lymphedema as a possible sequela of cancer treatment was either not included in manuals used by insurance companies to determine appropriate services, or it was not seen as "medically necessary." The issue remained silent therefore, and it took a great deal of momentum to start moving it along. A question remains about what might have happened without the possibility of cellulitis posing a health status threat, and leaving cosmesis as the primary issue. Would this progressive, chronic, potentially disfiguring condition be viewed as unworthy of treatment if there were less severe "medical" sequelae?

✧ ADVOCACY TO PROMOTE ACCESS

Advocacy efforts to promote access to treatment for lymphedema focused primarily on education and awareness, and targeted medical and health professionals, those in the insurance industry, and individuals with lymphedema or at risk for lymphedema. Advocacy has numerous definitions; however, the one most fitting for this case emphasizes giving a voice to a specific issue. In this case, there were numerous people (mostly women with breast cancer and who suspected they had lymphedema) who had communicated with physicians and insurers alike regarding the need for better identification and management of lymphedema. However, I feel one of the major factors ensuring I would be listened to was that a physician (friend and colleague) was affected with this disorder and, after hearing her compelling story, it was difficult for other parties not to act. There were a number of other initiatives where health professionals linked arms with women with breast cancer and lymphedema, presenting to medical directors of insurance companies or joining efforts in the physical demonstration of what treatment actually consisted of and looked like.

The advocacy required to raise the level of consciousness and education about lymphedema needed to be multifaceted and broad-based. There was some discussion about whether blame should be cast between the radiation oncologists and breast surgeons for "causing" lymphedema. Although several physicians did not find this to be the case, advocacy efforts toward developing a better knowledge base of the treatment needed to be undertaken.[10,30] Information about the natural progression of the disorder was not well understood and needed to be communicated with physicians, nurses, insurers, and those at risk for or affected by lymphedema. The notion of being upfront and sharing both what was known and what was not known about lymphedema was particularly important in gaining credibility and respect. In addition, once research efforts were begun in the community, patient advocates were consulted about the direction and methods of research. As noted in a National Lymphedema Network newsletter:[31]

Advocates participate in dialogues addressing the formation of research study ideas to keep scientists focused on studies that will result in improvements in treatment or that will address health concerns often overlooked and misunderstood—like lymphedema. Current issues in research make patient representative involvement very important. With strict limitations in available resources, it is no longer acceptable to do research only for the sake of science. Advocates provide a human focus and defend the human perspective when they are incorporated into scientific dialogue."[31]

✧ ETHICS AND EVIDENCE-BASED PRACTICE

As mentioned earlier, the research base for the measurement and treatment of lymphedema is not extensive; therefore, the ability to use compelling evidence in important clinical decision making and ethical arguments was, and continues to be, difficult. Evidence-based practice is defined as "integrating individual clinical expertise" with the "conscientious, explicit and judicious use of current best evidence in making decisions about the care of individual patients."[32]

The APTA Guide for Professional Conduct and Code of Ethics supports this through Principle 6:[20]

A physical therapist shall maintain and promote high standards for physical therapy practice, education and research.

The AOTA Code also addresses this in Principle 4:[21]

Occupational therapy personnel shall achieve and continually maintain high standards of competence (duties).

From an ethical perspective, evidence-based practice allows for more informed decisions by physicians, health care professionals and patients alike, as well as promoting the utilization of the best practices in health care.[33] In the 1980s, Caplan cautioned rehabilitation professionals of the paradox in advocating for improved access and funding for rehabilitation services, while at the same time doing little to seek this funding or become engaged in efforts that would accurately assess levels of need as well as demonstrate that the techniques and practices of rehabilitation are efficacious.[2] As Purtilo advocates, use of aggregate and evidence-based data, combined with individual stories and cases, can make convincing and compelling arguments to society about the value of physical therapy service that is being rendered.[22]

As Holm discusses, the strength of our evidence provides the level of confidence we find ourselves having in our clinical decisions.[34] In 1998, using Sackett's levels of evidence, Megens and Harris analyzed the research literature for the effectiveness of physical therapy in the management of lymphedema following treatment for breast cancer.[35] Sackett's 5 hierarchical levels of evidence were used with level 1 having the highest power and generally consisting of large randomized controlled trials, and descending to level 5 being generally descriptive and comprising case series without controls.[32] Based on 13 studies that were assessed, the following was found: 1 study was evaluated at level 2; 5 studies at level 3; and the remaining 7 studies were evaluated at level 5. Several therapeutic recommendations were issued based on these results; however, caution was urged when following

them, as it was felt that none of them were supported by strong definitive studies. The overall recommendation made was that more vigorous research is needed.

Lack of level 1 and 2 studies can make decision making difficult and render a health professional with less confidence than one would enjoy. Gray suggests:[36] "… the absence of excellent evidence does not make evidence-based decision making impossible; in this situation what is required is the best evidence available, not the best evidence possible." And that appears to be the current state of affairs, until the research base, particularly level 1 and 2 studies grows in the field of lymphedema. Perhaps the most frequently criticized area of lymphedema education and prevention has to do with the 18 steps to prevention put forth by the National Lymphedema Network.[12] The prevention and control measures are suggestions, collected primarily anecdotally by lymphologists, patients, and lymphedema therapists. Many of the measures focus on such things as knowledge of various triggers of lymphedema as well as protection of the skin, and use of the limb for activity. Currently researchers are hoping to provide an evidence base to most if not all of these measures; however, that endeavor is in progress and not complete at this time. The concern and danger, therefore, is that individuals who may be at risk for lymphedema may not practice these precautions and resume their regular lifestyle, because the precautions are not evidence-based.

Several lymphedema physician experts have publicly countered this type of thinking. Dr. Horst Weissleder feels that "the biggest problem we have is based on ethical practice. It is nearly impossible to perform evidence-based scientific studies (which are essential for reimbursement) comparing the effectiveness of different treatment methods."[10] His reason for this belief is due to the fact that effective treatment would possibly need to be withheld. Dr. Michael Foldi, medical director of the Foldi Lymphedema Clinic in Germany, states that:[37] "I must declare that I regard medicine as a natural science and that I agree with this principle (i.e. evidence-based medicine). Nevertheless, there are cases in which 'anecdotal observations' are in harmony with scientific facts and established knowledge, are looking for evidence by prospective, random clinical studies but are prohibited by ethical considerations."[37]

Petrek describes the underpinnings of the 18 steps as being based on "intuitive reasoning."[9] She cautions that we need to use individual patient factors as well as treatment factors as the determinants of preventative strategies as each person's anatomy varies greatly. She also raises the issue that disseminating information about precautions may be "counterproductive" as overprotection for some may lead to underuse and weakness.

In returning to Sackett's five levels of evidence, with much of lymphedema evidence being at levels 4 and 5, there is a body of knowledge residing within experts and standards of practice. Holm argues that this "evidence within the practitioner" is accepted within level 5 and that "when we use opinion-based evidence, we are grounding our clinical reasoning and therapeutic decisions and actions in the advice of experts, established practices, continuing education information, or reference texts by known leaders in the field."[34]

✦ ACTION INITIATIVES

Given all of these challenges and unknowns, we envisioned a long-term campaign to raise awareness and knowledge about lymphedema for providers and patients, as well as begin to create an avenue for research and changes in health care policy. We specifically targeted it to nurses, primary care physicians, oncologists, breast surgeons, radiation oncologists, general internists as well as physical, occupational, and radiation therapists, insurers, and patients. From 1997 through 2002 three specific initiatives were launched in an effort to achieve our goals.

Educational Efforts:

✦ We made educational presentations at grand rounds, medical office meetings, support groups, informal lunch meetings, etc. Small grants were obtained for teleconferencing with leading experts in lymphedema with broadcasts to the more remote, rural health care facilities and

consumer groups; we wrote and published several articles in hospital weeklies as well as local community newspapers. We conducted radio interviews at different times of day to improve listener access. What has now become a yearly breast cancer conference was established with educational offerings on lymphedema. As experience, skill, and research developed, presentations at national and international conferences also have been made. A full-day course for nonlymphedema therapists (physical, occupational, and radiation) as well as nurses and physicians who see individuals with cancer and possibly lymphedema has been developed and delivered. (The primary goal in developing this course, as mentioned earlier, was to provide the fundamental knowledge about lymphedema so that appropriate referrals could be made, but as importantly, so that harm from traditional therapapeutic treatment would not be rendered.) We opened a lymphedema clinic (currently it is held at the medical center 1 day each week, filled to full capacity). In a word, we undertook an all-out attempt to have people recognize what lymphedema is and that there is treatment for it.

Advocacy Efforts:

✦ As mentioned previously, we held meetings with medical directors and case managers of insurance companies; at times, in concert with individuals with lymphedema, so that case results could be shared or demonstration of care provided. These meetings were front-loaded with pertinent professional and research articles forwarded to the respective office for review prior to the meeting. We engaged in an honest sharing of the evidence for practice as well as what is not known, with an openness and willingness to participate in research studies as well as collaborate with the insurers to arrive at the most efficient and effective modes of documentation, communication, etc.

✦ We launched efforts with state legislators regarding lack of Medicare payment for compression garments.

✦ We made efforts to encourage timely referrals to certified therapists for people with lymphedema as well as for those at particularly high risk for lymphedema, so that appropriate examinations and follow-up could be offered. This involved responding to querying phone calls from nurse practitioners, physician assistants, physicians as well as from physical and occupational therapists who were not trained in lymphedema care. We helped them problem-solve whether a referral was needed or not.

Research/Practice Efforts:

✦ In 1999, after the level of consciousness and knowledge about lymphedema had started to rise, a new problem arose. With physicians and other health care professionals better able to identify and diagnose lymphedema, more people with lymphedema or at risk for it were being referred to the few lymphedema therapists in the state. In an effort to help remedy this problem, we obtained a grant and a lymphedema educational course offered at the university was developed for the purpose of training physical and occupational therapists and nurses. As a result of this course, 24 health care professionals became certified in lymphedema care. These people were selected not only for their interest, but as importantly for their geographic location within the state, the goal being that any patient would not have to travel more than 1 hour for care.

✦ Since 1997, we have received several research grants to begin inquiry about the incidence, educational needs, rehabilitation sequelae, and use of complementary/alternative medicines by women with both breast cancer and lymphedema. These grants have totaled approximately $65,000 and the hope is that we will gain more information from these preliminary investigations that will serve as a springboard to obtain further funding for more in-depth studies. Four articles have been published in professional journals as a result of these initial investigations. As well during this time, we have received grants for educational teleconferences and to assist women who are uninsured or underinsured for accessing. These grants have totaled nearly $80,000.

✦ SUMMARY

In summary, much work still needs to be done in order to optimally meet the medical, psycho-social, and rehabilitation needs of individuals with lymphedema. It is a somewhat rare occurrence that a group of therapists would encounter the depth and breadth of ethical, social, economic, and medical issues surrounding a somewhat obscure medical condition. It has been challenging, rewarding, and energizing to mark small measures of progress in this endeavor, while acknowledging that there is much more work to be done. As initially indicated, however, in today's health care climate there are people with even more common conditions in need of rehabilitation services who are "at risk" for necessary, adequate, and effective care. In order for the principles of justice, beneficence, and access to be served for all individuals seeking rehabilitation services, a collective, professional sense of will, determination, and action needs to be mobilized. Perhaps a new characteristic should be added to the list of professional responsibilities, that of moral tenacity, for it takes a keen focus, strong footing, an alliance of talented and convicted colleagues, and an unwavering commitment to move along a path of influencing health policy and practice.

References

1. Purtilo R: Managed care: Ethical issues for the rehabilitation professions. Trends Health Care Law Ethics. Winter/Spring10(1–2):105–118, 1995.
2. Caplan AL, Callahan D, and Haas J: Ethical and policy issues. In Rehabilitation Medicine, Hastings Center Report Special Supplement 7(4):S1–S20, 1987. Copyright 1987 The Hastings Center. Reprinted by permission. This article originally appeared in the Hastings Center Report. vol 17, no.4, p 3.
3. Martone M: Decision making issues in the rehabilitation process. Hastings Cent Rep 31(2):41, 2001.

4. VAVALT, Vodder School: Lymphedema: Information for Physicians and Patients. Educational Pamphlet. 1995.

5. Benner P: The phenomenon of care. In Toombs SK (ed): Handbook of Phenomenology and Medicine. Kluwer Academic Publishers, Boston, 2001, 351–369.

6. Centers for Disease Control. Cancer Facts and Figures. Available at: http://www.cdc.gov/cancer, 2003.

7. Ball AWR, Fish S, and Thomas JM: Radical axillary dissection in the staging and treatment of breast cancer. Ann R Coll Surg Engl 74(2):126–129, 1992.

8. Paci E, et al: Long-term sequelae of breast cancer surgery. Tumori 82:321–324, 1996.

9. Petrek J, Pressman P, and Smith R: Lymphedema: Current issues in research and management. CA Cancer J Clin 50(5):292–307, 2000.

10. Weissleder H: Personal e-mail communication. 2003.

11. International Society of Lymphology: The diagnosis and treatment of peripheral lymphedema: Consensus document of the International Society of Lymphology. Lymphology 36:84–91, 2003.

12. National Lymphedema Network Web Site. Prevention information. Treatment/Diagnostic Centers. Available at: http://www.lymphnet.org. Accessed December 10, 2003.

13. Reynolds J: Lymphedema: "An orphan" disease. PT Magazine June:54–63, 1996.

14. Foldi M, and Foldi E: Lymphoedema: Methods of Treatment and Control; A Guide for Patients and Therapists. Gustav Fischer Verlag, New York, 1991.

15. Purtilo R: Professional responsibility in physiotherapy: Old dimensions and new directions. Physiotherapy 72(12):579–583, 1986.

16. Glaser JW: Three realms of ethics: An integrating map of ethics for the future. In Purtilo R, Jensen GM, Royeen CB (eds): Educating for Moral Action: A Sourcebook in Health and Rehabilitation Ethics. FA Davis Co, Philadelphia, 2005.

17. Romanella M, and Knight-Abowitz K. The "Ethic of Care" in physical therapy practice and education: Challenges and opportunities. J Phys Ther Educ 14(3):20–25, 2000.

18. Pellegrino ED: What is a profession? J Allied Health August:168–176, 1983.

19. Hack LM: 2001 Polly Cerasoli Lecture: The Virtuous Spirit. J Phys Ther Educ 15(3):3–8, 2001.

20. American Physical Therapy Association: APTA Code of Ethics and Guide for Professional Conduct. Available at: http://www.apta.org/PT_Practice/

21. American Occupational Therapy Association: AOTA Code of Ethics. Available at: http://www.aota.org/general/coe/asp. Accessed Decemer 10, 2003.

22. Purtilo RB: A time to harvest, a time to sow: Ethics for a shifting landscape. Phys Ther 80(11):1112–1119, 2000.

23. United Nations General Assembly: Universal Declaration of Human Rights. 1948.

24. President's Commission on Health Needs of the Nation. 1953.

25. President's Commission for the Study of Ethical Problems in Medicine and Biomedical Research. 1983.

26. Dowling P: Access to medical care: Do physicians and academic medical centers have a societal responsibility? In Dula A, Goering S (eds): The Ethics of Healthcare for African Americans. Praeger Press, Westport, CT, 1994, pp 124–144.

27. Beauchamp T: Justice in access to health care. In Beauchamp T, and Walters L (eds): Contemporary Issues in Bioethics. ed 6. Thomson Wadsworth, Belmont, CA, 2003.

28. U.S. Census Bureau Web Site: U.S. Department of Commerce. Available at: http://www.census.gov.prod/www/abs/popula.html. Accessed December 14, 2003.

29. Gostin L: Securing health or just health care: The effect of the health care system on the health of America. St. Louis Univ Law J 1:7–43, 1994.

30. Harlow S: Personal e-mail communication regarding lymphedema. 2003.

31. Railey E: Lymphedema Advocacy: Who's speaking for you? Lymph Link-National Lymphedema Network 14:1–2, 2002.

32. Sackett D, et al: Evidence-based medicine: What it is and what it isn't. Br Med J 312:71–72, 1996.

33. Kerridge I, Lowe M, and Henry D: Ethics and evidence based medicine. Br Med J 316:1151–1163, 1998.

34. Holm MB: 2000 Eleanor Clarke Slagle Lecture. Our mandate for the new millennium: Evidence-based practice. Am J Occup Ther 54:575–585, 2000.

35. Megens A, and Harris S: Physical therapist management of lymphedema following treatment for breast cancer: A critical review of its effectiveness. Phys Ther 78(12):1302–1311, 1998.

36. Gray J: Evidence-Based Healthcare: How to Make Health Policy and Management Decisions. Churchill Livingstone Inc, New York, 1997.

37. Foldi M: Are there enigmas concerning the pathophysiology of lymphedema after breast cancer treatment? Nat Lymphedema Newsletter 10:1–4, 1998.

12

Disparity in Practice: Healing the Breach

Laurita M. Hack, phd, mba, pt, fapta

A b s t r a c t

In this chapter, I offer the hypothesis that it is the institutional imperative (the ethical choices made in the institutional realm) that leads to the reflexive behavior we so often see in clinicians and to the disconnect we see between espoused ethical beliefs and actual behavior. I also present concepts of profession as a special form of occupation, on work done to define best or expert practice in these fields, and on the work being done in the occupational and physical therapy areas to more clearly define practice. I conclude with the organizational changes that I recommend as well as some recommendations for possible research on these issues.

✧ INTRODUCTION

As I have talked with students and colleagues about ethical practice and moral behavior I have been struck by several disparities. One is the disparity between being *reflective* and being *reflexive*. By reflective, I mean exercising thought or judgment.[1] Certainly, philosophers and ethicists across the ages have offered examples of reflective thought about the translation of moral standards into ethical behavior, as is well documented in Gabard and Martin's chapter on good judgment and moral reasoning.[2] Yet, the behavior of many practicing clinicians seems almost purely reflexive, by which I mean reacting in response to the pressure of the moment.[1] The popular press is replete with examples of the behavior of people from all walks of life acting in ways that upon reflection they might have identified as unethical. But in the absence of that reflection these human beings make poor choices. Of even more concern are the lists of health care providers who are sanctioned by their licensing boards. Almost all of these sanctions are in response to behavior that could easily be described as unethical.[3] The presence of such behavior in the clinical practices of occupational and physical therapy is widely discussed, if not carefully documented.

A second disparity is the seeming reversal of attitudes and values shown by students once they become practicing clinicians. Based on personal experience and conversation with other people teaching in this area, I offer the following observations. They are not intended to characterize the behavior of all students and clinicians in occupational and physical therapy, but this description does seem to resonate with others as occurring all too often. In the classroom, most students seem open and receptive to discussions about ethics and seem able to make judgments about the ethical implications of various clinical behaviors, as demonstrated by their classroom conversations, and their written work, such as case analyses. Yet these same students when placed in actual clinical situations do not always act in a manner consistent with their stated views in the classroom. And when faced with the choice between what they learn about hypothetical ethical behavior from classroom faculty and what they see as typical clinical behavior from their clinical instructors, they often opt for the real world behavior, even when it flies in the face of the ethical values they espouse in the abstract.

A third disparity is the short shrift we give to the impact the organization has on the performance of occupational and physical therapists. Glaser has discussed the three realms of ethics, especially as applied to health care.[4,5] He describes these as the realm of the individual, the realm of the institution, and the realm of society. He goes on to describe the interconnection among these three realms. Each exists in relationship to the other, and actions within each realm must be understood to fully comprehend an ethical situation, especially in the area of health care. An individual's actions are colored by the decisions made at the institutional level, which are in turn colored by the decisions made at the societal environment. Certainly, individual actions also affect institutional actions and institutional actions affect societal actions. This model makes clear that we need to understand the impact each realm has on the other.

There is a sturdy body of literature with descriptive, normative, and prescriptive commentary on the individual's ethical responsibilities in clinical practice.[6–10] There is also a similar body of literature on the perceived problems in America's health care system related to distributive justice, access, accountability, and similar issues.[11–13] There is a growing body of literature that examines the impact of institutional change on physical therapy practice. Although there is reference in this literature to therapists' sense of loss of control, ethical considerations are not fully developed.[14–18]

Yet, it is this institutional realm that may best explain the first two disparities that I have identified. It is the institution that sets the day-to-day norms for behavior by individual clinicians. Certainly, the institution and the individual act within the context of society's choices related to the structure and function of the health care system. And certainly, the individual brings a personal ethic that is brought to bear on the clinical care choices he or she makes. But it is the institutional imperative that most strongly shapes the options available to each clinician. For example, it is most often institution policies and actions that decide which patients (Please substitute the word client here, if that better represents the person to whom you provide services.) will be sought out, how many of these patients should receive care in any given time period, where that care will be given, which people are available to assist in that care, the relationships among various caregivers, and when the patients will no longer be available for care.[19]

I believe these areas of disparity are directly related to each other. I offer the hypothesis that it is the institutional imperative (the ethical choices made in the institutional realm) that leads to the reflexive behavior we so often see in clinicians and to the disconnect we see between espoused ethical beliefs and actual behavior. To fully test my hypothesis would require organizational change and well-designed evaluation research to measure the effect of that organizational change.

The remaining portion of this chapter will present concepts of profession as a special form of occupation, on work done to define best or expert practice in these fields, and on the work being done in the occupational and physical therapy areas to more clearly define practice. I will conclude with the organizational changes that I recommend and some recommendations for possible research on these issues.

The Profession as a Special Form of Occupation

The concept of profession has it roots several centuries ago, but became a defined sociological construct in the early 20th century. The early work focused on the definition of profession as a particular type of occupation, identifying the hallmarks of such occupations and using the prototypical occupations of medicine, law, and divinity as the particulars from which the general was drawn.[20,21] That work evolved into the concept that the profession was an ideal state, not necessarily achieved by any occupation universally, and then many occupations could be said to be in some state of professionalization.[22] Later, the entire concept of profession and professionalization came under criticism from many corners. Marxist-based sociologists saw the concept as only furthering unnecessary and harmful class distinctions. Feminist scholars saw the entire concept as both paternal in the relationships it lead to between the member of the profession and the intended client, and not supportive of the career paths chosen by women.[23]

It is useful to return to the original distinctions made between occupations in general and professions in particular, however, to understand the special ethical or moral obligations that occupational and physical therapists, as do all health care professionals, have to their patients. There are two major characteristics of a profession: the use of a complex advanced body of knowledge to provide service to clients or patients in a fiduciary relationship. Although it is true that to be an ethical clinician, one must demonstrate mastery of the body of knowledge, it is the latter characteristic, service in a fiduciary relationship that is the focus of my discussion. In popular use, the term fiduciary has come to be associated with those professionals who provide money management as a service, but it is important to reclaim this term as descriptive, even prescriptive, of the ethical standard for our relationships with our patients.

The term fiduciary comes from the Latin to mean confidence or trust. As a noun, fiduciary is defined as, "One who occupies a position of such power and confidence with regard to property of another that the law requires him or her to act solely in the interest of the person whom he or she represents."[24] By substituting the word "health" for "property," the applicability to ethical matters becomes apparent. If we are perceived by society as a fiduciary, which is what occurs when society accords us the rights and responsibilities of being members of a profession, then we must place our patients' trust in us as our first obligation, as the thing we must most carefully earn and preserve. We must recognize that what we hold in trust for and with our patients is a very precious commodity indeed, their health. We must also recognize that this is a very personal relationship between the individual therapist and the individual patient. It is not a relationship that allows other parties to interfere in it. We also cannot allow other professional and personal goals to interfere. The responsibility is to "act solely" in the best interests of the patient. If we make any other choice, then we have violated the personal trust relationship and have thus lost the right to expect that the public, collectively, will continue to accord us the opportunity to be regarded with trust and respect.

Lessons Learned from the Experts

In work done to identify and describe expert practice in physical therapy, Jensen and colleagues have offered a model of expert practice that states that experts have an integrated philosophy of practice that arises out of mastery in and integration of four domains: knowledge, clinical reasoning, movement, and virtue.[25] These clinicians demonstrated a passion for seeking knowledge rooted in their actual practice, a complex clinical reasoning process that took into account the full range of factors necessary for good clinical decision making, an exquisite sense of the movement of their own bodies and their patients' bodies, and moral standards that were demonstrated through acts of moral courage.

Similarly, Mattingly and Fleming have described the clinical reasoning processes of occupational therapists.[26] They describe the clinical reasoning process of occupational therapists as having a dual focus: at times focusing on a biomedical orientation toward disease (the body as machine) and at other times having an anthropological-type concern with the patient's illness experience (the lived body). The occupational therapists studied spoke often of the tension between these two perspectives, as well as the opportunities to blend them. They displayed a commitment to working with their clients to allow them "to transcend the physical limits that they thought would now govern their lives."

Other health professions have sought to determine what experts think about the ethical standards that should be considered the norm for the particular profession. For example, Shelton defines thoughtfulness, fair mindedness, respect of differences, and commitment to professional values as the four virtues all physicians should possess when they leave medical school.[27] Tan, building on work done by the American Board of Internal Medicine, identified a list of eight virtues that physicians should display: altruism, accountability, excellence, duty, service, honor, integrity, and respect for others.[28] The American Board of Internal Medicine has gone so far as to say that this is what they would expect from their members.

Standards from the Professions

The professional associations in both occupational therapy (American Occupational Therapy Association, AOTA) and physical therapy (American Physical Therapy Association, APTA) have developed documents that describe the behavior expected of their members and that also serve as a guide for behavior among all practitioners of the professions. These documents include standards of practice, codes of ethics, guides for ethical conduct, accreditation criteria, and other policies and positions adopted by their governing bodies.[29,30]

In physical therapy there has recently been an effort to define the professional standards that would be expected of members of a doctoring profession. The American Physical Therapy Association brought together a group of 18 experts for a Consensus Conference on Professionalism in Physical Therapy. The outcomes of the conference were the development of a document on professionalism and its implications for professional education and practice that identified the core values of the profession. The seven core values that were identified are accountability, altruism, compassion/caring, excellence, integrity, professional duty, and social responsibility. For each core value listed, the model explicates these values by providing a core value definition and indicators that describe what the physical therapist would be doing in practice, education, and/or research if these core values were present.[31]

This conference was set in the context of Vision 2020, adopted by the APTA House of Delegates in 2000. The vision statement is:

Physical therapy, by 2020, will be provided by physical therapists who are doctors of physical therapy and who may be board-certified specialists … Consumers will have direct access to physical therapists in all environments for patient/client management, prevention, and wellness services. Physical therapists will be practitioners of choice in clients' health networks and will hold all privileges of autonomous practice. Physical therapists may be assisted by physical therapist assistants who are educated and licensed to provide physical therapist-directed and -supervised components of interventions. Guided by integrity, life-long learning, and a commitment to comprehensive and accessible health programs for all people, PTs and PTAs will render evidence-based service throughout the continuum of care and improve quality of life for society. They will provide culturally sensitive care distinguished by trust, respect, and an appreciation for individual differences. While fully availing themselves of new technologies, as well as basic and clinical research, physical therapists will continue to provide direct patient/client care. They will maintain active responsibility for the growth of the physical therapy profession and the health of the people it serves.[32]

These documents all demonstrate the emphasis in the professional organizations on describing the normative behavior by the professions and expected of all practitioners.

Describing the Breach

A breach is defined as a gap that results when something or somebody leaves and as a failure to obey, keep, or preserve something, for example a law, a trust, or a promise.[33] I submit that the actual behavior seen among some clinicians some of the time represents both parts of this definition. Something happens as students and new graduates gain experience, which causes them to leave behind the ethical principles they espoused as students, and therefore to violate the fiduciary trust that patients have a right to expect from them. A breach has, indeed, occurred.

One source of documentation for the exis-

Table 12.1 ✧ **Core Values at-a-Glance**		
CORE VALUES	DEFINITION	SAMPLE INDICATORS*
Accountability	Accountability is active acceptance of the responsibility for the diverse roles, obligations, and actions of the physical therapist including self-regulation and other behaviors that positively influence patient/client outcomes, the profession, and the health needs of society.	• Acknowledging and accepting consequences of his/her actions. • Adhering to code of ethics, standards of practice, policies/procedures that govern the conduct of professional activities. • Communicating accurately to others (payers, patients/clients, other health care providers) about professional actions. • Participating in the achievement of health goals of patients/clients and society. • Seeking continuous quality improvement (QI). • Maintaining membership in APTA and other organizations. • Engaging in political activism.
Altruism	Altruism is the primary regard for or devotion to the interest of patients/clients, thus assuming the fiduciary responsibility of placing the needs of the patient/client ahead of the physical therapist's self interest.	• Placing patient's/client's needs above the physical therapists'. • Providing pro bono services. • Providing physical therapy services to underserved and underrepresented populations. • Providing patient/client services that go beyond expected standards of practice. • Completing patient/client care and professional responsibility prior to personal needs.
Compassion/ Caring	Compassion is the desire to identify with or sense something of another's experience; a precursor of caring. Caring is the concern, empathy, and consideration for the needs and values of others.	• Understanding the socio-cultural, psychological, and economic influences on the individual's life in their environment. • Being an advocate for patient's/client's needs. • Communicating effectively both verbally and nonverbally with others taking into consideration individual differences in learning styles, language, and cognitive abilities, etc. • Designing patient/client programs/interventions that are congruent with patient/client needs. • Being aware of and suspending where appropriate, one's own social, cultural, and sexual biases.
Excellence	Excellence is outstanding physical therapy practice that consistently uses current knowledge and theory while understanding personal limits, integrates judgment and the patient/client perspective, challenges the status quo, and works toward development of new knowledge.	• Internalizing the importance of using multiple sources of evidence to support professional practice and decisions. • Participating in integrative and collaborative practice to promote high-quality health and educational outcomes. • Conveying intellectual humility. • Demonstrating high levels of knowledge and skill in all aspects of the profession. • Using evidence consistently to support professional decisions. • Demonstrating a tolerance for ambiguity. • Engaging in acquisition of new knowledge throughout one's professional career. • Sharing one's knowledge with others. • Contributing to the development and shaping of excellence in all professional roles.

(continued)

Table 12.1. ✧ **Core Values at-a-Glance** *(continued)*		
CORE VALUES	DEFINITION	SAMPLE INDICATORS*
Integrity	Integrity is the possession of and steadfast adherence to high moral principles or professional standards.	• Abiding by the rules, regulations, and laws applicable to the profession. • Adhering to the highest standards of the profession (practice, ethics, reimbursement, honor code, etc). • Using power (including avoidance of use of unearned privilege) judiciously. • Resolving dilemmas consistently based on core values. • Being trustworthy. • Taking responsibility to be an integral part in the continuing management of patients/clients. • Recognizing the limits of one's expertise and making referrals appropriately. • Choosing employment situations that are congruent with practice values and professional ethical standards. • Acting based on professional values even when the results of the behavior may place oneself at risk.
Professional Duty	Professional duty is the commitment to meeting one's obligations to provide effective physical therapy services to individual patients/clients, to serve the profession, and to positively influence the health of society.	• Demonstrating beneficence by providing "best care." • Facilitating achievement of health and wellness goals. • Preserving the safety, security, and confidentiality of individuals in all professional contexts. • Participating in professional activities beyond the practice setting. • Promoting the profession of physical therapy. • Mentoring others to realize their potential. • Taking pride in one's profession.
Social Responsibility	Social responsibility is the promotion of a mutual trust between the profession and the larger public that necessitates responding to societal needs for health and wellness.	• Advocating for the health and wellness needs of society including access to health care and physical therapy services. • Promoting cultural competence within the profession and the larger public. • Promoting community volunteerism. • Understanding of current community-wide, nationwide and worldwide issues and how they affect society's health and well-being and after the delivery of physical therapy. • Providing leadership in the community. • Participating in collaborative relationships with other health practitioners and the public at large. • Ensuring the blending of social justice and economic efficiency of services.

*Some indicators have been deleted from the original document due to space considerations.
Source: Adapted from American Physical Therapy Association, Report from the Consensus Conference on Professionalism, 2003.

tence of this breach is frequent and often impassioned conversation within both professions about the lack of consistency seen in the behavior. This is most clearly seen in the proliferating listservs that provide forums for discussion among clinicians with similar interests. Here practitioners share their frustrations with the behavior of their colleagues and decry the low standards of ethical behavior that they observe.[34] This is a typical example of a comment on one of these listservs in physical therapy.

I'm saying that standards are not "guidelines", they are just what they say: standards. If one is not a member of their professional organization, there is a better than even chance that one is not even aware of what their standards are, let alone how to apply them. There really is no point in being careful about how we define professionalism, the horse has left the barn on that issue. Professionalism is really not the fuzzy term that we might sometimes make it out to be. Our standards exist, they apply to all professionals, and we are bound to uphold them or bear the consequences. We can certainly affect or change those professional standards, but only if we are members of our professional organization.

We must be careful not to extrapolate too far from these anecdotal reports, but they do appear with regularity and frequency and seem to produce resonance among the other participants on the listservs.

There are reports in the research literature that identify the presence of tension placed on the therapists' ethical values by the organization, even though they do not clearly specify the nature of the tension nor the results on ethical behavior of this tension or conflict.

Triezenberg, Barnitt and Partridge, in describing ethical reasoning in occupational and physical therapists in Great Britain, identify issues of power between managers and the therapists as a source of conflict and conclude that "the most significant influence (on ethical standards and actions) was the context of the dilemma with social forces."[35,36] We have further evidence of the extent of the breach in anecdotal reports from students as they return to their academic settings following clinical education experiences.[37]

The sociological literature, the research literature, and the professional literature are replete with clear, specified behavioral expectations for clinical practice. Clinicians are given directive after directive about their behavior. Yet these normative behaviors are not seen consistently in clinical practice. I do not mean to imply by this discussion that I think students or academic faculty are particularly more moral and ethical than clinical practitioners. Quite the opposite—I believe that most people choose the health professions as a career because of a sincere desire to help people and their own natural proclivity is toward honoring our fiduciary relationship with our patients.

I believe that the disparity occurs through the press of the practice environment. Institutional polices and practices have diminished or even removed control over practice from the actual practitioners and placed it in the hands of people with very different imperatives. Health care administrators are in the highly unenviable position of having to do more with less in the growing managed care environments. The growth of for-profit chains of facilities has added responsibility to the shareholder as an imperative that often supersedes the responsibility to the patient.[36] These imperatives lead administrators to decisions that are not in the best interest of patients, decisions with implications for patient care they often don't even comprehend. This is a widespread phenomenon, affecting all areas of practice. It is this phenomenon that leads me to my recommendations.

Recommendations for Change

I postulate that we will not see widespread adoption of the normative behaviors described in the literature until professional leaders take the challenge and responsibility of bringing about change in that middle realm, the institution within which each therapist practices.

Those researchers who have documented actual practice in occupational and physical therapy have also noted this issue of the tension between individual intent and institutional mandates. Mattingly and Fleming, in discussing occupational therapy, say, "Conflicts over how involved the therapist should be in the personal life of the patient seemed to arise in a variety of forms and caused discomfort regarding the therapist's role and place in the institutional setting. This was especially difficult for therapists when they felt that their personal or professional values regarding good patient care conflicted either with individual persons or with stated or perceived institutional policies or implicit norms."[26]

Jensen and colleagues also report that their subjects felt conflict.[25] They reported examples of physical therapists who left practice situations because they could not affect the changes they deemed necessary for patient care. One subject risked professional alienation to report illegal and unethical behavior by her colleagues. Another subject reported a dramatic episode of defying the routine care being implemented for her patient. Their subjects talked often about their need to gain control over the practice environment in order to practice in the manner their patients needed.

In the concluding chapter of their text, *Expertise in Physical Therapy Practice*, Jensen and colleagues discuss the implications of their data and model for the practice of physical therapy.[25] We particularly discuss ways to restructure the environment as a means to accomplish change. These recommendations are derived from observation of and direct commentary from experts on what they needed, sought, and constructed for themselves in their practice environments. As one of the authors of this work, I continue to believe that these recommendations are sound and need implementation.

While speaking of the responsibility of clinicians to seek and use knowledge, we offer this advice:

- ✦ Our practice environments must find mechanisms to provide what has become perhaps the scarcest resource of all—time.[25]

- ✦ The learning component most desired by clinicians and most strongly emphasized by our therapists, however, is the opportunity to interact regularly with other clinicians who are also questioning and reflecting.[25]

- ✦ Therapists should engage in repetition of a specific skill to gain motor control, as in, "I should practice my manual muscle testing positions." Therapists also should incorporate the use of their own movement and the patient's movement into their conception of the practice of physical therapy.[25]

- ✦ Perhaps the most important thing we can learn from these therapists is to set high standards for other therapists. When lesser behavior is observed in colleagues, it must not be tolerated. A cultural norm that requires advocacy, generosity, and compassion can be established. People's personal values cannot be changed, but their behavior can be altered, or they can be made to feel so uncomfortable that they choose to leave.

Most of these recommendations will be best met when occupational and physical therapists control their own practices. We must move out from under the administrative control of people who are not members of our professions. We must claim the fiduciary relationship with our patients as the prime imperative in our decisions. We must seek autonomy, not in its negative sense of isolation from others, but in its positive sense of placing control where control should be—with the health care practitioners with whom patients trust their health.

Recommendations for Future Research

Obviously, my views are just that, my views. In addition to working toward the changes described above, we must also seek out and develop the evidence that helps us describe current practice and the results of change. Currently, we do not seem to really understand the clinical imperatives that appear to drive people who once expressed support for ethical behavior toward behaviors that seem antithetical to these ethical standards. Swisher, in an analysis of the ethical literature in physical therapy, points out that the literature has failed to keep pace with the growing autonomy in physical therapy practice. She identifies the following question as one of many that need to be answered, "What organizational, contextual, or policy factors act as barriers or resources to ethical behavior?"[36] This can certainly be seen as an overarching area of research that includes many specific questions:

+ What are the actual ethical values of students in physical therapy?

+ Do they support the ethical principles put forward by classroom faculty mainly because they want to please those faculty members (for a variety of reasons)?

+ Do they support the actual behavior demonstrated by clinical faculty mainly because they want to please those faculty members (again for a variety of reasons)?

+ If the answer to these two questions is yes, what role do students' actual personal values play in making ethical decisions in the future?

+ What are the actual ethical values of practicing clinicians?

+ Are the professional behaviors identified through activities such as APTA's Consensus Conference really reflective of the practice community?

+ What barriers do clinicians identify to acting on their own ethical proclivities?

+ Does the breach exist? If so, how wide and widespread is the breach?

+ How does any particular organizational change affect clinician behavior?

I believe similar types of questions could apply in occupational therapy. Perhaps once we know more about the real ethos that arises from our professional cultures, we will have better ideas on how to heal the breach between actual behavior observed in individual clinicians and the normative behavior espoused by the professions collectively.

References

1. Lexico Publishing Group: Dictionary.com. Available at: http://dictionary.reference.com. Accessed December 12, 2003.
2. Gabard DL, and Martin MW: Physical Therapy Ethics. FA Davis Co, Philadelphia, 2003.
3. Pennsylvania Department of State: Pennsylvania Department of State. Available at: http://www.dos. state.pa.us/DOS/site.default.asp. Accessed December 12, 2003.
4. Glaser JW: Three Realms of Ethics: Individual, Institutional, Societal, Theoretical Model and Case Studies. Rowman & Littlefield Publishers, Lanham, MD, 1994.
5. Glaser JW, and Hamel RP: Three Realms of Managed Care: Societal, Institutional, Individual: Resources for Group Reflection and Action. Rowman & Littlefield Publishers, Lanham, MD, 1997.
6. Purtilo R: Ethical Dimensions in the Health Professions, ed. 3. WB Saunders Company, Philadelphia, 1993.
7. Beauchamp TL, and Childress JF: Principles of Biomedical Ethics, ed 4. Oxford University Press, New York, 1994.
8. Swisher LL, and Krueger-Brophy C: Legal and Ethical Issues in Physical Therapy. Butterworth-Heinemann, Boston, 1998.
9. Sim J: Ethical Decision Making in Therapy Practice. Butterworth-Heinemann, Oxford, 1997.
10. Lo B: Resolving Ethical Dilemmas. Williams & Wilkins, Baltimore, 1995.
11. Ginzberg E: Health Services Research: Key to Health Policy. Foundation for Health Services Research, Cambridge, 1991.
12. U.S. Department of Health and Human Services: Healthy People 2010. Available at: http://www.healthy-people.gov/Publications. Accessed December 17, 2003.
13. Institute of Medicine: Crossing the Quality Chasm: A New Health System for the 21st Century. National Academy Press, Washington, DC, 2001.
14. Lopopolo RB: The effect of hospital restructuring on the role of physical therapists in acute care. Phys Ther 77:918–936, 1997.
15. Lopopolo RB: Hospital restructuring and the changing nature of the physical therapist's role. Phys Ther 5(1):38–44, 1999.
16. Miller PA, and Solomon P. The influence of a move to program management on the practice of physical therapy. Phys Ther 82:449–458, 2002.
17. Blau R, et al: The experience of providing physical therapy in a changing health care environment. Phys Ther 82:648–657, 2002.
18. Griffin S: Occupational therapists and the concept of power: A review of the literature. Aust Occup Ther J 46:24–34, 2001.
19. Crabtree JL: The self under siege: Warring constructs of individualism versus communitarianism and autocratic versus democratic models of governance in rehabilitation settings. In Purtilo R, Jensen G, and Royeen C (eds): Educating for Moral Action: A Sourcebook in Health and Rehabilitation. Philadelphia: FA Davis Company, Philadelphia, 2005.
20. Freidson E: Profession of Medicine: A Study of the Sociology of Applied Knowledge. Dodd, Mead and Company, New York, 1972.
21. Strauss AL: Professions, Work, and Careers. The Sociology Press, San Francisco, 1971.
22. Vollmer HM, and Mills DL: Professionalization. Prentice Hall, Englewood Cliffs, NJ, 1966.
23. Larson M: The Rise of Professionalism. University of California Press, Berkeley, 1977.
24. http://merriamwebster.com/egi_bin/dictionary.
25. Jensen GM, et al: Expertise in Physical Therapy Practice. Butterworth-Heinemann, Boston, 1999.

26. Mattingly C, and Fleming MH: Clinical Reasoning: Forms of Inquiry in a Therapeutic Practice. FA Davis Co, Philadelphia, 1994.

27. Shelton W: Can virtue be taught. Acad Med 74(6):671–674, 1999.

28. Tan SY: Medical professionalism: Our badge and our pledge. Singapore Med J 41(7):312–316, 2000.

29. American Physical Therapy Association: Guide to Physical Therapist Practice. ed 2. American Physical Therapy Association, Alexandria, VA, 2003.

30. Moyers PA: The Guide to occupational therapy practice. Am J Occup Ther 53(3):1–48, 1999.

31. American Physical Therapy Association: Consensus Conference on Professionalism and a Doctoring Profession. Alexandria, VA, 2002.

32. Massey BJ: APTA Presidential Address: Making vision 2020 a reality. Phys Ther 83:1023–1026, 2003.

33. Microsoft Incorporated: Microsoft Word Dictionary. 2000;Version 9.0.1.

34. Yahoo: Yahoo.com/health groups. Available at: http://health.groups.yahoo.com/group/. Accessed December 17, 2003.

35. Triezenberg HL: Examining the moral role of physical therapists. In Purtilo R, Jensen G, and Royeen C (eds): Education for Moral Action: A Sourcebook in Health and Rehabilitation. FA Davis Co, Philadelphia, 2005.

36. Swisher LL: A retrospective analysis of ethics knowledge in physical therapy (1970–2000). Phys Ther 82(7):692–706, 2002.

37. Mostrom E: Teaching and learning about ethical and human dimensions of care in clinical education: Exploring student and clinical instructor experiences in physical therapy. In Purtilo R, Jensen G, and Royeen C (eds): Educating for Moral Action: A Sourcebook in Health and Rehabilitation. FA Davis Co, Philadelphia, 2005.

13

Enhancing Professional Accountability: Inquiry into the Work of a Professional Ethics Committee

MARY ANN WHARTON, MS, PT

Abstract

A major agenda for ethics educators is to identify effective ways that ethics can be integrated into occupational therapy and physical therapy curricula in order to empower students to become mindful and reflective practitioners. The goal of ethics education is to produce clinicians who value the importance of ethics and incorporate ethical decision making in every patient interaction. To help achieve this goal, each profession has endorsed a code of ethics that articulates the values of the profession to the public it serves and has an established mechanism to hold practitioners accountable for adhering to ethical standards. The most important mechanism is a profession-wide ethics committee. Understandably, these professional ethics committees, which are a part of the larger professional associations in many health professions, have the potential to serve a valuable role in fostering professional accountability and ethical practice. An important first step in promoting this potential is to be clear about the appropriate roles and responsibilities of such ethics committees. To help assess the roles and responsibilities of the state ("chapter") components of the American Physical Therapy Association (APTA) Ethics and Judicial Committee, I interviewed a number of current chairpersons of the state committees. These interviews explored the structure and function of each state's Chapter Committee, as well as its interaction with the APTA. The goal of the study was to delineate the scope of responsibilities that are currently under the purview of Chapter Ethics Committees with the intent that such knowledge can be used to enhance their mission and function.

The practice of physical therapy and occupational therapy in today's complex health care environment demands that clinicians balance technical knowledge and expertise with clinical reasoning. Expert practice further demands that clinicians embrace commitment, caring, concern, and ethical problem solving when making clinical judgments.[1] A major agenda for ethics educators is to identify effective ways that ethics can be integrated into occupational and physical therapy curricula in order to empower students to become mindful and reflective practitioners. An emerging theme is that the goal of ethics education is to produce clinicians who value the importance of ethics when interacting with patients and who incorporate ethical decision making in every patient interaction. An underlying assumption is that each profession endorses a code of ethics that articulates the values of the profession to the public it serves and has an established mechanism for holding practitioners of that discipline accountable for adhering to ethical standards. An additional assumption is that professional ethics committees established by each discipline have the potential to serve a valuable role in fostering professional accountability and ethical practice. Although that seems to be a reasonable assumption, a closer look at the Chapter Ethics Committees developed for the physical therapy profession by the American Physical Therapy Association (APTA) reveals that there is not clear consensus from chairs of these committees about their mission and role. The focus of this chapter is to explore the mission and role of Chapter Ethics Committees established within the American Physical Therapy Association, and to discuss implications for the American Occupational Therapy Association's Commission on Standards and Ethics. The chapter is based on a study I conducted that had three primary goals: (1) to establish the structure and function of Chapter Ethics Committees, (2) to delineate the scope of responsibilities of Chapter Ethics Committees; and (3) to enhance understanding and knowledge of the influence that these committees can have on promoting professional accountability. Although this chapter focuses primarily on discussion about the Chapter Ethics Committees established by the physical therapy profession, the intent is that occupational therapy and other disciplines can benefit from this information to enhance the mission and function of their ethics committees, too.

✦ CODES OF ETHICS AND ETHICS COMMITTEES

Thomas Percival, a philosophically trained English physician, is credited with publishing the first book on medical ethics in 1803. His vision of professional ethics shifted the primary responsibility for caring for the sick from the individual practitioner, which had been the traditional focus of medical morality, to the collective responsibility of the medical profession. He presumed that professions would develop codes of ethics that would be autonomously enforced by ethics committees through professional self-regulation. His belief was that the shift in focus

from the individual practitioner to the profession could enhance the ability of the medical profession to advocate for the interest of patients and the public, and challenge administrators and governments who promulgated regulations that failed to serve the needs of patients.

The American Medical Association (AMA) adopted Percival's notion of professional ethics when it defined a code of ethics in 1847 and formed its first ethics committee in 1850. The AMA Code of Ethics was the first adopted anywhere by a national professional association.[2] Other health care professions followed suit with the adoption of their own codes of ethics and establishment of ethics committees. Today, a code of ethics is recognized as one credential that supports the claim that a group should be designated with professional status. Most health professions embrace the concept of using a code to define professional ethics as a means of self-regulation and autonomy, and adopt a code of ethics as one hallmark of professionalism.[3]

Ethics Documents in the APTA

In 1935, APTA recognized the importance of the ethical dimension of practice when it adopted its first Code of Ethics and Discipline. This Code provided a formal statement that acknowledged the ethical obligations of association members.[4] It defined the limits of professional practice by noting, "diagnosing, stating of the prognosis of a case and prescribing of treatment shall be entirely the responsibility of the physician. Any assumption of this responsibility by one of our members shall be considered unethical."[5] The Code also articulated statements about advertising for services, and provided guidance for professional behaviors that prohibited criticism of doctors, co-workers, or predecessors. Finally, it gave authority for disciplinary action for offenders to the Executive Committee of the association.

Since 1935, the APTA Code of Ethics has been revised several times to reflect contemporary societal and practice standards and respond to the increasingly sophisticated demands of a complex health care delivery system. The current version of the APTA Code of Ethics, adopted by APTA's House of Delegates in

June 2000, sets forth principles of ethical practice for the physical therapist and it includes a preamble and 11 principles.[6] These principles are shown in Table 13.1.

A companion document, the APTA Guide for Professional Conduct, serves as an interpretation of the principles, and provides guidance for ethical conduct. The preamble of the APTA Code of Ethics states that the ethical principles articulated in the code are binding on all physical therapists. The intention of the language in the preamble is to strengthen the understanding that the association's code is the primary source of ethical guidance for all physical therapists, and makes all physical therapists legally re-

sponsible for behavior that is consistent with the recognized ethical standards of the profession. The 11 principles of the code contain patient-centered statements of the ethical values of the APTA, and incorporate concepts of virtue ethics. Two principles focus on the rights of patients to receive confidential, compassionate, and trustworthy care (Principles 1 and 2). Four principles require physical therapists to exercise sound professional judgment, maintain professional competence, promote high standards, and engage in ethical business practices (Principles 4 through 7). Two principles address societal responsibility by stating that physical therapists shall strive to effect changes that ben-

Table 13.1 ✧ American Physical Therapy Association Code of Ethics Adopted by House of Delegates, June 2000

PREAMBLE

This Code of Ethics of the American Physical Therapy Association sets forth principles for the ethical practice of physical therapy. All physical therapists are responsible for maintaining and promoting ethical practice. To this end, the physical therapist shall act in the best interest of the patient/client. This Code of Ethics shall be binding on all physical therapists.

PRINCIPLE 1

A physical therapist shall respect the rights and dignity of all individuals and shall provide compassionate care.

PRINCIPLE 2

A physical therapist shall act in a trustworthy manner towards patients/clients, and in all other aspects of physical therapy practice.

PRINCIPLE 3

A physical therapist shall comply with laws and regulations governing physical therapy and shall strive to effect changes that benefit patients/clients.

PRINCIPLE 4

A physical therapist shall exercise sound professional judgment.

PRINCIPLE 5

A physical therapist shall achieve and maintain professional competence.

PRINCIPLE 6

A physical therapist shall maintain and promote high standards for physical therapy practice, education and research.

PRINCIPLE 7

A physical therapist shall seek only such remuneration as is deserved and reasonable for physical therapy services.

PRINCIPLE 8

A physical therapist shall provide and make available accurate and relevant information to patients/clients about their care and to the public about physical therapy services.

PRINCIPLE 9

A physical therapist shall protect the public and the profession from unethical, incompetent, and illegal acts.

PRINCIPLE 10

A physical therapist shall endeavor to address the health needs of society.

PRINCIPLE 11

A physical therapist shall respect the rights, knowledge, and skills of colleagues and other health care professionals.

efit patients in laws governing physical therapy, and that physical therapists shall endeavor to address the health needs of society (Principle 3 and 10). One principle directs physical therapists to provide accurate information to patient and consumers regarding physical therapy services (Principle 8). One mandates respect for the rights, knowledge, and skills of colleagues and other health care professionals (Principle 11), and one principle defines a standard of accountability by enjoining therapists to protect the public and the profession from unethical, incompetent, and illegal acts (Principle 9). It is this principle that places responsibility on all physical therapists to adhere to the ethical principles and to enforce accountability by all members of the profession.

In contrast to the first APTA Code of Ethics that directs physical therapists to practice under the direction and supervision of the physician, this current version of the Code of Ethics expands the notion of professionalism to recognize the ability of practitioners to practice autonomously and to make independent judgments. It reinforces the concept that the primary authority for professional judgment lies solely with the physical therapist. It delineates that the decisions made by the therapist should always be in the best interest of the patient and should never be compromised by personal, business, or professional relationships. With these statements, this code supports the notion that physical therapy is making a claim for professional status. Also in contrast to the first Code of Ethics, the current one shifts its focus from conduct of the individual to statements that provide guidance for ethical conduct that is rooted in the concept of societal justice. Specifically, the principle that addresses fair and just remuneration in light of society's limited resources reflects an attempt to provide guidance for the challenges of providing services in a delivery system driven by economic resources. In addition, the principle that directs physical therapists to advocate for just and fair laws and regulations to govern health care delivery and the principle that directs therapists to meet the health needs of society, including consideration for the provision of pro bono services, make direct statements about professionalism, and promote the notion that physical therapists

must be responsive to the health needs of individuals who lack resources to pay for services.

Complementing the APTA Code of Ethics is the APTA Standards of Ethical Conduct for the Physical Therapist Assistant.[7] These standards are shown in Table 13.2.

APTA adopted this set of seven standards to govern the ethical conduct of the physical therapist assistant while assisting the physical therapist in the provision of services. Similar to the Code of Ethics, it is binding on all physical therapist assistants. Standards address the rights of patients/clients to be respected and receive compassionate care and direct physical therapist assistants to act in a trustworthy manner when providing physical therapy services (Standards 1 and 2). Two standards instruct the physical therapist assistant to work only under the direction and supervision of a physical therapist, and to comply with laws and regulations that govern physical therapy practice (Standards 3 and 4). Additional standards guide the physical therapist assistant to achieve and maintain competence, and to make judgments that are commensurate with their educational and legal qualifications (Standards 5 and 6). The final standard directs the physical therapist assistant to protect the public and the profession from unethical, incompetent, and illegal acts (Standard 7).

Ethics Documents in the AOTA

The American Occupational Therapy Association has similarly embraced a code of ethics to promote and maintain high standards of behavior in occupational therapy.[8] These principles are shown in Table 13.3.

AOTA specifies that the principles set forth in its code apply to occupational therapy personnel at all levels. In this respect, it differs from APTA, which establishes its code for physical therapists and defines Standards of Conduct for the physical therapist assistant. The current AOTA Code identifies seven principles. Principles 1 and 2, which are based on the ethical principles of beneficence and nonmaleficence, direct practitioners to demonstrate concern for recipients of services and to avoid harm. Principle 3 directs practitioners to respect the rights of recipients of occupational

Table 13.2 ✧ American Physical Therapy Association Standards of Ethical Conduct for the Physical Therapist Assistant Adopted by the House of Delegates, June, 2000

PREAMBLE

This document of the American Physical Therapy Association sets forth standards for the ethical conduct of the physical therapist assistant. All physical therapist assistants are responsible for maintaining high standards of conduct while assisting physical therapists. The physical therapist assistant shall act in the best interest of the patient/client. These standards of conduct shall be binding on all physical therapist assistants.

STANDARD 1

A physical therapist assistant shall respect the rights and dignity of all individuals and shall provide compassionate care.

STANDARD 2

A physical therapist assistant shall act in a trustworthy manner toward patients/clients.

STANDARD 3

A physical therapist assistant shall provide selected physical therapy interventions only under the supervision and direction of a physical therapist.

STANDARD 4

A physical therapist assistant shall comply with the laws and regulations governing physical therapy.

STANDARD 5

A physical therapist assistant shall achieve and maintain competence in the provision of selected physical therapy interventions.

STANDARD 6

A physical therapist assistant shall make judgments that are commensurate with his or her educational and legal qualifications as a physical therapist assistant.

STANDARD 7

A physical therapist assistant shall protect the public and the profession from unethical, incompetent, and illegal acts.

---

therapy services, based on the ethical principles of autonomy, privacy, and confidentiality. Principles 4 through 6 invoke occupational therapy personnel to achieve and maintain high standards of competence, comply with laws and association policies guiding the profession, and provide accurate information regarding occupational therapy services. Finally, principle 7, grounded in the ethical principle of fidelity, directs occupational therapy personnel to treat colleagues and other professionals with fairness, discretion, and integrity.[8]

APTA and AOTA Documents Compared

A comparison of the current APTA Code of Ethics and Standards of Ethical Conduct for the Physical Therapist Assistant and the AOTA Code of Ethics shows that each profession is bound by similar principles to guide ethical conduct. Each profession's current code of ethics shifts from a focus only on ethical con-

duct of the individual practitioner to include statements about professionalism and social justice. Each document focuses on the responsibility of practitioners to respect patient rights. Each document also contains broad statements that are based on the ethical principles of beneficence and nonmaleficence, patient autonomy, privacy, and confidentiality. Each document directs practitioners to maintain professional competence and to comply with laws, regulations, and association policies that govern practice. Finally, each document recognizes the importance of respecting the rights, knowledge, and skill of professional colleagues and prescribes a framework for ethical and collegial professional relationships.

The ultimate responsibility for ethical conduct of physical therapy and occupational therapy practitioners and enforcement of the APTA and AOTA documents lies within each profession's defined self-regulatory process. Each organization has devised a system that is based on the structure of that discipline's professional

PREAMBLE

The American Occupational Therapy Association's Code of Ethics is a public statement of the common set of values and principles used to promote and maintain high standards of behavior in occupational therapy. The American Occupational Therapy Association and its members are committed to furthering the ability of individuals, groups, and systems to function within their total environment. To this end, occupational therapy personnel, including all staff and personnel who work and assist in providing occupational therapy services (e.g., aides, orderlies, secretaries, technicians), have a responsibility to provide services to recipients in any stage of health and illness who are individuals, research participants, institutions and businesses, other professionals and colleagues, students, and to the general public.

The *Occupational Therapy Code of Ethics* is a set of principles that applies to occupational therapy personnel at all levels. These principles to which occupational therapists and occupational therapy assistants aspire are part of a lifelong effort to act in an ethical manner. The various roles of practitioner (occupational therapist and occupational therapy assistant), educator, fieldwork educator, clinical supervisor, manager, administrator, consultant, fieldwork coordinator, faculty program director, researcher/scholar, private practice owner, entrepreneur, and student are assumed.

Any action in violation of the spirit and purpose of this Code shall be considered unethical. To ensure compliance with the Code, the Commission on Standards and Ethics (SEC) establishes and maintains the enforcement procedures. Acceptance of membership in the American Occupational Therapy Association commits members to adherence to the Code of Ethics and its enforcement procedures. The Code of Ethics, Core Values and Attitudes of Occupational Therapy Practice (AOTA, 1993), and the Guidelines to the Occupational Therapy Code of Ethics (AOTA, 1998) are aspirational documents designed to be used together to guide occupational therapy personnel.

Principle 1

Occupational therapy personnel shall demonstrate a concern for the well-being of the recipients of their services. (beneficence)

Principle 2

Occupational therapy personnel shall take reasonable precautions to avoid imposing or inflicting harm upon the recipient of services or to his or her property. (nonmaleficence)

Principle 3

Occupational therapy personnel shall respect the recipient and/or their surrogate(s) as well as the recipient's rights. (autonomy, privacy, confidentiality)

Principle 4

Occupational therapy personnel shall achieve and continually maintain high standards of competence. (duties)

Principle 5

Occupational therapy personnel shall comply with laws and Association policies guiding the profession of occupational therapy. (justice)

Principle 6

Occupational therapy personnel shall provide accurate information about occupational therapy services. (veracity)

Principle 7

Occupational therapy personnel shall treat colleagues and other professionals with fairness, discretion, and dignity. (fidelity)

organization. APTA has a complex, tiered system comprising a national association and 52 chapters; 1 chapter for each state, the District of Columbia, and Puerto Rico. APTA bylaws define the mechanism to oversee enforcement of the Code of Ethics for members of the association and to promote ethical practice for all physical therapists regardless of association membership.[9] The association bylaws prescribe a national Ethics and Judicial Committee that is charged to interpret and propose revisions to the ethical principles and standards of the association, promote activities to disseminate ethics information, and adjudicate members for violations of principles and standards. APTA bylaws also obligate the 52 chapters of the association to investigate ethical complaints in accordance with APTA's Procedural Document on Disciplinary Action.[10] This document, originally adopted by the House of Delegates in 1979 and most recently amended in 1999, outlines a relationship between the national Ethics and Judicial Committee and the Chapter Ethics Committees. Specifically, it details the process that must be taken to adjudicate members who have been charged with violations of the ethical standards, and provides timelines for each step in the process. This link between the bylaws and the procedural document provides the only reference to the responsibility of a Chapter Ethics Committee by the APTA. There is no standard that mandates the formation of Chapter Ethics Committees, per se, and no expectation that these committees foster ethical practice through education or consultation. In contrast to APTA's tiered system, AOTA has established a national system for overseeing ethical practice of members and enforcing ethical conduct through its Commission on Standards and Ethics (SEC). Therefore, there is no corollary to APTA's Chapter Ethics Committees within the AOTA. Similar to the Procedural Document for Disciplinary Action, AOTA has developed Enforcement Procedures for the Occupational Therapy Code of Ethics.[11] Membership in AOTA commits members to adherence to the AOTA Code of Ethics and its enforcement procedures. AOTA's enforcement procedures do not specifically address an obligation for nonmembers to adhere to the Code of Ethics, but it can be inferred that, similar to physical therapists, all occupational therapists should maintain these ethical standards of practice.

✧ ROLES OF ETHICS COMMITTEES IN HEALTH CARE

Inherent in a profession's adoption of a code of ethics is the notion of autonomy and self-regulation by the profession's ethics committees. A review of the literature reveals that little has been written about the purpose, function, or efficacy of these ethics committees. However, several articles were identified that discuss the role of *hospital* ethics committees, each suggesting that the institution's committee is to provide education and consultation, and to assist in developing policies that promote ethical standards of practice. They suggest that many such committees are struggling with their roles and responsibilities as health care delivery faces more barriers in terms of management, managed care, reimbursement, and social accountability.[12–14] In addition, I identified one article that reported on a survey of ethics committees in *state nurses associations*. This survey, conducted in 1987 and never replicated, identified that 36% of state nurses associations at the time of the survey had either an ethics committee or some alternate mechanism to handle ethical issues. The purposes of the state committees were similar in that they specified a relationship to the American Nurses Association Code for Nurses, and promoted mechanisms for education, resource identification, and promotion of quality care and ethical practice. Although the major activity of these nurse ethics committees was educational, several committees also identified affirmative and disciplinary actions as a purpose of the state committee.[15]

Triezenberg reported results of a survey of members of APTA's Ethics and Judicial Committee, which has the authority to enforce the APTA Code of Ethics and Standards of Ethical Conduct.[16] Although this survey identified 16 issues that addressed ethical considerations in physical therapy practice, it did not identify the role or mission of the national or state committees in promoting ethical physical therapy practice relative to these issues. No investigators have reported on the mission and role of Chapter Ethics Committees established within the association. Similarly, no articles were identified that studied the mission and role of AOTA's Commission on Standards and Ethics.

✧ A STUDY OF THE MISSION AND ROLE OF APTA'S CHAPTER ETHICS COMMITTEES

Ethics committees have the potential to play an important role in fostering professional accountability and ethical practice of both physical and occupational therapists. In addition to adjudicating practitioners who violate ethical standards, ethics committees could play critical roles in education of members, nonmembers, and the public. Although this seems to be a reasonable assumption, a review of the literature reveals that there is no published information that identifies the mission or roles of ethics committees within the physical or occupational therapy professions. Therefore, a qualitative study was conducted to explore the mission and role of the Chapter Ethics Committees established within the American Physical Therapy Association. There were three primary purposes of this study. The first purpose was to determine how APTA Chapter Ethics Committees are structured and how they function and partner with the APTA Ethics and Judicial Committee to enhance professional accountability. The second purpose was to delineate the scope of responsibilities that are currently under their purview. The third purpose was to enhance understanding and knowledge of the impact that Chapter Ethics Committees can have on promoting professional accountability. Interviews were conducted with a purposeful sample of 6 current Chapter Ethics Committee chairpersons derived from a list of 15 potential participants identified by members of APTA's Ethics and Judicial Committee. In order to obtain a diverse sample for the study, the members of the Ethics and Judicial Committee were asked to develop the pool of potential participants based on one or more of the following criteria: (a) Individuals who served as chair for a Chapter Ethics Committee for a minimum of 1 year to 5-plus years; (b) Range of chapter size (small to large); (c) Chapters in geographically diverse locations; (d) Chairs of Chapter Ethics Committees who, in the collective opinion of the Ethics and Judicial Committee, have varying degrees of skill (highly effective to struggling to be effective).

To maintain confidentiality of the subjects, the names of the 15 Chapter Ethics Committee chairs and their chapter affiliation were listed randomly, without indicating which criteria were used for inclusion in this pool. Individuals identified on the list were contacted in the order that they appeared, until a sample size of six[6] Chapter Ethics Committee chairpersons was

achieved. This manner of selection allowed for refusal to participate by the committee chairs, and selection of final participants based on availability and willingness to participate. Prior to conducting interviews, each individual who consented to participate signed an informed consent. Once the purposeful sample was obtained, telephone interviews were conducted with the Ethics Committee chairpersons to determine how each Chapter Ethics Committee is structured and how they function and partner with APTA's Ethics and Judicial Committee to enhance professional accountability. The remainder of this chapter summarizes and discusses comments from these interviews, and provides suggestions and recommendations for ethics educators to enhance the mission and roles of Ethics Committees in physical and occupational therapy professions.

Background and Experience of Chapter Ethics Committee Chairs

The Ethics Committee chairpersons interviewed were asked to outline their background and training in ethics. Five of the six stated that they had no formal background in ethics and that their primary experience with ethics came through association activities. One chairperson had training through workshops conducted at Rushworth Kidder's Institute of Global Ethics. Three stated that they have responsibility for teaching ethics in physical therapy curricula. Years of experience on Chapter Ethics Committees ranged from 2 to 12 years, with 4 of the chairpersons holding long-standing, consecutive appointments for 10 to 12 years.

Essential Roles and Responsibilities for Chapter Ethics Committees

Each subject stated that authority for their Chapter Ethics Committee was derived from provisions in their chapter bylaws. However, they noted that the bylaws primarily addressed appointment, term of office, and responsibility to investigate complaints following APTA's procedural document. Even in the absence of specific directives, the committee chairs overwhelmingly expressed their opinion that the primary responsibility of their committee is to protect the public, defend the ethical standards of the association, and hold members of the association accountable for ethical practice. Each committee chair mentioned the obligation to follow the procedural document, although there were differences in interpretation of the exact steps outlined in this document. Significantly, all six chairs cited the ability of the committee to conduct fair investigations of reported violations of ethical practice as a major accomplishment of their committee.

Four of the committee chairs discussed dissemination of information and education as secondary responsibilities of their respective committees. Activities undertaken by their committees included newsletter articles in chapter publications and education sessions held at chapter meetings. One committee chair stated that his committee uses the chapter web site to publish notices about changes in the APTA Code of Ethics or Standards and to keep members informed of activities undertaken by his committee. One committee chair makes presentations to students enrolled in the physical therapy programs.

Most committee chairs questioned the effectiveness of engaging in education of chapter members, noting that there is no concrete way of measuring the efficacy. They stated that they could track how many individuals attended an educational session or received a publication, but do not have a system in place to determine whether these activities change ethical practice. One committee chair stated the belief that it is not the responsibility of the Chapter Ethics Committee to educate members about ethical practice, and that ethics education should be part of the curriculum for entry level and transition doctoral programs in physical therapy. This individual questioned whether members of a Chapter Ethics Committee would be comfortable enough to provide education.

Only one committee chair initially mentioned providing consultation to members and the public as a secondary role and activity undertaken by his committee. When prompted, however, the majority of committee chairs stated that they do engage in some consultation activities. The consultation services are primarily limited to providing information when inquiries are made about potential ethical situations. These inquiries generally are initiated by physical therapists who are questioning what is the right thing to do in a certain clinical practice situation. One barrier to providing more consultation activities, perceived by most of the committee chairs, is that their committee does not promote this activity and, therefore, it is not recognized as a responsibility of the committee by physical therapists or by the public.

Relationship of Chapter Ethics Committees to APTA's Ethics and Judicial Committee

The majority of Chapter Ethics Committee chairs stated that they currently have a positive relationship with the APTA Ethics and Judicial Committee, one that supports and enhances the ability of their committee to achieve its goals. All of the chairs stated that the primary interaction with the Ethics and Judicial Committee is about specific cases, and that the primary contact is with legal counsel rather than individual committee members. They cited examples of consulting with legal counsel to clarify policy and to obtain advice regarding adjudication of particular cases. The committee chairs attribute the positive relationship between the committees to improved communication regarding cases, and to perceived softening and leniency of recommendations for issuing sanctions and enhanced respect for Chapter Ethics Committee decisions by the APTA Ethics and Judicial Committee. The committee chairs believe that the relationship between the committees facilitates their ability to adjudicate cases fairly.

Several committee chairs discussed the newly implemented liaison program initiated by the APTA Ethics and Judicial Committee as a positive step in enhancing the national committee's relationships with the Chapter Ethics Committees. In 2002, a member of the national committee was assigned to contact each chapter committee chair and establish a liaison relationship. Only one chapter committee chair stated that she had not been contacted by her liaison.

Committee chairs overwhelmingly stated that this program could serve as a valuable resource for enhancing committee activities, citing possibilities of training programs, shared responsibility for developing educational programs and newsletter articles, and timely updates regarding current issues and changes in the APTA Code of Ethics and Standards of Practice. They specifically noted that periodic memos or bulletins to Chapter Ethics Committee chairs from liaisons or from the APTA Ethics and Judicial Committee staff would be invaluable in improving communication and keeping the chapter committees informed.

Two Chapter Ethics Committee chairs discussed the Ethics and Judicial Committee/Chapter Ethics Committee breakfasts as a helpful mechanism to enhance relations between the national and chapter committees. These breakfasts, typically held at the association's annual meeting, consist of an educational program followed by an opportunity to discuss issues and exchange ideas. Although not intended as specific training sessions, they have served a valuable role in updating and informing chapter committee chairs of current ethical issues and procedural matters.

Typical Problems Hindering Chapter Ethics Committee Function

The majority of chairs identified procedural matters as problematic, hindering the function of their Chapter Ethics Committee. Specifically, they cited difficulty in meeting the procedural document deadlines in a timely manner when adjudicating a case as the primary problem. The chairs stated that it was not always reasonable to gather the required documentation, conduct the investigations, hold necessary hearings, and finalize the adjudication process within the deadlines set forth by the procedural document. Most committee chairs felt that their chapters provided adequate budgets to allow communication and meetings to enable fair and equitable adjudication of cases. Only one chair stated that there was no budget for the committee. A secondary factor hindering timeliness was committee members'

diverse geographic locations within their respective chapters, making it difficult to schedule and conduct face-to-face meetings.

Another hindrance stated by several committee chairs is committee members' inexperience and lack of specific training in ethics. The chairs stated that experience in ethics is not a requirement for committee appointment. Suggestions were given for more specific direction from chapter bylaws to committees, development of Committee Policy and Procedures manuals, increased consultation from Ethics and Judicial Committee liaisons, and training for Chapter Ethics Committee members by the Ethics and Judicial Committee.

Perceived Barriers That Hinder Chapter Ethics Committees

The Chapter Ethics Committee chairs discussed a number of barriers that they discern as hindering their committee's ability to enhance ethical physical therapy practice. The primary barrier identified by the majority of the chairs is the perceived unwillingness of therapists to follow through with ethical complaints. Chairs reported that individuals would inquire about ethical practice, but would stop short of filing an ethical complaint to initiate the disciplinary process. The committee chairs speculated on a variety of reasons for this situation: Several believed that members are unwilling to disclose and get involved in the process; another stated that he believes it is fear of the actual process, namely, the disclosure aspects and the prospect of participating in a hearing.

Another barrier is perceived apathy of therapists and lack of interest in ethics. It was the opinion of one chair that practitioners are overwrought with the day-to-day issues and the critical thinking and decision making that occur in physical therapy practice because of today's complex health care environment. Consequently, this chair believes that clinicians are not interested in understanding the ethical context of that decision making.

The final barrier hindering effective promotion of ethical practice, cited by several committee chairs, is inexperience of committee members and limited knowledge of what activities should be undertaken by the committee. Individuals who discussed this mentioned the need for a closer relationship with the APTA Ethics and Judicial Committee, and stated that they were hopeful that having an appointed liaison from the National Committee could facilitate overcoming this barrier.

✦ DISCUSSION/STUDY OF RESULTS

The interviews conducted with six Chapter Ethics Committee chairs provide valuable insight into their perception of the mission, role, and function of the American Physical Therapy Association's Chapter Ethics Committees. A summary of the subjects' responses is provided in Table 13.4.

These interviews provide valuable lessons for ethics educators instructing students and clinicians about the ethical dimensions of physical therapy practice. The Chapter Ethics Committee chairs stated almost universally that they had no formal background or education in ethics prior to assuming positions on the ethics committees. Furthermore, they all cited inexperience and lack of formal ethics training as a barrier hindering Chapter Ethics Committee function. Enhancing ethics education must begin in physical therapy curricula. At this level, future practitioners can begin to develop the knowledge, skills, attitudes, and values that will prepare them to analyze ethical situations in clinical practice and appreciate the importance and need for a lifelong study of ethics. The implication is that clinicians who learn to incorporate ethical problem solving into every clinical decision will develop a repertoire of skills to enhance ethical decision making. These clinicians will, in turn, foster ethical practices and become more proficient and comfortable in making ethical decisions.

Clinicians who have enhanced training in ethics and who develop an appreciation for lifelong acquisition of knowledge and skills will be better prepared to assume leadership roles on ethics committees. Although education was not initially reported as a primary role for Chapter Ethics Committees, when clinicians value the

Table 13.4 ✦ Study of the Mission and Roles of APTA's Chapter Ethics Committees (CEC) Summary of Chapter Ethics Committee Chairpersons' Interview Responses

Background and Experience of CEC Chairpersons

- No formal background or education in ethics
- Primary ethics experience is through Association activities

Essential Roles and Responsibilities of CEC Chairpersons

- Adjudicate APTA members for violations of ethical conduct
- Disseminate information and educate practitioners and students
- Provide consultation to members and the public

Relationship to APTA's Ethics and Judicial Committee

- Positive relationship, with primary purpose of clarifying policy and obtaining legal advice regarding adjudication of cases
- Liaison program viewed as a means of educating ethics committee members and developing education programs

Typical Problems Hindering CEC Function

- Procedural matters, especially timeliness in adjudicating cases
- Inexperience and lack of formal training in ethics

Perceived Barriers Hindering CEC Function

- Unwillingness of therapists to follow through with ethical complaints
- Perceived apathy of therapists and lack of interest in ethics
- Inexperience of committee members
- Limited knowledge of activities that should be undertaken by the committee and lack of specific directives in Association Bylaws and policies

importance of ethics education, an assumption is that they will view the responsibility to disseminate information and educate practitioners and students as a more essential role and responsibility of their position on an ethics committee. In this context, ethics committees can assume a crucial role in providing ongoing ethics education for clinicians.

One barrier limiting the role of ethics committee members as educators is that they have no concrete way of measuring the efficacy of educational efforts. They state that they can ascertain how many individuals attend educational sessions or receive publications, but they do not have a mechanism to determine whether learning was effective. One consideration for educators might be to assist in developing outcome studies that could be used by the ethics committees to indicate whether these activities facilitate ethical practice.

Another barrier precluding ethics committees from providing educational services is the inexperience of committee members as educators. An immediate solution to this barrier is to strengthen the relationship between Chapter Ethics Committee and APTA Ethics and Judicial Committee members. The liaison program discussed above, initiated in 2002, is an important first step. One outcome may be facilitation of learning opportunities. Joint programs, newsletters, or bulletins could be developed to address current concepts in ethical practice and keep committee members informed.

The Chapter Ethics Committee chairs universally identified adjudicating members for violations of ethical practice as a primary responsibility of their committee. This fact is supported by the literature on ethics committees, and is consistent with the notion that a hallmark of professionalism is development of a code of ethics that a professional association enforces through self-regulation. Clearly, the APTA, by adopting the Procedural Document for Disciplinary Action, has outlined a detailed mechanism for enforcing the ethical principles articulated in the APTA Code of Ethics. Although Chapter Ethics Committee chairs cited logistic problems with following the steps outlined in this document, they feel that they are adequately prepared to adjudicate cases in a fair and just manner. Overwhelmingly, they

express a current interest in providing education regarding appropriate ethical conduct to individuals prior to initiating the disciplinary process. They also feel that they could include recommendations for ethical practice and education as a condition of compliance for violators, and thus not limit the sanctions to punitive measures that may not change behavior.

Another significant barrier hindering Chapter Ethics Committee function is the perceived apathy of therapists and lack of interest in ethics. One potential solution is to enhance appreciation for the importance of incorporating critical thinking and self-assessment, including personal moral convictions, into case studies. By addressing these issues in the context of clinical scenarios, students will begin to understand and appreciate that patient management requires skill in identifying and solving ethical problems that have an impact on patient interaction. With experience in case analysis, the students should be able to transition these skills into clinical education and ultimately, into clinical practice. Coupled with knowledge of the code of ethics, this self assessment and knowledge will foster the ability of clinicians to make ethical decisions in the context of clinical practice in today's complex health care environment. Other ideas are to encourage students to articulate and critically examine their reactions to the ethical dimensions of practice by keeping a journal where students can document patient stories and their reactions.

This can foster a lifelong practice for self-reflection that could be instrumental in developing expertise in ethical analysis.

The final, and perhaps most significant, barrier identified by Chapter Ethics Committee chairs as hindering their committee's ability to enhance ethical practice is the perceived unwillingness of therapists to follow through with ethical complaints. It is unrealistic to expect ethics education to change an individual's moral compass. However, ethics education can significantly influence the willingness to disclose of those individuals who fear the process. For individuals with strong moral values, knowledge of the process and experience in participating in the steps delineated by the professional association for enforcement of the APTA Code of Ethics may increase their comfort and enhance their willingness to become whistleblowers. An effective educational tool might be to develop a mock scenario in which an unethical practice is reported and the adjudication steps are completed. Providing clinicians with pertinent cases may heighten their awareness of the importance of professional self-regulation.

This discussion reflects on the study of Chapter Ethics Committees established by the American Physical Therapy Association and the impact that ethics education can have in enhancing their mission and role. However, these same lessons can apply to the Commission on Standards and Ethics of the American Occupational Therapy Association. Even though the structure of the committee differs, it can be assumed that the mission and roles are similar.

❖ CONCLUSION

Ethics education has the potential to make a profound impact on enhancing professional accountability and facilitating the mission and role of ethics committees. If ethics educators are better prepared to facilitate knowledge and understanding of ethical practice, future practitioners should be able to better assume the role of ethicist in professional endeavors. Practitioners will have greater knowledge and understanding of the Code of Ethics and the principles and theories of ethical practice. Most importantly, physical and occupational therapists should be more capable of mindful and reflective analysis of contemporary moral problems that arise in clinical practice. Enhanced ethics education can also assist in achieving the more altruistic goal of greater adherence by physical and occupational therapists to ethical standards of practice. Increased knowledge and understanding of ethical practice will provide a sound foundation for physical and occupational therapists to value and uphold standards. Familiarity with disciplinary procedures may make it more comfortable for physical and occupational therapists to report instances of unethical conduct among their peers.

References

1. Jensen GM, et al: Expert practice in physical therapy. Phys Ther 80(1):28–43, 2000.
2. Baker R, and Emmanual L: The efficacy of professional ethics: The AMA Code of Ethics in historical and current perspective. Hastings Cent Rep 30:513–516, 2000.
3. Purtilo R: Codes of ethics in physiotherapy: A retrospective view and look ahead. Physiother Pract 3:28–34, 1987.
4. Purtilo R: The American Physical Therapy Association's Code of Ethics. Phys Ther 57:1001–1006, 1977.
5. American Physiotherapy Association: Code of Ethics and Discipline. American Physiotherapy Association, 1935.
6. American Physical Therapy Association: APTA Code of Ethics and Guide for Professional Conduct. Available at: http://www.apta.org/PT_Practice/ethics_pt/pro_conduct. Accessed November 2003.
7. American Physical Therapy Association: Standards of Ethical Conduct for Physical Therapist Assistants. American Physical Therapy Association. Available at: http://www.apta.org/PT_Practice/ethics_pt/ethics_pt_assistant. Accessed March 29, 2004.
8. American Occupational Therapy Association: AOTA Code of Ethics. Available at: http://www.aota.org/general/coe/asp. Accessed December 10, 2003.
9. American Physical Therapy Association: Bylaws of the American Physical Therapy Association. American Physical Therapy Association, 2003.
10. American Physical Therapy Association: Procedural document on disciplinary action of the American Physical Therapy Association. American Physical Therapy Association, 1999.
11. American Occupational Therapy Association: Enforcement procedures for the Occupational Therapy Code of Ethics. American Occupational Therapy Association, 2002.
12. Nelson WA: Evaluating your ethics committee. Healthcare Exec 15:48–49, 2000.
13. Hoffman PB: Improving ethics committee effectiveness. Healthcare Exec 16:58–59, 2001.
14. Pharr E: The hospital ethics committee: Bridging the gulf of miscommunication and values. Trustee 56:24–28, 2003.
15. Pinch WJ, and Miya PA: Ethics committees in State Nurses' Associations: Report on the national status. Hosp Ethics Comm For 1:167–177, 1989.
16. Triezenberg HL: The identification of ethical issues in physical therapy practice. Phys Ther 76:1097–1107, 1996.

14

Neuroethics: The New Millennium View

IVELISSE LAZZARINI, OTD, OTR/L

Abstract

Over the past 2 years, the scientific community has demonstrated an increased interest in the relationship between ethics and neuroscience. The emerging field of neuroethics is a distinctive area of philosophy that examines the rights and wrongs of the treatment of human brains. Advances in neuroscience hold exciting prospects for the treatment of neurological diseases, but our increasing ability to manipulate the brain poses serious questions. Our understanding of how the brain works is about to be transformed, with enormous social, legal, and ethical implications. Health care professionals have a moral obligation to become informed of the potential ethical quandaries generated by new knowledge in brain science.

Neuroethics is an emergent field concerned with the benefits and possible harms of modern research pertaining to the human brain and related legal, social, and ethical implications. The exponential advances in neurotechnology paired with scientists' unparalleled ability to manipulate and monitor the human brain are moving brain research and its clinical applications beyond the scope of purely medical use. Neuroscientists, like geneticists and nuclear physicists before them, are becoming increasingly aware of the potential ethical implications of their research. Individuals' freedom and right to medical treatment, biologic determinism, discrimination, and social responsibility are issues that have been familiar to scholars in the scientific, medical, and, to some extent, allied health communities, but their importance has escalated in the past few years with the astounding progress made in brain sciences (Fig. 14.1).[1]

The rising knowledge in brain sciences is shaping a range of domains, such as health care delivery and policy, education, the judiciary, and economics among others. In addition, as neurotechnology (a set of tools, technology, or products), nanotechnology, biotechnology, information technology, and cognitive science converge, powerful tools with the potential to considerably enhance human performance as well as transform society are being developed. Consequently, there are many questions that will require serious clinical and academic reflection from the scientific, philosophical, and rehabilitative points of view.

Among the pressing neuroethical issues arising from advances in neuroscience relevant to the rehabilitation professions are the potential to enhance cognitive functioning and change emotional states. Also critical are the implications for informed consent and protection of patients' rights to privacy. As technology evolves, providing access to a full spectrum of human mental states underlying behavior, it is likely that

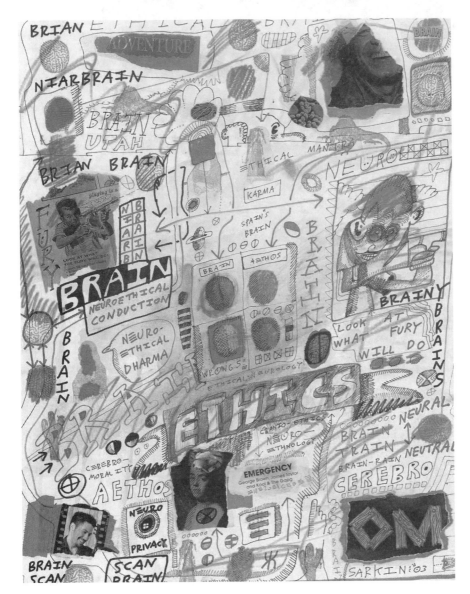

Figure 14.1 ✧ Reprinted with permission of the author: Jon Sarkin.

our common clinical practice of identifying certain behaviors as normal, moral (right versus wrong) and ethical (good versus bad) will change. Thus, new knowledge concerning neuronal brain dynamics, synchronization, and activity patterns may prompt clinicians to redefine what is normal and hence change treatment interventions. It is likely that discoveries in neuroscience will soon make it possible for individuals to enhance their cognitive capacity, change their emotional states, and amplify their sensory perceptions.[2,3] What implications could

this have for the future of clinical practice? At this time it is not clear how these changes will influence clinicians' views and the interplay between clients and therapists. Moreover, as neuroscientific discoveries enhance the capacity for memory recall and accelerate adult learning, how will this change practitioners' views and approaches toward rehabilitation services? Ultimately, as it becomes possible to safely extend the senses of sight, hearing, and taste, how will this influence individuals' decision making and rehabilitation choices?

This chapter elucidates the importance of neuroethics relating to the practice of rehabilitation, discusses some of the possible implications and concerns of the broader social consequences of neuroscientific advances and ultimately solicits the attention of educators and practitioners alike to engage in provocative and proactive discussions about the influences neurotechnology will have in rehabilitation. The proposed views have been influenced by the proceedings of two major conferences held in 2002: "Neuroscience Future" sponsored by the Royal Institution in London and the "Neurocthics: Mapping the Field" sponsored by the Dana Foundation in collaboration with Stanford University and University of California, San Francisco, and by the author's knowledge in cognition, nonlinear brain dynamics, and occupational therapy practice.

✧ EMERGING ISSUES IN NEUROETHICS

Neuroethics overlaps the familiar field and traditional concerns in bioethics; however, it is not merely an extension or subdivision of bioethical issues. In the last two decades, the field of bioethics experienced the rise of modern genetics. Just as ethical issues have been a part of discourse in genetics from the onset, it is now time to pay attention to ethics in neuroscience. And, whereas the ethics of genetics was in many ways a new conversation, the philosophical discussion of mental function and behavior follows an ancient tradition that both informs and complicates the up-and-coming field of neuroethics.

Control or Alteration of the Mind and Brain

In the context of neuroethics, there are emerging issues about the control or alteration of the mind and brain that are rapidly becoming the most challenging scientific and public discourse of modern time. Although debate about the brain and its product—behavior—dates back to ancient philosophy, neuroethics embodies the examination of theoretical and practical issues in the neurological sciences that have moral and social consequences in health care practice and in the public domain. Technical and medical interventions ranging from neuroenhancers (drugs or other technology) to the implications for human self-understanding in areas such as the nature of ethical judgment and the character of personal responsibility are among the present quandaries debated in the field of neuroethics.[4-6]

Motivation, Cooperation, and Competition

New inquires in neuroscience also focus on human motivation, cooperation, and competition, brain differences in violent people, genetic influences on brain structure and function, and ultimately, human reasoning and social attitudes.[5,6] Neurotechnology is demonstrating the intimate connection between individuals' social behavior and the variability of brain activity and pattern formation, generating debate and discussion about the interplay between ethical behavior and neuroscientific knowledge. Presently, brain imaging technologies are mapping the neural substrate of overall brain disorders, helping scientists understand and define mental illnesses from the bottom up.[7] Research in neuroscience demonstrates that integration of moral behaviors is dependent on late myelinating neural tissue in the ventromedial frontal cortex as well as in several other brain regions and systems.[8,9] This improved understanding of brain mechanisms underlying diverse behaviors has unique and potentially dramatic implications for our perspective on ethics and for society.[10]

Emotion and Cognition

Ethicists and scientists alike are beginning to reflect on the work of neuroscience in areas such as emotion and cognition as it pertains to decision making, education, conduct, moral vision, policies, psychiatry, college admissions, economics, corporate hiring, and the judiciary.[11,12] These broad inquiries warrant the introduction of a new area of intellectual and social discourse because individuals and organizations will adopt these new tools. It is important not to view neuroscientific advances as merely drugs or technology that alter the human condition. Instead we must consider them as tools neuroscience is developing that will help us go beyond the examination of traditional ethical issues on individual self-determination as well as enhance our present knowledge of cognitive processes.

Given this information, what does it mean for behaviors such as complying with rehabilitation interventions, the law, self-control, and differences in cultural behavior?

As brain sciences advance, it is important to have a moral framework to help guide the use of this new knowledge. Technology and industrialization had an impact on the course of civilization. The emerging tools and advances in neuroscience and neurotechnology will create new forms of social organization, categorization, and a renewed understanding of social justice.[9,12,13] Neurotechnology's capacity to allow individuals to influence their emotional, cognitive, and sensory states represents the most transformative force that human society will experience in the next 25 years.[9,14] Thus, it should be reflected throughout our education and clinical practice agendas.

✧ NEUROETHICS: BROADER ISSUES AND IMPLICATIONS

Neuroethics is emerging as the vehicle to understanding some important implications of neuroscience and the new devices it affords. We are in the midst of profound and important changes in our ability to manipulate the brain. The dawning age of neuroscience promises not only new treatments for mental illnesses like Alzheimer's disease and other traumatic brain injuries, but also enhancements to improve memory, boost intellectual capacity, and fine-tune our emotional responses.[8,12,14] It is expected that the next two decades will be the golden age of neuroscience.[15]

Concerns About Justice

We are on the verge of rapid growth of information in neuroscience. Consequently, present mechanistic understanding of brain function for society will require integrating neuroscientific knowledge with ethical and social considerations. Advances in neuroscience have the potential to create or ameliorate serious social injustices. Neuroscience may soon be able to screen people's brains to evaluate their mental health. This information may be accidentally shared with employers or insurers with detrimental implications. Faulty personalities may be improved with drugs or implants on demand to the benefit of the individual.

For the past 10 years or so, the field of ethics has been concerned with the danger of illicit use of human genetic information. However, what is more worrying is an inappropriate use of the information enclosed in our brains, which we believe contains the essence of our most inner desires and sense of self—thought, memories, and feelings. If we think inappropriate dissemination of personal information can create havoc, what about illicit manipulation of higher brain functions in mildly, cognitively/emotionally impaired, or nonconsenting individuals? Moreover, in pursuing the freedom of neuroscientific research at a molecular level, what policies or framework will guide the appropriate use of the knowledge acquired for the benefit of the whole? Furthermore, responding to societal pressures for faster and better outcomes, will healthy individuals be justified in enhancing their senses and cognitive functioning with drugs that are used to treat specific illnesses? Through functional brain imaging, scientists believe they may help predict who will be prone to future drug abuse, to tell lies, or to suffer from diseases, such as Huntington's disease, Alzheimer's disease, or multiple sclerosis.[12]

Privacy

Though brain scientists are nowhere near being able to read the mind, their mounting success at mapping brains is sparking neuroethical discussions that echo recent bioethical debates about preserving the privacy of people's genes. Presently, functional brain imaging helps scientists understand the relationship between particular areas of the brain, by charting which regions experience increased blood flow or metabolism or electromagnetic activity over time. It is a step beyond CAT (computed tomography) scans, or CT scans, which can map the brain's structure but not its functions.[16] Consequently, the pressing issue holding the potential for an even more serious controversy in neuroethics is about "brain privacy," i.e., the ebb and flow of brain activity and its consequences.[12] The controversy concerns the issue of tinkering directly with the brain, which is ultimately the organ from which all ethical reflections arise.

Understanding of Human Nature

Neuroscientific advances have the potential to transform our understanding of human nature. In the near future, scientists may be able to make predictions about an individual's behavioral tendencies, including health risks accompanied by cognitive impairments, success for employment, addictions, or propensity for violent behavior. Neuroscience could potentially define the boundary between what society views as normal and determined to be pathological. Children, for example, are being placed on medicines such as Ritalin for conditions that worry many but are not clear-cut brain diseases. Who should receive neurological enhancers, and how? What will be the role of rehabilitation practitioners? How will these choices and changes in what is socially acceptable affect rehabilitation services and ultimately our ability to advocate for our patients?

How we use current and future neuroscience knowledge will shape rehabilitation practice and society. If learning can be accelerated and attention intensified through neuroenhancers, should such drugs be available to all, or should resources be devoted to transforming the environment of the classroom without the need for rehabilitation interventions? How will

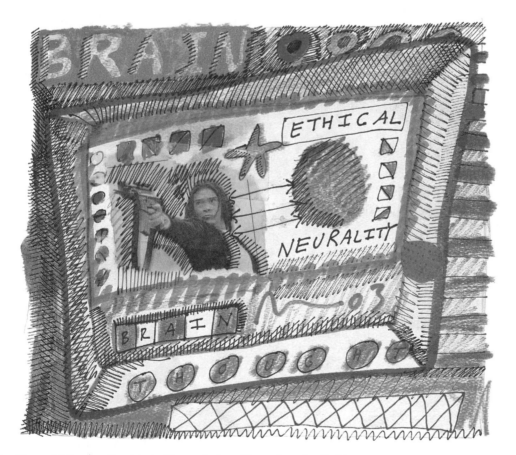

Figure 14.2   ✧   Reprinted with permission of the author: Jon Sarkin.

practitioners and educators reconcile the new knowledge about brain function, behavior, and the causes of mental dysfunction related to the present ethical and social metaphors that allow our society and clinical practice to work efficiently (Fig. 14.2)?[17,18]

Guilt and Innocence

Soon, brain imaging might be able to pinpoint brain abnormalities in those accused of breaking the law, thus changing our perceptions of guilt and innocence. It has been predicted that the first time neuroethics will become a real-life issue will be in the realm of the legal system. Lawyers have already used neurotechnology to absolve their clients of criminal responsibility on the basis of mapping brain function.[19] Brain fingerprinting is used to monitor the electrical activity in a person's brain in response to images from a crime or other specific events.[20] In March 2001, an Iowa District Court judge ruled that the science behind brain fingerprinting, a concept called the P-300 response, met the legal standards for admissibility in court.[20] If this is the case, how should our professional analysis and assessments about moral and legal responsibilities change to accommodate this fact? What do we do with this information? How will these techniques be used as they become mainstreamed? What policies and laws will regulate these activities? None exists at the present time.

Authenticity and Responsibility

One need not project very far into the future to see how ethical influences of neuroscience will invariably affect issues previously thought to be only in the realm of ethics of professional and clinical practice. On issues of authenticity and responsibility, some scientists are of the opinion that neurological enhancements or brain altering chemicals render people less authentic.[21] However, some individuals already using these types of neurological enhancements will contest this premise. In the book *Listening to Prozac*, the author chronicles some dramatic transformations in the personalities and attributes of his patients. Some patients referred to their life as being in a drugged state until they started taking Prozac.[22] What is more, the same question acquires a different twist when one considers the false dichotomy between biologic and nonbiologic enhancements. Consider a person who undergoes a profound spiritual transformation (religious or not) and emerges from the experience with a more optimistic and appealing personality. Is she no longer her "real" self? Are spiritual experiences a form of neurological enhancements?

Some neuroscientists fear that neuroenhancements will undermine individuals' responsible moral behavior and free will. Preliminary research studies suggest that an array of violent criminals do have altered brain function.[9,23] As a result, as scientists increase their understanding of brain function the legal system will be forced into making adjustments in how we punish those who break the law.[1,20] A rapist, a pedophile, or a murderer might plead their innocence on the grounds that their "amygdala made them do it" or that their "free will" was compromised.[24] The precedent exists because the legal system already mitigates criminal punishment when an offender can convince a jury that his or her degree of mental illness or diminished capacity precluded his or her judgment.[1,25] In 1989, Kenneth Parks was acquitted of murder after he stabbed his mother-in-law to death while he was sleepwalking.[26,27] His lawyer argued he was in a state of noninsane automatism and was not aware of his actions. With no free will, he could not be guilty.

There might be other ways in which the discoveries about brain function can be dealt with in the legal system with less damaging results to social order. One possibility could be that the offender agrees to take a neurological enhancer (a pill or otherwise) that corrects the brain deficit he claims forced him to commit the crime. The judiciary system already holds people responsible when their drug use causes harm to others. A useful example is the law against drunk driving. Perhaps in the near future, the legal system will hold people responsible if they fail to comply with neurological enhancers prescribed that would help prevent them from behaving in harmful ways.

Summary

Increased understanding of brain function and human development will help redefine issues such as decision making, life and death, abortion, education, judiciary, termination of life support, mental illness, and rehabilitation interventions among others.[8,19,28] Thus, the growing understanding of mind-brain relationships and our ability to assess its physiological relationship with functional neuroimaging begs for a redefinition of what is considered higher cognitive functions.[8,29] The new tools and neuroscientific technologies (from neurological enhancers to implantable brain chips, neuroimaging techniques, and brain scan lie detectors) offer new ways to alter and explore our understanding of human cognition. The questions are: What is safe? What is ethical? Moreover, how will all these affect rehabilitation interventions and our treatment outcomes?

✧ BRAIN, MIND, AND NEUROENHANCERS

Cognition-enhancing drugs affect our most intimate organ involved in awareness of the world around us and inside us—our brain. But the connection between the brain and the mind is not obvious, nor is it well understood. Neuroscientists are productively engaged in the quantification of brain functions, but analysis of the mind is largely left to theoreticians, theologians, and philosophers.

The brain-mind dichotomy exemplifies the difficulty in quantifying the subjective. Brain science, at the present time, is still highly quantitative and/or mechanistic. Mind science on the other hand is qualitative and/or theoretical. When philosophers and scientists talk, they make assertions; however, their perspectives come from significantly different epistemological sources. Neurological enhancers in any form must therefore involve issues that are beyond the present limitations of our modern biochemical and mechanistic science. In other words, neuroscience technology and its neurological enhancers are as much a subjective issue as a technological one. They can be used to achieve technological goals, such as altering neurotransmitter levels, or for subjective goals, such as increasing alertness or enhancing sexual responses. Just because we do not know exactly how we achieve these subjective ends does not mean that they are not real. If neurological enhancers boost human values, let us recognize and acknowledge that fact. To the extent that they pose risks, let us be cautious and become well educated and informed to contribute to a deeper understanding of our clients' needs and choices.

✧ COGNITION AND EMOTION

Although still in its infancy, the ethics of neuroscience as it pertains to cognition or moral cognition is expected to be the most important area of scientific inquiry for the way in which we deal with ethical issues in clinical practice in the 21st century.[1,8,14] Numerous scientists are asking how ordinary everyday life decisions are made in the brain. How are ethical decisions similar to or different from other types of mundane decisions? How are values characterized?

For centuries, we have considered moral or cognitive reasoning as pure rational thought. Studies using magnetic resonance imaging technology demonstrate that moral deliberation is not free of sentiments, passions, or emotions.[9,14] As a consequence, emotions and feelings themselves are part and parcel of what we are, privately and publicly. Neuroscientific research strongly demonstrates that emotions are an essential element of viable practical reasoning about what a person will do. Individuals whose affects are flat or lacking due to brain injury may be incapable of judging or evaluating between courses of action.[9] Emotion prompts and guides our everyday choices.[8,9] In this manner, neuroscience reinforces Hume's insight that "reason is an ought only to be the slave of the passions."[30]

Certainly moral agents come to be morally and practically wise not through pure cognition but by developing moral beliefs and habits through life experiences.[8] Our moral reactions are sharpened through watching and hearing about which actions are rewarded and which are punished; we learn to be moral the same way we learn language.[8] Hence, society's perennial presumption that individuals are responsible for their actions and its consequences are empirically necessary for an individual's learning, both cognitively and emotionally.[8]

What does this mean? It means that it is neurologically impossible to separate our emotions from our conscious activity, unless individuals have experienced a traumatic brain injury or brain cancer, whereby the structural function of the brain has been damaged. What's more, neuroscientific studies underscore the undeniable facts that not only are emotions inseparable from conscious activity, but emotion also plays a significant role in assisting reason to make choices.[9,31] As identified by Damasio,[14] emotion and reason are continuous processes because emotions are the beginning of reasoning having an inherent rationality within a broad number of contexts, and are quite meaningful for the individuals who exhibit them. It means that for the virtue ethicist, understanding of moral behavior as doing the right thing, for the right reason, maintained by the right feelings[14] demonstrates a quintessential *neurological* truth! Unfortunately, at present, clinical assessment within rehabilitation services do not account for this truth.

Rehabilitation services, for the most part, are using assessment tools that measure cognition in traditional ways: stripped of emotional content. However, as demonstrated by neuroscience, emotion is not only the loop of reason but also the package of reactions well preserved in evolution.[14] Hence clinicians and theoreticians must realize that in neural reality there is a continuum between reason and emotion instead of two entirely different categories. Perhaps in trying to be terribly objective about our assessment tools we have used the traditional bifurcations of emotion and reason to create an interesting psychoneural distinction that does not exist.[8] How then do we promote the scientific value and efficacy of emotion in treatment interventions? How do we overcome the outdated belief that emotion is an insignificant part of treatment interventions and is undermined, downplayed, and placed in second agenda?

When we speak about neurological conditions, whether Alzheimer's disease, a stroke, a traumatic brain injury, or schizophrenia, metaphorically we imply that these conditions are monolithic. We refer to these neurological conditions (e.g., sense feelings in others and decision making) as permanent impairments.[14] In fact, all of these conditions can at times change depending on the context and circumstances and the brain's high degree of redundancy, which affords the possibility of compensating by other brain structures. To deny the impact of neuroscience advances relating to emotion and its role in moral cognition implies unsuccessful clinical interventions, lack of responsible professional behavior, and ultimately, the neglect for human life.

At present, the field of bioethics predominantly speaks about deterministic ethics, emphasizing issues of free will, determinism, and criminal responsibility. Even though these issues are of tremendous importance, neuroscience may affect society in many other crucial ways that are not captured in the areas mentioned above.[19] One of the limitations encountered by traditional bioethics is the depiction and belief that human choices, actions, and behaviors are entirely rational, free from emotional concern and attachment. This is far from scientific validation. As emotional mental states dictate the well-being of individuals, it is impossible for clinical practitioners to view them from the perspective of such scientific deterministic facts. As previously pointed out, what is reason without emotion and vice versa?

✧ INFORMED CONSENT AND RIGHT TO TREATMENT

Policy related to researchers' use of individuals with impaired decision making capacity is one of the most important areas in neuroethics.[15] Researchers generally consider policy issues regarding informed consent a boring and uninteresting kind of problem, thus neglecting it.[15] As a result, state legislatures are in charge of making decisions about who counts as a legally authorized representative. This is problematic because it has a direct effect on the kind of research institutions will support and promote.

Consent is an ongoing process that should involve education of the potential research participant and when necessary, family members. Researchers must exercise greater caution to safeguard as well as enhance participants' understanding of the study, including its risks and benefits.[10,15] One growing concern proposed by neuroethicists is that new technologies and those who exercise them should be cautious to prevent the marginalization of people with disabilities, individuals at risk, and those unable to make informed decisions.[10,15] Children and individuals who are disabled with impaired decision making capacity are the most vulnerable and prone to being exploited.[10] Special care must be taken in the informed-consent process and throughout research protocols when individuals demonstrate mild-to-moderate cognitive or emotional impairments that might affect their decision making capacity.

In the case of individuals suffering from Alzheimer's disease, clinicians can recognize and follow the well-defined current standards of practice for those with considerable cognitive impairments (i.e., next of kin or competency evaluations for legal adjudication of guardianship). However, in other cases treatment and consent for clinical research is vexed with imprecise standards. We have a slippery slope when deciding if individuals with moderate-to-severe cognitive or emotional impairments should be treated. Although for most cases federal guidelines exist, there is limited agreement from one institution to the next, leaving the decision making to institutional review boards (IRBs), whose composition, knowledge, and skills can at times be ambiguous. The slope gets even more slippery in the case of those who experience mild cognitive deficits. At first glance, they appear to be normal. Most therapists have the tendency to think that these individuals can make decisions about clinical care; whether or not to participate in research; and most importantly, understand the implications of their actions. Research however demonstrates that apart from having memory impairments, they have no understanding for the long-term effects of their actions.[9,32] What does this mean and why is it important? It means

that neuroscientists cannot only measure cognitive capacity but as technology continues to be refined, questions about statistically aberrant behaviors will be addressed, thus exploring what these abnormalities mean for the neural basis of moral reasoning.[33] It is important because if today we have a slippery slope in terms of deciding if we treat or do not treat individuals with Alzheimer's or other traumatic brain injuries, tomorrow they may not have a chance. It will all depend on the ethics and moral principles of what is valuable, acceptable, and consistent with society standards.

In time and with the advances in neurotechnology, scientists may be able to clearly discern between normal and abnormal patterns of brain activity. Therefore, it is imperative that clinicians performing research pay close attention and get involved in legal consent and right to treatment issues to help develop policies that will safeguard individuals' needs as well as promote much needed research.

✧ SUPPORTING THE PATIENT'S RIGHT TO CHOOSE

The acceptance of risk is a political and ethical issue in these modern times. Many therapists, in their authoritarian wisdom, deem that risks must be eliminated and crusade to that end. They do not do so to lower risks to themselves (that is already within their power). They do so to lower the risks of others. This motivation is a natural extension of the role of therapists in which they must protect patients from dangers patients do not recognize. In addition, just as some therapists hold back their patients through overprotection, many politicians and health care insurers allocate huge resources to combating increasingly smaller risks, marginalizing and hindering the patient's right to choose.

Neurological enhancers are not likely to be exempt from such actions. Neurological enhancers and technology may indeed pose significant risks as well as a significant potential for abuse. Most human activities and technologies do. Where the line will ultimately be drawn between use of neurological enhancers and access to their benefits will be a part of the role clinicians need to consider in their daily practice. Despite the present lack of exposure to the subject matter in professional educational programs, it is the responsibility of rehabilitation professionals to stay informed of new scientific trends and discoveries. Only then can they advocate and provide their clients with professional and well-informed advice. In addition, therapists should support the right of adults to decide for themselves what is in their best interest and the best course of action to achieve their goals. Doing so requires knowledge and awareness of available resources and the risks each entails.

✧ PHARMACOLOGY-RELATED CHALLENGES

Brain research is giving rise to a rapidly growing class of drugs known as psychopharmaceuticals.[4] These drugs promise to increase memory retention, even out the rough spots in our moods, and focus our attention when performing complex tasks. Some of the drugs include Prozac to fight depression and Ampalex to treat schizophrenia or memory deficits. In the future, medications may enhance the mind by boosting memory. Scientists predict that compounds developed to treat Alzheimer's disease will lead to substances that boost cognition.[19] A case in point is compound CX516. CX516 is an ampakine that improves memory in elderly individuals and patients with schizophrenia.[34] Ampakine affects and enhances the activity of AMPA-type glutamate receptors, complexes of proteins that are involved in communication between neurons.[34] Glutamatergic transmission between neurons is by far the brain's most abundant communication system.[35] When a neuron releases glutamate and binds to the AMPA receptor, Ampakine compounds increase or magnify the effect of glutamate, thereby amplifying normal brain signals.[36]

Although the statistical and predictive aspect of neuroscientific data is extremely important, rehabilitation professionals have a deeper ethical understanding to pursue. That is, rather than deal with pharmacological neuroenhancers only within the narrow contexts of cog-

nition, intelligence, and memory, therapists must also deal with them in regards to all aspects of human performance. Any drug (or nutrient) that enhances aspects of mental performance can be considered a neurological enhancer. When therapists speak of cognitive or neurological enhancement, they should include the entire myriad of mental functions that go into making us what we are, including such obvious aspects as intelligence and memory, but also aspects of meaningful daily living activities, such as habits, routines, and occupations. This is because much of our knowledge of physiological reactions of the immune system is paired with knowledge of neuroendocrine regulation. These are all vital aspects of human health and well-being, which are related to the functioning of the brain and the survival of the mind. After all, when the ongoing brain mapping of the body is entirely absent or momentarily suspended, a radical interruption in the flow of body information that supports our feelings occurs, obliterating our thoughts of objects and situations.[9] In the ethical principle of do no harm, these are fundamental issues for professional and scientific reflection.

Rehabilitation practice, for the most part, is concerned with individuals' quality of life, ability to perform daily activities safely, and mental health. Cognitive deficits and therefore pharmacologically induced enhancement therapy raise new questions for rehabilitation practice. How will we approach those who, although "healthy" in our eyes, believe they can do better? How will notions of what we considered "normal" change based on drug therapy enhancement? And, how will present tools and assessments used to measure cognitive impairments inevitably change?

Presently, we know that the loss of cholinergic neurons is responsible for many of the cognitive deficits in Alzheimer's disease.[16] Discussions around the use of memory enhancement medications are already on the way, not only to improve memory in those with fatal illness, but also to improve the memory of healthy individuals. Memory enhancement is of prevalent interest in middle-age and beyond, when the normal process of memory loss is first noticeable in healthy individuals. At any rate, the aging of the baby boomers and their unwillingness to go quietly into the night provides a big incentive for drug companies to come out with compounds that will help this cohort think more clearly.

Rejuvenation of memory function in healthy individuals is a form of memory enhancement with broad appeal. Many drug companies are presently directing enormous research efforts to the development of memory-boosting drugs. These drugs target various stages in the molecular cascade that underlies memory formation, including presynaptic neurotransmitter release (such as donezipil) and postsynaptic effect known as ampakines.[34] These drugs are being used for the treatment of dementia and what we labeled as "mild cognitive impairments," which is more severe than normal age-related cognitive decline.

Today, no pharmaceutical company has yet targeted normal memory for enhancement but there is reason to believe that some of the drugs under development would work for that purpose as well. For example, in clinical trials healthy human subjects treated with ampakine showed improved performance in several memory tests.[11,37] If this happens, will rehabilitation practitioners' views and ways of treatment change for those who do not have access to enhancement drugs? Will we deem individuals as poor rehabilitation candidates based on the lack of accessibility to drug enhancement therapy treatment? Will it mean that acute care interventions will only be offered to those with full access to the array of technological and pharmacological advances rendering the less fortunate to nursing homes and the like? Does it mean that practice will hold a double standard for the haves and the have nots?

❖ OVERALL IMPLICATIONS OF NEUROETHICS IN CLINICAL PRACTICE

Neuroscience discoveries and predictions can have major effects in the practice of rehabilitation as well as in society. The information provided by neuroimaging tests has serious consequences for individuals' future access to care, employment, insurance, family relations, and for that matter, personal happiness.

The practice of rehabilitation is presently driven by evidence-based practice. Evidence-based practice calls for the need to demonstrate how clinical interventions aid to facilitate individuals in returning to normal and productive social lives. How would practitioners determine intervention effectiveness based on a double standard of practice wherein one client is coping with traditional treatment interventions while others have access to enhancement drugs? Will practitioners determine treatment interventions based on drugs that enhance brain activity and therefore reduce length of treatment interventions to measure rehabilitation outcomes, thus, limiting access to care to those who do not? How do we guarantee a fair and equitable right to treatment to those unable to access these drugs? How would normal cognitive capacity be defined and by whom? After all, what is normal if it is not a slippery term. I think of it as a distribution and not as a point.[13]

❖ CONCLUSIONS

The future of neurosciences will bring new ways of enhancing, manipulating, and mapping the brain. The drive behind neuroscientific research is a humanitarian one—finding ways to help individuals who are disabled—and indeed it raises the hope that maybe one day cognitive deficits will be a thing of the past, or that people with paralysis will be able to control complex devices with their minds. However, all of these discoveries will reduce the range of ways that it is acceptable to be. If more healthy adults use memory enhancers does it mean to our society that we are all more confident, assertive, resilient people? What does it mean for rehabilitation practice? How do we serve our moral and ethical duty of do no harm in the face of individuals' inequitable access to enhancing drugs and therefore, care? It seems that neuroscience and its byproduct, neuroethics, will set a new pace reaching well beyond our present scientific methods and applications.

Brain science can provide us with better therapeutic efficacy, and even better predictive power. In return, these outcomes will significantly change the way we look at our patients and the way we view and understand our clinical practice. In the past, rehabilitation professionals have seldom, if ever, played an active role in these demanding and pressing ethical issues, focusing instead on everyday ethics and relationship-centered ethics. Thus, it is crucial that therapists actively engage in the already present and upcoming debates posed by the field of neuroethics. In addition, the importance of this area for future research requires that physical therapists and occupational therapists have a superior and sophisticated understanding of ethics so that they can obtain the necessary skills to sort through complicated problems that arise at the boundaries of neuroscience and ethics.

Therapists have a special responsibility in the area of neuroethics. This responsibility derives in part from their obligation to clients, many of whom stand to be affected by neurotechnological developments. Of particular concern are the issues of distributive justice and responsibility. Throughout history, dating back to Aristotle, Western ethics have considered individuals as moral rational agents whose decisions are divorced from emotional content.[8] Moreover, we have shared the moral understanding that responsibility is linked to control. Neuroethics however challenge these notions in two ways. First, ethical and emotional behaviors are linked. Hence, we need to take emotion seriously and integrate it in some way with our current models. Second, new research demonstrates that our behavior is not always subject to our control.[9]

Therapists might be inclined to assume that individuals' intact social knowledge and practice of social problem solving prior to the onset of brain damage would be sufficient to ensure normal social behavior and therefore be accountable for their actions. Nevertheless, this is not the case. The realistic knowledge about social behavior requires the brain structures of emotion and feeling to work normally.[14] Sadly, the individuals' perception of right or wrong, good or bad is substantially and chronically at variance with what is considered social normal behavior.

Educators must create a milieu to facilitate the integration of the necessary skills and knowledge for clinical practitioners to tackle the ethical issues presented by new technolo-gies. Critical examination of the legal and social concerns of neuroscientific advances is necessary to understand its effect in the future of rehabilitation services. It is important to underscore the imperative need for educators and practitioners to engage in a scholarly discourse that explores and proposes a moral framework that can help guide the utilization of the new scientific advances and knowledge that neuroscience brings about.

References
1. Kennedy D: Are there things we'd rather not know? Paper presented at: Neuroethics: Mapping the Field, 2002, San Francisco, CA.
2. Borod JC, et al: Neuropsychological assessment of emotional processing in brain-damaged patients. In Borod JC (ed): The Neuropsychology of Emotion. Oxford University Press, New York, 2000.
3. Borod JC, ed.: Neuropsychology of Emotion: An Overview and Research Directions. Oxford University Press, New York, 2000.
4. Hyman S: Ethical issues in pharmacology: research and practice. Paper presented at: Neuroethics: Mapping the Field, 2002, San Francisco, CA.
5. Parens E: How far will the term enhancement get us as we grapple with new ways to shape our selves? Paper presented at: Neuroethics: Mapping the Field, 2002, San Francisco, CA.
6. Wolpe PR: Neurotechnology, cyborgs and the sense of self. Paper presented at: Neuroethics: Mapping the Field, 2002, San Francisco, CA.
7. Mobley W: Summary of the conference. Paper presented at: Neuroethics: Mapping the field, 2002, San Francisco, CA.
8. Churchland P: The engine of reason, the seat of the soul: A philosophical journey into the brain. MIT Press, Cambridge, MA, 1995.
9. Damasio A: Looking for Spinoza: Joy, Sorrow, and the Feeling Brain. Harcourt, Inc, New York, 2003.
10. Hall Z: Mapping the future of neuroethics. Paper presented at: Neuroethics: Mapping the Field, 2002, San Francisco, CA.
11. Greene J, et al: An fMRI investigation of emotional engagement in moral judgment. Science 293:2105–2108, 2001.
12. Caplan A: No-brainer: Can we cope with the ethical ramification of new knowledge of the human brain? Paper presented at: Neuroethics: Mapping the Field, 2002, San Francisco, CA.
13. Greely H: Neuroethics and ELSI: Some comparisons and considerations. Paper presented at: Neuroethics: Mapping the Field, 2002, San Francisco, CA.
14. Damasio A: The neural bases of social behavior: Ethical implications. Paper presented at: Neuroethics: Mapping the Field, 2002, San Francisco, CA.
15. Moreno JD: Gaging ethics. Paper presented at: Neuroethics: Mapping the Field; May 13–14, 2002, San Francisco, CA.
16. Kolb B, and Whishaw IQ: An Introduction to Brain and Behavior. Worth Publisher, New York, 2001.

17. Freeman W: Societies of Brains: A Study in the Neuroscience of Love and Hate. Lawrence Erlbaum Associates, Inc., Hillsdale, 1995.

18. Freeman W: Neurodynamics: An Exploration in Mesoscopic Brain Dynamics. Springer-Verlag, New York, 2002.

19. Winslade WJ: Traumatic brain injury and legal responsibility. Paper presented at: Neuroethics: Mapping the Field, 2001, San Francisco, CA.

20. Farwell LA, and Dunchin, E: The "Brain Detector": P300 in the Detection of Deception. Psychophysiology 24:434, 1986.

21. Fukumaya F: Our Posthuman Future: Consequences of the Biotechnology Revolution. Farrar, Straus & Girous, New York, 2002.

22. Kramer PD: Listening to Prozac. Penguin, New York, 1993.

23. DuVal G, et al: What triggers requests for ethics consultations? J Med Ethics 27:124–129, 2001.

24. Rolls E: Neurophysiology and functions of the primate amygdale, and the neural basis of emotion. In Aggleton JP (ed): The Amygdala: A Functional Analysis. Oxford University Press, New York, 2002.

25. Farwell LA, et al: Specific memory deficit in elderly subjects who lack A P300. Psychophysiology 23:589, 1985.

26. Broughton R, et al: Homicidal somnambulism: A case report. Sleep 17(3):253–264, 1994.

27. LexUM: R. vs. Parks. Montreal LtatCotUo. Supreme Court Reports. LexUM [internet]. Accessed January 20, 2004.

28. Moreno JD: Neuroethics: An agenda for neuroscience and society. Nat Rev Neurosci 4(2):149–153, 2003.

29. Blank RH: Brain Policy: How the New Neuroscience Will Change Our Lives and Our Politics. Georgetown University Press, Washington, DC, 1999.

30. Foot P: Virtues and Vices and Other Essays in Moral Philosophy. Blackwell: Oxford: University of California Press, Berkeley, 1978.

31. Nussbaum M: A Classical Defense of Reform in Liberal Education. Harvard University Press, Cambridge, 1999.

32. Albert M: Ethical challenges in Alzheimer's disease. Paper presented at: Neuroethics: Mapping the Field, 2002, San Francisco, CA.

33. Illes J, Kirschen MP, and Gabrieli J: From neuroimaging to neuroethics. Nat Neurosci 6(3):205, 2003.

34. Ingvar M, et al: Enhancement by an ampakine of memory encoding in humans. Exp Neurology 146:553–559, 1997.

35. Czubayko UP, D. Fast synaptic transmission between striatal spiny projections neurons. Graybiel AM. PNAS. Available at: http://www.cortexpharm.com/pdfs/COR_Lynch_11–02 pdf. Accessed January 20, 2004.

36. Lynch G: Memory enhancement: the search for mechanism-based drugs. Nat Neurosci 5(Suppl):1035–1038, 2002

37. Yesavage JA, et al: Donepezil and flight simulator performance: Effects on retention of complex skills. Neurology 59:123–125, 2002.

15

The Ethics of Client-Centered Care Models*

PANELPHA L. KYLER, MA, OTR, FAOTA

A b s t r a c t

Ethical concepts within health professions support the efficacy of inclusion of families and the recipients of care into discussions regarding health- or education-related decisions. Health professions often use the language of client-centered and family-centered care, to imply a partnership in the decision making process. Called by a variety of names and written about in a variety of ways, client-centered, family-centered, autonomy, and deliberative decision making all share the universal standard of substantive inclusion of the primary individual and his or her family as part of the decision making process.

Client-centered care viewed from the medical community is one of several models for practitioner-client relationships. Models for physician-client relationships include: the paternalistic model in which the physician acts as the client's guardian; the informative model that assumes a clear distinction between facts provided by the physician and the client's views; the interpretive model where the physician helps the client articulate his or her values in determining the medical intervention, and the deliberative model where the physician discusses health-related values that are affected by the client's disease or treatment.[1] The important variations of the models are concepts regarding client autonomy and the physician's (practitioner) role as technical expert, teacher, healer, guardian, or advisor. Emanuel and Emanuel noted that if the aim of the physician (practitioner) is to help the client determine the best health-related value, a deliberative model could be used.[1] In this model the physician acts as a teacher or friend engaging the client in a dialogue about options. What lessons may be learned from these physician-based models? Are they synonymous with occupational and physical therapy's concepts of client-centered care? This article will explore the ethical concepts inherent in client-centered care, family-centered care, and the physician-based deliberative model.

✧ INTRODUCTION

In this article I discuss the various definitions of client-centered versus family-centered care and indicate how inclusion of the individual or family may or may not take place within each model. Intertwined in these brief discussions are the ethical issues that we need to view through the lens of professionals and recipients of services. Initially I shall describe the goals for client-centered care and for family-centered care noting that all

*Developed in part for the U.S. Department of Health and Human Services, HRSA Grant #1 D37 HP 00824–01. Leadership Institute in Ethics Education for OT and PT Educators.

of the varieties of models for client–health professional participation have some degree of questions and concerns that must be considered prior to implementation. Finally, I shall discuss the application of the model of choice to the health professions of occupational therapy and physical therapy.

Concepts of Inclusion: Client-Centered Care

Client-centered care (Fig. 15.1) is a concept that speaks to a universal standard of substantive inclusion of the primary individual as part of the decision making health care process.[1-7]

The terminology has come to education and health care from a variety of sources, but all share the motivational features of trying to establish a relationship that will provide a good outcome in keeping with the desires and values of the client. The client-centered approach focuses explicit attention on models designed to involve the individual collaboratively in contrast to previously prevalent expert-driven approaches.[1,4,5] Client-centered approaches, emphasize professionals as agents of the individual who intervene in ways to help the individual act as autonomously as possible, protect that person's integrity, and strengthen family functioning. Adopting a client-centered approach often requires the professionals to apply a shift in attitudes as they try to deliver good quality services. Many health professionals and other staff members assumed that they, as health care experts, know what is best for clients. An orientation to the client-centered approach recognizes that clients' concerns and preferences are valid and important. Individuals come to the decision making process recognizing their preferences, values, goals, and expected outcomes. This approach also recognizes a contemporary vision of inclusion and dialogue among all parties that is a give-and-take and

accepts the decision making process as one where individuals make decisions based upon a dialogue and input by the health providers and individuals.

Concepts of Inclusion: Family-Centered Care

The family-centered (Fig. 15.2) approach is somewhat similar and yet markedly different from the client-centered approach.

A family-centered approach engages the familial unit in the decision making process. The familial unit can be seen as a "group of individuals with interrelated lives such that changes in one family member affect all other members."[8] It should be noted that concepts of family are to some degree controversial and changeable. Embedded in the complex relationships of families and their obligations to the person about to make a health care decision are issues regarding social, financial, emotional, and rehabilitative risks and burdens as they may affect the family unit and the individual. Family-centered care requires health care professionals to consider whether the family as a unit has enough information to make a decision, whether the family is properly motivated, and whether the treatment decisions are in accord with what the client would elect.[9] This approach also requires a communication process that considers multiple receivers of the message and the beneficial versus the benign motivation of the family. Family-centered care may have some unintended consequences in that clients are especially vulnerable, in many cases have been placed in a health care facility, and are not always in the position to defend their interests fairly. The clients have unique views and treatment decisions affect them in a very vivid and concrete way that does not affect the family members.[10] The imposition of family values on the uniquely personal perspective of the individual and his or her values and concepts of health is difficult and not always a tidy process. Issues of personal privacy, implied coercion, and integrity filter throughout the family-centered care concept. Hardwig noted, "A fundamental assumption of medical ethics: medical treatment ought to serve the interests of the client. This of course implies

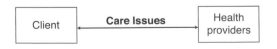

Figure 15.1 ❖ The client-centered approach with direct communication between the client and provider.

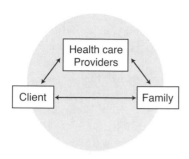

Figure 15.2 ✦ The family-centered approach wherein communication is among the health provider, client, and family.

that the interests of family members should be irrelevant to medical treatment decisions or at least never ought to take precedence over the interest of the client."[11] The family-centered process validates a dialogue method for a collective or common decision making practice. The family members must talk to one another and focus on the common good or common resolve for the good of the recipient of care and the family unit.

Concepts of Inclusion: Physician Deliberative Model

In 1956, Szasz and Hollender proposed a "model of mutual participation" in which "essentially, the physician helps the client to help himself."[12] Szasz and Hollender noted that this model is a far cry from the then dominant models of "activity-passivity" where the patient/client passively takes the direction from the physician who is actively directing the treatment and "guidance-cooperation" where the physician provides guided step-down choices and the patient/client is cooperative in following those choices. These models were widely used in the management of chronic illnesses, such as diabetes, arthritis, and tuberculosis. They were not only preferable but essential. Nearly four decades later, Emanuel and Emanuel advocate a deliberative model of physician-client interaction that also requires the client's active involvement.[1] In the Emanuel deliberative model "the aim of the physician-client interaction is to help the client determine and choose the best health-related values that can be realized in the clinical situation."[1] In

both the Szasz and Emanuel models, the physicians (health professional) and clients are communicating on an adult-to-adult level versus a parent-infant or parent-child level. The communication processes are central to medicine and are grounded in a covenant of trust. Similarly communication is a core aspect to the therapist-client relationship where the therapist is involved with teaching or facilitating client learning. Enhancing cooperation or motivating clients is an essential aspect of the therapist's intervention.[13]

In 1996, Dr. Richard Glass noted that the client-physician relationship was under siege, thus causing distress resulting in a negative experience for both. He noted that there was tension between the science and the art of medicine.[14] Today, in the era of new technology, the ancient therapeutic art of listening is being ignored, thus leading to an empathy gap and poor collaboration. The Szasz and Emanuel models attempt to overcome the listening gap.[1,12] The deliberative model recognizes as obstacles that the values of the individual may be different than the values of the physician, and that once discussions occur they may easily metamorphose into unintended paternalism.[1] A classic example of value differences may include the value of individuals regarding the sick role concept versus the values of the physician toward getting people well. The physician, occupational therapist, or physical therapist may view illness from a biomedical model, where there are mechanistic malfunctions or a microbiological invasion; however, the person may view the sick role as a temporary, medically sanctioned form of deviant behavior. The individuals who may be in the "sick role" may be excused from their usual duties and are considered not responsible for their condition. The individual may be absent from the workforce and family duties, including offering others support and participating in decision making discussions.

✦ ETHICAL ISSUES

With the various models of inclusion—client-centered care, family-centered care, and the deliberative model—communication is critical. However, sometimes the communication is somewhat superficial and fails to actively consider the ethical issues that may have an impact on decision making processes and the anticipated health outcome. Ethicists have asked, "What about the family and what about the client?" These rhetorical questions help to focus the health provider on the outcome of intervention and to improve the client's adherence to treatment. The prevalent ethic of client autonomy fails to consider issues requiring the family to sacrifice their interests so the client may have the treatment she or he wants. Interests of families should not be irrelevant to the health care treatment decisions nor should they take precedence over the primary needs of the client.[11] In order to preserve the moral relevance of the family, a concept of collective decision making or family as beneficiary of the decision making, the deliberative model could be considered. Concepts of the common good pervade this thinking and provide the health care professionals with the added burdens of viewing an individual's needs through the lens of many and incorporating many voices into the conversation prior to the health care decision. In some cases, treatment considerations and options for the client are intensified by the added issues of familial interpersonal conflict and stress.[9] In some cases, these questions and concerns are ignored or not recognized as important because of the fundamental ethical concept of serving the interest of the client.

Traditional perspectives of trust and autonomy are included in client-centered and family-centered care. However, it is sometimes difficult for health care providers to view clients as fully able to participate and partner in the process of health care decisions when families have different and incompatible desires and interests. The concept of trust in the individual doctor-patient (client) relationship is a covenantal one, because the patient relies on the doctor in illness, medical decisions have a holistic character, and doctors display personal commitment.[15] These traits are still true today in the managed-care arena and are also true for the relationship other health professionals have with their clients. Others recognize that when working with a family the needs of the family must be assessed, but the way the intervention is deliv-

ered by the therapist should also allow the family to be enabled and empowered.[7-10] Within these working partnerships concepts of autonomy play out in a variety of ways. Dworkin noted that in medical ethics the concept of autonomy has played a major role, but has also undergone a shift from authority of the physician (paternalism) to one shared by physician and clients, to one giving the ultimate authority to the clients.[16] The concern embodied by this shift from authority of the physician to authority of the client is one of trust and trusting relationships. By whom and how much information is provided and how much confidence does one have in the information provider? Is the information skewed by personal values that are not in keeping with a health care decision making setting? Hence, in keeping with Emanuel's model of deliberative decision making, health care providers must come to the treatment process ready to accept clients as partners. They must also be ready to accept or at least not distort personal values that may be different than their own.

Howe indicates to clinicians that how care providers intervene is of critical importance. Telling the client what to do before earning their trust is a cardinal mistake and may cause future efforts to backfire.[17] Indeed, because of the importance of clients' outcomes, the deficiencies of any model that excludes clients is clear. The absence of the client's active involvement in the decision making process and the articulation of functional goals may affect treatment adherence.[13] Although the client-centered focus increases the emphasis on the quality of the therapeutic encounter between clients and the occupational or physical therapists, this focus may not provide for input from the family and not provide for deliberative decision making. The therapeutic intervention must be skillfully implemented and must include the client in the context of his or her life. If this focus is absent, the intervention may fail.

Failing to consider families and pay heed to familial conflicts with efforts to listen, mediate, or facilitate an acceptable health care decision is a clear indication that the family-centered care concept is disingenuous and not seriously taking the family into consideration.

Concepts of Inclusion: Partnership

Partnership brings with it the paradox of the juxtaposition of paternalism and autonomy. Partnership literature discusses the role of partnerships in client-centered care and family-centered care as part of an equation.[1,5,18] A partnership in the context of child health care differs from partnership in the adult context. In many cases, the parents are the advocates for the child, who often until reaching the age of majority has no legal voice. Parents act as case managers for their child, carrying information between the medical community and the educational community. They are often lobbying for full services, and see as their roles the changing of the professional's attitude regarding the abilities of their child with special health needs as well as helping their child experience options for self-determination in education and living. The roles are often played out within the context of client-centered or family-centered care. Partnership in the adult context has been defined differently and has been a source of contention within the medical community for years. Literature abounds with different perspectives regarding how to include, when to include, and why to include the appropriate decision maker in health care decisions.[1,19-21] Occupational therapy has taken on the topic of partnerships in the decision making process in a variety of ways; however, the literature that has gotten the most currency has been that which focused on client-centered care.[2,4,22] Physical therapy has also discussed concepts of partnerships relative to positive outcomes of interventions and they have often used the language of the patient-practitioner model.[23]

In the patient-practitioner collaborative model, the focus is on consideration of the physical therapy intervention based upon the patient's needs.[13] Without this consideration the practitioner may do a preliminary evaluation that focuses on diagnosis rather than the individual's experience with illness or the representation to the physical or occupational therapist of what went wrong.

However, client-centered care may well be, or may not be, the best approach to produce the best end results of treatment. Indeed, each of the above models—client-centered care, family-centered care, and the deliberative model— has pluses and minuses. Another model, the relationship-centered model (Fig. 15.3) may offer health providers an alternative to the current inclusion models.

✧ DISCUSSION

Each model provides something for health providers to consider. The individual and family perspectives are important components to the overall health and healing process. In many ways, occupational and physical therapies have viewed themselves as professions that embrace a client-centered approach; however, there is evidence that there can be differences between the perspectives of the clients and the professionals. Problems may arise in the definition of the health problem as it relates to function or the goals to be attained. In some areas, the occupational and physical therapy intervention is mandated by law, such as Individuals with Disabilities Education Act (IDEA: P.L. 101–476).Within IDEA, the focus changed from one that merely provided disabled children access to an education to one that strengthens the role of parents in educational planning and decision making on behalf of their children. Thus the family's involvement in partnership with the occupational or physical therapy practice is essential. In other areas, the occupational or physical therapy professionals are aware that those who are interested in obtaining additional knowledge may not be motivated to participate in actual decision making. The client-therapist relationship may more likely resemble the "physician-as-agent" model. In this case, the client (the knowledge-acquirer) provides some personal values to the therapist. By possessing the health knowledge and learning about clients' values and beliefs, the therapists may be the formulator of the final decision. Though the client may not actively pursue outside sources of information prior to the clinical visit, there still may be interest in learning more about the health condition or treatment decided on by the occupational or physical therapists.

The phrase relationship-centered care captures the importance of the interaction among

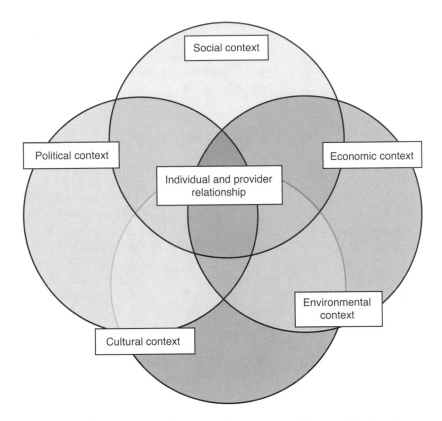

Figure 15.3   ✧   The relationship-centered approach includes consideration of the individual and internal as well as external influences in a fluid and changing manner.

people with their environment and other people as the foundation of any therapeutic or healing activity.[24] Relationship-centered care is an iteration of the older Szasz approach that considers mutual participation merged with the newer Emanuel approach that considers the best health-related values in a particular clinical situation. Determinants of health and illness lie not only within individuals, but also within our social, economic, environmental, cultural, and political contexts.[24] These contextual determinants are part of the family dynamics and are part of the external factors that influence decisions. We are coming to understand health not as the absence of disease, but rather as the process by which individuals maintain their sense of coherence (i.e., sense that life is comprehensible, manageable, and meaningful) and ability to function in the face of changes in themselves and their relationships with their families and their environment.[24]

In a relationship-centered approach there are multiple layers of communication and external factors that have an impact on the decision making process. These layers are flexible and one adds or subtracts depending upon the individual and his or her needs. This understanding challenges health professionals to identify the factors inhibiting healing and help the client and family strengthen and release healing power. Supportive family relationships are one of the factors promoting healing and the relationship between the health professional, the client, and family is another major factor in promoting healing. Just as the relationship has the power to do well, it also has the potential for harm if, for example, the client or family feels misunderstood, demeaned, or rejected.[24] These multiple determinants are important deliberative components. Health professionals' relationships with their clients and the clients' families are central to health care and are the vehicles for putting into action a paradigm of health that integrates listening, caring, deliberation, and decisions. This paradigm also focuses the health professionals' ethical obligation of acknowledging the unique factors at work within families and individuals as they go through any decision making process.

A fundamental tenet of both professions is to help achieve patient benefits. The concept of paternalism, that of a wise and caring father, comes down to us from the physician-client relationship that viewed the physician as a guardian with recognized, specialized knowledge who works tirelessly for the benefit of those in need of his care. Within medicine, strong paternalistic concepts have diminished in favor of the more inclusive concepts. Occupational therapy and physical therapy have revised their codes of ethics. Both professions have moved from traditional paternalistic codes of ethics to social justice codes built upon the tenets of beneficence, caring for the well-being of the recipients of therapy services. Both professions do recognize the importance of understanding clients in the context of their life experiences. As such, beneficence is a moral principle that occupational therapists and occupational therapy assistants, physical therapists and physical therapy assistants are expected to provide for and maintain. One comes to understand and embrace concepts of beneficence in clinical practice by providing a degree and level of recognition, understanding, and fidelity to those being served. As an example, it is important for occupational and physical therapists to understand and embrace elements of family-centered care, recognition that the family is the constant in a sick child's life while service providers may fluctuate. The sharing of ongoing, unbiased, and complete information during the course of occupational or physical therapy sessions in an appropriate and supportive manner is essential for client buy-in, as is recognition of the strengths of the individual and family and respect for different communication styles and different coping styles.[24] Occupational and physical therapies have to recognize that dialogues must take place in order for the clients and the families to gain benefit from the therapies.

A parallel to attaining comfort with the involvement of clients and recognition of their unique perspective on the therapeutic relationship is embedded in the road to cultural competency. The student section of the American Medical Association suggests the LEARN model guidelines for cultural competency.

Listen with sympathy and understanding to the patient's perception of the problem.

Explain your perceptions of the problem and your strategy for treatment.

Acknowledge and discuss the differences and similarities between these perceptions.

Recommend treatment while remembering the patient's cultural parameters.

Negotiate agreement. It is important to understand the patient's explanatory model so that medical treatment fits in their cultural framework.[25]

Each letter of this mnemonic indicates an action that is consistent with occupational and physical therapy practice and their codes of ethics. No matter what one's profession, the concepts embedded in respecting individuals and families requires occupational and physical therapists to be sensitive, reasoned, committed, and exhibit perseverance. This is the crux of a relationship-centered approach. Each therapy builds a relationship from the initial meeting whether it is a formal or informal interview, evaluation, or screening. It is the relationship with the clients in the context of those factors that is meaningful and important to the individuals and their sense of full participation. In some cases, it is just the client and in other cases it is the client in the context of a family unit. In addition, Rest, Bebeau, and others describe moral action as requiring four steps:[26]

Sensitivity: awareness of the potential ethical dimensions of a situation (e.g., the potential for conflicts of interest, options for action)

Reasoning: ability to identify that which is moral among competing options for action

Commitment: ability to choose moral values over personal ends

Perseverance: ability to persevere in spite of opposition (e.g., "everyone does it this way ...")

A combination of LEARN and the Rest and

Bebeau four steps for moral action offers steps or strategies for enhancing the client-therapist relationship.[25,26] In today's fast-pace delivery of therapy services, individuals or group practices may not have the time or the ability to take the time, for discussion of these four steps prior to or during formal or informal client conferences. Yet these components are essential for moving forward with a relationship-centered focus. As occupational and physical therapy think about their explanatory model for care, they must also think about the wants and needs of those they serve. They should also consider the ethical, social, and financial implications of services to the clients. The relationship-centered care approach considers the LEARN mnemonic and the moral action steps. Relationship-centered care fosters dialogue and is affirming or reaffirming for the clients. It thus captures the importance of the interaction among people as the foundation of any therapeutic or healing alliance, supports the ethical concepts within occupational therapy and physical therapy and supports the efficacy of inclusion of families and clients, the recipients of care, into discussions regarding health-related decisions.

✧ CONCLUSION

It is noteworthy that we tend to emphasize the relationship aspect with our clients. Central to our efforts is the development of a relationship or therapeutic alliance. There are several models for inclusion of the substantive voice of the individual or family into health care decision making processes. Occupational and physical therapists are familiar with client-centered care and family-centered care. However, the use of these models may at times pay short attention to the embedded ethical issues regarding lack of fluidity, influence of external factors, individual and group dynamics, and communication processes that may lead to implied paternalism and true lack of autonomy. Another model, the relationship-centered model based upon the work of Szasz and Hollender, offers occupational and physical therapists another approach to the inclusion of clients and families into the health care decision making processes. The relationship-centered approach asks us to be more open and consider the influences of internal and external drivers as they color the decision making processes. Most importantly, the relationship-centered model may be broadened by the basic knowledge of cultural sensitivity, as indicated with LEARN and broadened in ethical efficacy with the four-step moral action guide. This model is proposed to provide occupational and physical therapists with concrete steps to use in a variety of practice arenas—academic, research, and clinical practice.

In the end, I suggest to you that we must go beyond the diagnostic perspective and understand the challenges, which health professionals need to identify, inhibiting the healing. What is most important to health professionals and those we call our clients is a relationship grounded in ethical consideration and based upon the values of trust, communication, and respect. These qualities are part of a relationship-centered approach.

References

1. Emanuel EJ, and Emanuel LL: Four models of physician-patient relationship. JAMA 267(16):2221–2227, 1992.
2. Department of National Health and Welfare and Canadian Association of Occupational Therapy: Guidelines for the client-centered practice of occupational therapy. (H39-33/1983E). Department of National Heath and Welfare, Ottawa, ON, 1983.
3. Goetz AL, Gavin W, and Lane SJ: Measuring parent/professional interaction in early intervention: validity and reliability. Occup Ther J Res 22(4):222–240, 2000.
4. Law M, Baptiste S, and Mills J: Client-centered practice: What does it mean and does it make a difference? Can J Occup Ther 62:250–257, 1995.
5. Lawlor MC, and Mattingly CF: The complexities embedded in family-centered care. Am J Occup Ther 52:260–267, 1998.
6. Nachshen JS, and Jamieson J: Advocacy, stress and quality of life in parents of children with developmental disabilities. Develop Disabil Bull 28(1):39–55, 2000.
7. Sumsin T: Reflections on … client-centered practice: The truce impact. Can J Occup Ther 60:6–8, 1993.
8. Case-Smith J, Allen AS, and Pratt PN: Occupational Therapy for Children. ed 3. Elsevier Science Publishing Co Inc, 1996.
9. Hyun I: Conceptions of family-centered medical decision-making and their difficulties. Cambridge Quart Healthcare Ethics 12:196–200, 2003.
10. Nelson JL: Taking families seriously. Hastings Cent Rep 22(4):6–12, 1992.
11. Hardwig J: What about the family? Hastings Cent Rep 20(2):5–10, 1990.

12. Szasz TS, and Hollender MH: A contribution to the philosophy of medicine: The basic models of the doctor-client relationship. Arch Int Med 97:585–592, 1956.

13. Jensen GM, Lorish C, and Shepard KF: Understanding and influencing patient receptivity to change: The patient-practitioner collaborative model. In Shepard KF, and Jensen GM (eds): Handbook of Teaching for Physical Therapists. Butterworth-Heinemann, Boston, 2002, pp 323–350.

14. Glass RM: The patient-physician relationship. JAMA 275(2):147–148, 1996.

15. LaPuma J: Managed Care Ethics: Essays on the Impact of Managed Care on Traditional Medical Ethics. Hatherleigh Press, Hatherleigh, NY, 1998.

16. Dworkin G: Can you trust autonomy? Hastings Cent Rep 33(2):42–44, 2003.

17. Howe EG: Challenging patients' personal, cultural and religious beliefs. J Clin Ethics 13(4):259–273, 2003.

18. Klein BS: Reflections on … An ally as well as a partner in practice. Can J Occup Ther 62:283–285, 1995.

19. Wilkins S, et al: Implementing client-centered practice: Why is it so difficult to do? Can J Occup Ther 60.6–8, 2001.

20. Beisecker AE: Using metaphors to characterize doctor-patient relationships: Paternalism versus consumerism. Health Comm 5(1):41–58, 1993.

21. Kassirer JP: Adding insult to injury, usurping patients' prerogatives. N Engl J Med 308(15):898–900, 1983.

22. Clark FA, et al: Occupational science: Academic innovation in the service of occupational therapy's future. Am J Occup Ther 45(4):300–310, 1991.

23. Mostrom E: The wisdom of practice in a transdisciplinary rehabilitation clinic: Situated expertise and client centering. In Jensen GM, Gwyer J, Hack LM, and Shepard KF (eds): Expertise in Physical Therapy Practice. Butterworth-Heinemann, Boston, MA, 1999.

24. Roberts RN, Rule S, and Innocenti MS: Strengthening the Family-Provider Partnership in Services for Young Children. Brookes Publishing, Baltimore, 1998.

25. Berlin, EA, and Fowkes, WC: A teaching framework for cross-cultural care. West J Med 139: 934–938, 1983.

26. Rest JR, Bebeau MJ, and Volker J: An overview of the psychology of morality. In Rest JR (ed): Moral Development: Advances in Research and Therapy. Prager Publishers, Boston, 1986, pp 1–39.

16

Three Realms of Ethics: An Integrating Map of Ethics for the Future

John W. Glaser, STD

Abstract

The study of bioethics often, especially among health professionals, focuses on the health professional and patient (or other individual) relationship. This limited context serves important ends, but taken alone, distorts the true environment in which health professionals and others live and make moral decisions. A three-tiered partial paradigm of ethics designed to complement existing approaches is described in this chapter.

The first section of the chapter provides background information from many sources and introduces the notion of benevolence and beneficence as used in the paradigm. Benevolence is our inner attitude of "mind and heart relative to human dignity" and aims at affirming all that allows the human spirit to flourish. Beneficence refers to our specific external actions springing from benevolence but takes into account that hard choices must be made because the biddings of benevolence cannot always be realized toward all, due to practical constraints in our everyday lives within society. The foundation upon which benevolence and beneficence is based is the idea of human dignity as the inherent value that every person possesses by virtue of their individual and unique personhood. Some of the reasons we try to avoid hard choices are delineated.

The second and major section of the chapter describes three realms of beneficence or three realms of ethics—individual, organizational, and societal. The several dimensions at each level and the interaction among levels are described.

In the final section, the author provides conclusions and opportunities for further exploration within the three realms paradigm. He explores the potential of a "community of concern" and a shared common vision of community members, including two examples of moving from the individual to the societal realm as the basic orientation by which hard choices are analyzed and acted upon.

Health care ethics lacks a paradigm of ethics that integrates but also differentiates its various realms or dimensions. This is a costly lacuna that, in the judgment of many, leads to confusion and even significant harm to the enterprise of ethics.

Some 40 years ago, Catholic ethicist John Courtney Murray voiced a concern about the failure of Christian morality to recognize the "analogical character of the structures of life (personal, familial, political, social)."[1] Dennis Thompson raises a similar concern about levels of morality in his study of ethics in Congress. He comments, "the task of ethics reform ... should shift its focus from individual corruption to what is here called institutional corruption. ... Instead of simply generating more rules and mounting more investigations to prevent the familiar forms of individual corruption, we should put more effort into identifying the less familiar institutional forms and devising remedies appropriate to them."[2]

Richard Lamm identifies the same problem in medical ethics and warns that the current map of medical ethics "is leading to increasingly unethical public policy results. ... Medical ethics needs to be revised if it is to provide meaningful guides to future health policy. We need a new ethics map."[3]

In this chapter I address the concerns I share with Murray, Thompson, and Lamm to develop a paradigm that distinguishes and integrates three realms of ethics—individual, organizational, and societal. I want to clarify how and why all of these realms deal with the substance of ethics, but how there is need for significant distinctions between and among these realms. Figure 16.1 illustrates some basic features of this paradigm of layered and nested ethical unity and complexity.

The full picture of ethics includes a fourth realm—global ethics—which I will not discuss further because of the limited concerns of this chapter.[4,5] But I believe that the paradigm I am suggesting—a layered and nested *beneficence ethic*—calls for and is very compatible with this further dimension.

✧ ANOTHER MAP OF ETHICS?

A decade ago I offered this caution about mapping ethics, "Imagine that someone handed you a AAA road map of California and suggested that this represented the state. If you want to drive from Santa Ana to Sacramento, the statement is a valid one. But if you want to drill for oil, plant a vineyard, sell medical supplies, or run for public office, a map of California highways is the wrong map. I am concerned that too often in healthcare ethics we have taken one of many valid maps and treated it as if it were the one, true map of ethics."

Ethics, like friendship, marriage, or death, for example, is too rich a reality to fit into any simple, single conceptualization. As Samuel Johnson reminded us, "We are moralists perpetually, geometers only by accident." So morality is as broad and deep as life itself. It demands a correspondingly wide range of mental models and paradigms.

A strength of recent criticisms of medical ethics is their thrust to expand our understanding of ethics to better approximate the scope of reality. A weakness of some criticisms is that they give the impression that they have arrived with the true map. It seems obvious that the truth lies in no single map but in the complementarity of many essential maps.

This chapter intends to offer another *partial and complementary map* of ethics. It is only the beginning and more a sketch than a blueprint, but it is, I believe, a map that in its evolution and refinement will become increasingly useful in dealing with the growing challenges of our society and our organizations.

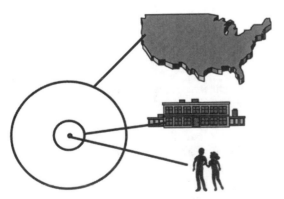

Figure 16.1 ✧   The figure illustrates some basic features of this paradigm of layered and nested ethical unity and complexity.

Human Dignity as Foundation of Ethics and The Moral Law

Our first step is to establish a common foundation of ethics that will then allow us to identify key differences and relationships within and between the three realms.

I propose that we think of ethics as *the disciplined and systematic effort to promote and protect human dignity*. As the starting point for ethics, I begin with the human experience that persons and their world are precious—they deserve our reverence, esteem, careful attention, and service. When we look to history we see that its moral heroes are persons who have brought sensitivity and passion to promoting human dignity.[6] Conversely, history's villains are consistently those who have disregarded and trampled the dignity of their fellow humans. Our experience further confirms that this is a moral *law*—much like the law of gravity—that we ignore at our own peril: to devalue and abuse the dignity of others leads inexorably to the erosion of our own humanity; to respect and champion human dignity correspondingly deepens our humanity.

By "human dignity" I mean the inherent value that every person possesses by virtue of their individual and unique personhood. This is what Kant points to with his notion that a person is an end and should never be treated as a means. It is what the U.S. Catholic bishops describe in religious terms, "The dignity of the human person, realized in community with others, is the criterion against which all aspects of economic life must be measured. ... When we deal with each other, we should do so with the sense of awe that arises in the presence of something holy and sacred."[7]

There are many perspectives from which we can view and describe this dignity including secular/philosophical and religious/theological; in terms of values and virtues; in terms of law and politics; in terms of ethics and aesthetics. The foundation for building this layered paradigm of ethics is the experienced value of human persons—"human dignity."

On the one hand, there is a clarity and simplicity about this foundation of ethics—respecting human dignity. On the other hand, we routinely experience how enormously difficult this can be—hence the need for the discipline of ethics. Because it will help develop my line of thought, I want to recall only two of the many reasons why respecting human dignity can be so tortuously difficult; first, human dignity is extremely complex; second, choices for human dignity here are choices against human dignity there.

Human Dignity is Extremely Rich and Complex

We are historical beings—placed in the flow of human history and developing individually through the "seven stages" of personhood. We are social and relational in a multilayered and evolving manner, from con-

ception to death. We are unique and individual. There are many schema for teasing apart this social/individual body-mind-spirit complexity. To mention only a few, we have Maslow's hierarchy of needs; we have the *Diagnostic and Statistical Manual of Mental Disorders* (DSM IV) categories of psychosocial deficits; we have the fields of human studies listed in a university's catalogue of course offerings. These and multiple other analyses remind us of the expanse and depth of this mystery that we refer to as human dignity.

Human Dignity and Finitude

Our hearts and minds create endless dreams but the reach of our serving hands is severely limited. Both philosophical and religious literature make a helpful distinction here between *benevolence* and *beneficence,* which can help us understand ethics and its service to human dignity.[8-10]

Benevolence refers to our *inner attitude* of mind and heart relative to human dignity. It aims at openness and affirmation of all human dignity; a readiness to cherish and reach out to all. Wherever there is human suffering, benevolence weeps; wherever the human spirit rises up in hope, so too does benevolence. *Beneficence* refers to our specific *external actions*, which spring from our disposition of benevolence. However, beneficence has no alternative but to make hard choices—decisions that serve human dignity here, in this way, at the cost of not serving dignity there, and in other ways.

Bruno Schüller illustrates this with the example of a physician who must cause her patient pain in order to provide needed care. He observes, "In such a situation one stands before two values that compete with one another. To realize one value a person must leave the other unrealized. One must then decide which of the values deserves priority. *If we look carefully we see here the characteristic and fundamental human condition: as a finite being, a person has only limited possibilities available for serving the neighbor's good. A person's actions cannot effectively benefit everyone, nor respond to any and every legitimate need and deficit. One must make a choice and decide which of those currently available possibilities deserves to be* selected. ... *In our daily lives we are not normally conscious of this constant choosing between competing values. In any case, we have become so accustomed to this unrelenting value preference that it hardly ever catches our attention* [emphasis added].[10]

The great Western thinker, Augustine of Hippo, provided a succinct statement of the key elements of this approach to ethics which I paraphrase in the following way: We must love everyone equally (benevolence), but since we cannot be of equal service to everyone (beneficence), we should choose those we will serve according to reasoned criteria (i.e., ethical methodology).

I want to emphasize that beneficence as I am using it here is radically different than its usage in bioethical discussions of the last decades. The prevailing bioethical understanding of beneficence interprets it as being virtually synonymous with a paternalistic attitude toward patients. Pellegrino and Thomasma comment, "This is the conception of beneficence still dominant in the minds of many physicians and patients; it still shapes the ethos and ethics of medicine. It is the conception, too, that is the focus of criticisms by proponents of autonomy who equate beneficence almost entirely with medical paternalism."[11]

The way I am using beneficence it does not carry any connotation of superiority or parentalism. Nor is it one of several moral principles; it is not a principle at all. Rather it is the fundamental action and reverential response of a finite moral agent to human dignity. The discipline of normative ethics (which is not the entirety of ethics) is the network of human systems and tools that individuals and communities use to discern where and how dignity should be served in a specific situation.

One might wonder why I would choose beneficence as a central concept when it is so burdened with negative connotations. I have done this because my intended meaning and the role of beneficence have a rich and long tradition measured in millennia. It has this longevity, I believe, because of the power it has to emphasize, integrate, and differentiate foundational realities of human moral existence. I prefer to work for the reestablishment of its profound and original meaning in Western thought, rather than leave it in its current diminished and blemished usage.

Hard Choices: An Overlooked Essential of Ethics

The insight that the fundamental situation of normative ethics always involves a hard choice—for some values to the detriment of others/for dignity here at the cost of dignity there—has found various expressions across millennia and traditions. Still, in my opinion, its cardinal importance has not been recognized and exploited for health care ethics. This is puzzling, and deserves some exploration before we move on.

Prominent authors—rather than identifying values-in-conflict as an essential dimension of ethical existence—explicitly identify this as an *occasional occurrence* in ethical experience. For example, we read, "Sometimes we confront two or more *prima facie* duties or obligations, one of which we cannot fulfill without sacrificing the other(s)."[12] Another author says, "It is clear that an increasing number of theologians insist on understanding moral norms within the conflict model of human reality. Conflicted values mean that occasionally our choices (actions or omissions) are inextricably associated with evil. Thus we cannot always successfully defend professional secrets without deliberately deceiving others..."[13] If, as I am claiming, such value conflicts are omnipresent, how might one explain that this very fabric of value existence and its centrality for ethics are so little noticed?

A partial explanation lies in Schüller's citation of Wittgenstein suggesting that "the aspects of things that are most important to us are concealed under their simplicity and their everyday nature. (One cannot notice the thing because it is always right in front of our eyes.)"[14] We can compare this to our breathing, to the structure of our mother tongue, to the rules of logic—we are inclined to notice these "infrastructures of life" only when they take the forms of aberrations or exaggerations. We only notice our breathing when we are "out of breath"; we spend weeks using our language without attending to its grammatical structure, until someone makes a grammatical mistake.

Then, too, most of the daily value conflicts are so disproportionate that their resolution is obvious and requires no explicit attention. Overlapping this consideration is the fact that macro life decisions—choice of profession, marriage, parenthood, and so forth—imply circles of subordinate micro-decisions that flow spontaneously from the priorities established in the macro-decision. Again, resolving the vast majority of our daily value conflicts takes place spontaneously and below the threshold of our attention. Further, our language usage and mental paradigms habitually direct our attention away from rather than toward this value conflict dimension of life. I think of an experience I had recently, which involved actions that could in certain circumstances qualify as battery, sexual assault, invasion of privacy, infliction of bodily pain, causing anxiety, and inflicting financial loss. How did I refer to this experience in my conversations? As my annual physical exam. That is, I name this actual conflict of values in terms of the preferred value(s) that I intend and that I judge to outweigh the disvalues involved. This is, perhaps, an essential characteristic of human perception and expression; and it points to a central task of ethics, namely to tease out hidden dimensions of life so that we can more consciously and responsibly take them in hand.

In this regard it is important to note how much language goes beyond being a mirror of life and functions as hammer and anvil of our conscious experience. Language shapes consciousness certainly as much as it reflects it.

Werner Stark suggests that we recognize the role of language as a mental grid. "We see the broad and deep acres of history through a mental grid. ... through a system of values which is established in our minds before we look out onto it—and it is this grid which decides ... what will fall into our field of perception."[15]

So we see that we can be *inattentive* to our finitude, but we cannot escape the hard choices that this finitude serves up, even in our sleep, or resting in our backyard.

Above we have looked at a basic understanding of ethics that I have characterized as *beneficence* (not used in its traditional bioethical meaning, but understood as) serving and protecting human dignity within the limited human condition. As Gustafson puts it, "the good is sought under the conditions of finitude."[16] My claim is not that this is the single best way to understand ethics, but that it is an excellent approach, for many reasons, and especially if we want to differentiate and integrate multiple levels of ethical complexity that are often conflated and seldom well integrated.

✧ THE THREE REALMS

In this section we will unpack the understanding of ethics-as-beneficence, and explore how beneficence spells itself out on three levels, individual, organization, and society (Fig. 16.2).

We will examine some key relationships between the three realms and finally make some limited applications.

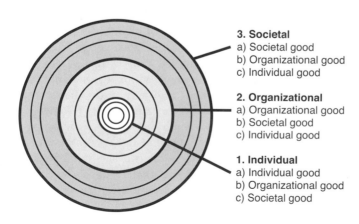

3. Societal
a) Societal good
b) Organizational good
c) Individual good

2. Organizational
a) Organizational good
b) Societal good
c) Individual good

1. Individual
a) Individual good
b) Organizational good
c) Societal good

Figure 16.2 ✧ Three Realms of Ethics/Beneficence

Individual Beneficence

The simplest realm of ethics/beneficence concerns individuals and their relationships: the relationships that exist within one individual between various values and needs. We can think of these values/needs in various ways— for example, in terms of Maslow's hierarchy of needs; or in terms of physical, emotional, mental, and spiritual. Individual beneficence grapples with differences in degree and intensity within and between these goods. For example, it must weigh the relative importance of intense physical good and moderate spiritual good. It attends to differences of probability and certainty; for example, between near certain emotional harm of a moderate degree and probable intellectual benefit to an extensive degree. It must attend to the whole range of comparable elements, such as long/short term, partial/ total, transient/abiding, direct/indirect, central/ peripheral.

This realm also deals with weighing and balancing the values/goods/ loyalties that stand in tension between two or more individuals. For example, we must weigh my privacy and your need to have information about me, or the need of one person's need for medical treatment and the danger of infection for the professional providing treatment. Again the issues of probability, long/short term trade-offs, degree and extent of harms and benefits all come into play.

Two issues are immediately evident: we are comparing apples and oranges—*all the time*; and there is no simple, math-like formula for weighing and balancing such "non-comparables." We can only marshal all the human powers of discernment—reasons, intuition, imagination, affect, humor; gifts of individuals, and the synergy of community (its centrality will be further discussed below); discipline and surprise, method and madness—to give ourselves the best chance to make such prudential judgments wisely and with consistency.

The first two decades of bioethics have dealt extensively with this realm of 1a. Most of this era's burning questions fit comfortably in this realm of individual good—patient autonomy, informed consent, privacy, patient rights, truth-telling, living wills, and confidentiality. George Amos, a pioneer and leading researcher in U.S. bioethics captures this focus and spirit when he says, "The core legal and ethical principle that underlies all human interactions in medicine is autonomy."[17]

But beyond the intra- and inter-individual issues are questions that treat sphere 1b: relationships of individuals to organizations. What responsibilities do patients, nurses, physicians have to their hospital? What trade-offs in income, safety, efficacy of treatment, and confidentiality can individuals be expected to make for the benefit of the institution?

Beyond this realm are issues in the sphere of l c: relationships of individuals to the common good of society. What personal benefits should I forego or burdens should I bear in order to make community benefits available or harms avoidable? For example, what limits on care, what delays or diminished quality should an individual accept in order that the whole community can be ensured of basic services?

So, in this realm of individual beneficence/ ethics there are three aspects: (1) within and between individuals; (2) from individuals toward organizations; and (3) from individuals toward the larger society

Organizational Beneficence

Normally, the use of the word beneficence has only individuals as its referent. The present analysis understands beneficence in terms of organizations as well. The social realities that I refer to as "organizations"—a family, a union, a business, a hospital, a religious community— have an identity, a purpose, a history, and character. They have vital systems that account for their vigor and health. They have commitments, claims, relationships, and responsibilities.

A primary object of organizational beneficence is the net organizational good—that is, a state of organizational vigor and development that enables the organization to maximize its purpose now and into the future. Those responsible for the organization must seek this net good just as individuals seek net good at an individual level. Obviously the resolution of beneficence choices, in terms of complexity and extent, increases exponentially at this level.

But such pursuit of the organizational good must also consider 2c: the individual good of those within the organization. For example, let us assume a demonstrated need for the good of a hospital to reduce its size. There are usually many ways to accomplish such a goal. The imperative of beneficence is to find the complex balance of burden/benefit distribution that serves organizational net good, but also attends to the needs of individuals.

An abiding central concern in this regard must be to create a workplace in which human dignity can flourish. In organizations this is accomplished primarily through organizational systems and structures. A simple rule of thumb to guide this effort says, "continuously improve systems and structures so that they make dignity-respecting behavior the easier, rather than the harder, thing to do."

Organizational beneficence must also attend to 2b: the common good of the society within which the organization exists. For health care institutions not only provide health services, they are also a powerful cultural force and agent. By their presence, their promotional efforts, their budgets, and their services health care institutions have a significant influence on what the general population thinks, hopes, and demands in terms of health care. Hospitals not only respond to but also create demand in the general public about what to expect of a hospital by way of service, convenience, and opulence. Health care institutions are significant forces in shaping public apathy, energy, and indignation. In an over-bedded community, a hospital could even have to face the subordination of its institutional good to the good of the community, resulting in its consolidation with another institution or even its dissolution. Beneficence in the sphere of 2b sustains a consciousness of the organization's impact on the larger society and insists that as the organization pursues its own net good, it does so constrained by this consideration: how can we best achieve the net good of the organization while also promoting the common good of society? Ethics on this level rejects the adage, what's good for General Motors is good for America.

In daily operations these issues of organizational/institutional ethics are commonly thought of as "operational questions," "organizational issues," "financial concerns," "management issues," or "marketing programs." They are that. But in the terms of our discussion they must also be identified as issues that have an impact on human dignity and, therefore, vital issues of ethics.

Societal Beneficence

The third realm of an ethic of beneficence is that of society. This realm deals with the common good of society. The *Hastings Center Report* defines the common good as "that which constitutes the well-being of the community—its safety, the integrity of its basic institutions and practices, the preservation of its core values. It also refers to the telos or end toward which the members of the community cooperatively strive—the 'good life,' human flourishing, and moral development."[18]

Garrett Hardin offers a helpful illustration of the common good and how it differs from and can conflict with the good of individuals. He asks us to think of a group of herdsmen who share a common grazing pasture. As long as there is enough pasture to feed the cattle and rejuvenate itself for the future, each individual herder can pursue personal aggrandizement without jeopardizing the common good. But at some point the danger of overgrazing emerges if each individual continues to increase the size of his herd. As long as the horizon of reflection remains individual—"what benefit comes to me from adding one more animal to my herd?"—the problem can neither be identified in a timely way nor resolved. Hardin says, "Therein is the tragedy. Each man is locked into a system that compels him to increase his herd without limits—in a world that is limited. Ruin is the destination toward which all men rush, each pursuing his own best interest in a society that believes in the freedom of the commons. Freedom in a commons brings ruin to all."[19] This echoes the comment of Lamm at the beginning of this chapter, that bringing the categories of individual ethics to societal problems "is leading to increasingly unethical public policy results."

Societal beneficence is another term for the ethics of the commons. It knows that the common good is not achieved by some invisible hand as we each pursue our own individual good. Societal beneficence brings heart, mind, imagination, and hands to the nurturing of this common good.

Attending to the commons involves balancing the many conflicting needs/ goods of the commons—education, housing, defense, health care, art, infrastructure, and so forth. Being unable to meet any one or all of these societal needs fully, we seek a reasonable balance among them. The major task of societal beneficence is continually to attend to this balance by correcting historical aberrations, adjusting to new forces and circumstances, and creating new opportunities so that society can be the environment of dignity's flourishing.

A further dimension of societal ethics concerns the balance within the essential institutions of societal common good—education, health, housing, and so forth. For example, achieving the "health care good" of society involves finding the appropriate balance among competing health care needs, such as prevention and cure, acute and chronic care, research and education, administration and direct service.

The primary goal of societal ethics is not to attend to the unique and specific goals of each individual but to so structure society and allocate resources that the fabric of society in which individuals and institutions exist can be an environment of human flourishing in the present moment and into the future. But in seeking this primary goal of the common good of society, the good of individuals and the good of organizations must also be attended to. As in the other two realms of beneficence the concern must look in three directions: 3a, primarily to the common good, to the net good of society as a whole; secondarily to 3b, the good of organizations; and 3c, the good of individuals.

✧ DETERMINING THE PRIMARY LEVEL OF ETHICAL CONCERN

Most issues have ethical significance on all three levels and need to be addressed on each level appropriately. For example, informed consent has ethical concerns on the levels of individual, institution, and society. This issue deserves ethical inquiry. On the individual level, what should this physician disclose to this patient/family in this set of circumstances? On the institutional level, what policies, procedures, educational programs, patient brochures, quality assurance mechanisms, ethics committee activities should a hospital have to promote informed consent in the institution? On the societal level, what professional standards, federal regulations, state laws should be in place to promote a general practice of informed consent?

But hardly ever are these levels of equal importance. Some questions are primarily "institutional questions," with the individual/societal levels being secondary and/or tertiary considerations. Other issues are primarily issues of individual ethics, and still others are essentially issues of societal ethics.

For example, the decision to downsize an institution is primarily a question of *institutional ethics*. This means that the decision results from a careful examination and weighing of the good of the institution: for the good of the institution, is this drastic step necessary? What other alternatives must be tried? For how long? How should it be done? What follow-up is required for those terminated and the survivors? So, even though many individuals will suffer harm from such a decision, it can be the institution's ethical responsibility to move forward with a reduction in force. An important benefit of the beneficence understanding of ethics is that it demands that we explicitly note and attend to the values that are determined to be of lower priority in this instance.[20]

But the question of participation in an experimental treatment is primarily a question on the *individual level*. This question should be resolved in terms of the individual patient's best interest, as defined by the patient. One cannot justify forcing patient participation because the hospital's experimental program will greatly benefit, or because future generations will benefit. Those are considerations that an individual could include in their calculus on the individual level but could not justify an institution's coercive action.

The question of national health policy is an ethical issue on the *societal level*. For the sake of the common good of the United States many institutions—e.g., insurance companies, hospitals, universities—and many individuals—e.g., patients and clinicians—will have to accept serious burdens and limits set to their expectations and practices in order for society to create a reasonable and just health care system.

One of the fundamental starting points for ethical discussion will be to determine which level, if any, is the preeminent level of ethical importance. This presents us with a set of ethical questions that we seldom ask explicitly and clearly in current discussions. For example, in the extensive discussion of California's Proposition 161 (the proposition that would have authorized active euthanasia and physician-assisted suicide), most discussions went forward as if this were primarily an issue of individual ethics with some secondary questions on the societal level—primarily formulated in terms of prevention of abuse. There would have been a different series of discussions had we all presumed that Proposition 161 was essentially a question of societal ethics—or even if we had begun by asking which level deserved to be primary.

How does one establish the preeminent level? Although the fullness of this consideration can only emerge from the community addressing these difficult questions over time, the following suggestions are an invitation to take up this challenge. I will phrase these in terms of ethical presumptions (I cast these in terms of *societal* ethics, but with appropriate changes, similar presumptions could be formulated concerning individual and institutional ethics).

A question is presumed to be one of societal ethics if:

- ✦ it has serious consequences for future generations;
- ✦ it involves interdependence of major societal institutions—political, economic, educational, legal, etc.;
- ✦ it demands sacrifices from significant numbers on behalf of others;
- ✦ it has disproportionate impact on identifiable groups of persons;
- ✦ it requires extensive studies of multiple

disciplines to reasonably represent its complexity;

- ✦ it has an impact on significant institutions—schools, businesses, groups of professionals, etc.;
- ✦ it requires organization and integration of such complexity that individuals and institutions cannot accomplish it adequately;
- ✦ it endangers the already marginalized;
- ✦ it involves long-standing cultural assumptions;.
- ✦ its center concerns pivotal mysteries of life—sexuality, partnering, aging, dying, etc.
- ✦ its success requires broad, coercive measures.

These modest suggestions invite critique and modification; they point to the kind of ethical collaborative work that should rank high on the list of priorities for the future.

✧ UNITY AND DIVERSITY OF BENEFICENCE ACROSS THE THREE REALMS

It is important to emphasize the fundamental unity of beneficence/ ethics across these spheres, but also to recognize its diversity.

Unity

The emphasis on unity and the interdependence of these spheres on one another is a major strength of the Three Realms model. Too often our language masks this unity instead of emphasizing it. Authors often distinguish "morality" from "public policy," the "abstract order of ethics" from the "concrete order of jurisprudence," the "moral order" from "public policy." This inconsistent language confuses and fragments our ethical efforts. We need to develop a conceptual world and language that first emphasizes the unity of morality as we move across these spheres. Absent this foundation, we reinforce the common error that the "authentic world of ethics" resides in the realm of individual good and that beyond such real ethics lies only the ethical "outback" of politics, common sense, and law. Especially in U.S. culture, we further make the mistake of approaching all ethical questions with the conceptual tools, moral imagination, and methodology adequate only for the simplest level of ethical reflection. Such misperception blunts our awareness of the most demanding areas of ethics, and tends to fragment our moral intellect and imagination. A major strength of the three-realm paradigm resides in its emphasis on the unity of ethical reality.

Diversity

But beneficence/ethics across these realms is *analogous, not univocal,* and this involves significant differences between these spheres with relationships of interdependence that are not always parallel or reciprocal in every way. A suggestive sketch of some differences would include the following:

1. All things being equal, as we move from realm 1 to 3, the ethical reality becomes exponentially both more significant and more complex.

2. Methods, concepts, and principles are presumed not to have the same importance, relevance, and adequacy on one level as they do on another (for example: The principle of autonomy has an importance on level 1a that it does not sustain on level 2a, and is relativized still more on level 3a), nor does this mean that individuals must be honest, but organizations or societies need not be honest. It does mean that telling the truth, the whole truth, and nothing but the truth is not simply the same for individuals, organizations, and society.

3. Conclusions reached on one level do not lead to necessary conclusions on another level. (For example, to demonstrate that active euthanasia could be an ethically reasonable option in an individual case does not lead with any logical necessity to substantive conclusions on the organizational level and even less so on the societal level.)

4. Substantial deficits on a higher level cannot be adequately compensated for by interventions on a lower level. (For example, it is not possible to correct a substantially unjust health care system merely by multiplying the activity of individual hospitals or health professionals.)

5. The ethical character of the higher spheres tends to powerfully define the limits on ethical behavior in the sphere(s) below. (For example, the injustices of a societal system, such as Medicaid, will tend to inhibit just behavior of institutions and professionals by punishing those who attempt to behave beyond the boundaries drawn by the system.)

6. Professional education in different fields tends to develop awareness/unawareness to different levels of beneficence. (For example, in the United States professional training for social work tends to open awareness to the full range of beneficence more than does professional training for law.)

7. Different cultures can predispose their members to emphasize one level of beneficence over the others. For example, according to a statement by Fox and Swazey that for the Chinese "the bedrock and point of departure of medical morality lie in the quality of these human relationships: in how correct, respectful, harmonious, complementary, and reciprocal they are."[21] We would expect this culture to emphasize social beneficence more than individual beneficence. By contrast, the proclivity in U.S. culture is to make the perspective of the individual realm dominant, if not exclusive. This cultural predisposition finds expression in statements that rely on autonomy.

8. Most issues of health care ethics have significance on all three levels, but more often than not an issue has a primary level of ethical significance that constitutes the ethical center of the issue. The other spheres should be resolved relative to this ethical center. For example, refus-

ing treatment is primarily a question of individual ethics, but institutions and society need to make structural protection and facilitation of this refusal a real possibility. On the other hand, developing a reasonable national health policy is essentially an issue of societal ethics, where individuals and institutions must subordinate their specific interests to the greater good of society.

This is a beginning list of some obvious differences that exist between these realms of ethical reality. Here again we meet an area where significant work remains to be done in understanding such differences across these spheres.

✧ FURTHER EXPLORATIONS

At the heart of beneficence is community. The very term beneficence emphasizes that we are essentially social beings—persons-in-relationships. It implies that the natural state of persons is reciprocal, responsive, and engaged. It understands self-giving as essential and self-realizing; it sees the love imperative primarily as an invitation to become, not as a constraint on being. The three-tiered model of beneficence symbolizes how thoroughly individuals are embedded in layers of social reality—individuals exist within networks of mediating organizations and these in turn are woven into a matrix of society. Community is the ocean in which we swim.

Exploring the "Community of Concern" Presumption

In a beneficence ethic there is a presumption that the privileged agent of ethical discernment is the "community of concern."[22] Certainly, individual ethics makes sense and existential ethical decisions are always made by individuals. But as the three-layered paradigm makes clear at a glance, most ethical terrain involves community. Beyond this, making normative ethical judgments involves the weighing of complex and subtle values and this emerges primarily from experience of these values—

from a pool of experience wide and deep enough to do justice to the issue at hand. Here we are on the wrong track if professionals' views of patient experience are taken for patient experience; if men represent the experience of women; if doctors mediate nurses' views; if administrators speak for the general public. To weigh complex values, we need complex, first-hand experience, as well as adequate analysis of that experience.

Gathering the key elements of this first-hand experience is what the "community of concern" is all about. This is a formal concept to be materially specified by the issue at hand. *The community of concern is constituted by whatever group is necessary to be in experiential touch with all the essential facets of a beneficence question.* Lacking the full community of concern, we are in ethical trouble from the start. No individual or partial group, regardless of ethical fiber or training, can substitute for the full community of concern.[22]

A historical example illustrates this. As late as 1866 the Holy Office of the Roman Catholic Church declared, "Slavery itself ... is not at all contrary to the natural and divine law. ... For the sort of ownership which a slave owner has over a slave is understood as nothing other than the perpetual right of disposing of the work of a slave for one's own benefit." It was not until 1891 that the Vatican formally condemned the institution of slavery as a moral evil. We can imagine how differently the reality of slavery would have been understood, and how much more quickly it would have been condemned, if slaves had been empowered partners in that discernment process.

This historical example illustrates *the importance of having all persons relevant to an issue, present and empowered in the discernment process about that issue.* There is a tendency that haunts us humans when we face complex value issues; we tend to accept the de facto empowered group as adequate for the discernment at hand. Why is this?

I think a central cause is what I call unconscious, constricted, and stratified consciousness. Our consciousness is unavoidably constricted—we don't know important things, but we don't know that we don't know. Further, this constricted consciousness is stratified—the systems and structures of life tend to cluster us with others who share our ignorance and the ignorance of our ignorance. Being such a community of compassionate but unaware constricted consciousness, we experience little reservation about the depth or breadth of our vision and little urgency to expand the community of discernment.

If we aim to improve the ethical culture of our organization we will go a long way by first recognizing the fact of our constricted consciousness and our strong tendency to be untroubled by this; second, by building a culture in which decision makers at all levels live by this credo: *In this organization, decisions start with defining and gathering the community of concern.*

From this perspective, hospitals represent a moral minefield. Hospitals are highly structured along lines that stratify, fragment, and compartmentalize. Such a structure is ethically inhibiting, viewed from the perspective of the community of concern because it keeps like-minded groups reflecting within their limited field of experience. Perhaps the ethics committee movement's greatest contribution can be to introduce a new paradigm of reflection and empowerment into the highly compartmentalized health care structure.

One of the first questions asked by an ethic of beneficence will be, do we have the right community for this issue? If not, what persons do we need to give us the necessary fullness of perspective?

Exploring a Shared Common Vision of Community Members

A key difference between a gathering of special interest advocates and a community of concern is that the latter share a deeper vision that binds them and their differing perspectives into a coherent whole. There may be strong differences on various perspectives of the issue, but stronger still are their grounding meanings and priorities. Selecting the community of concern involves finding persons who share this deeper vision or are capable of being called to it. This deeper vision demands attention and

resources. It is not simply a given. Elsewhere I have explored how a superficial agreement about justice can hide a deeper level of strong disagreements.[23] A community of concern needs to nurture its shared vision, to test its consensus, to sharpen its definitions, to deepen it, to revise it. Neglect of this deeper vision erodes the community's ability to ethically discern.

Tools of Community Enablement

The community of concern needs to be enabled to harness the complexity of values and disvalues, deeper vision and complementary perspectives. For this we need cognitional tools and process tools.

Cognitional Tools

Philosophical and theological ethics can help us understand the importance and role of definitions, distinctions, concepts, principles, and paradigms. These disciplines can provide formal understanding of these elements and material content for application. These disciplines can also suggest methodologies for harnessing this complexity of elements and moving it progressively to closure.

But evaluative knowledge involved in beneficence is more than abstract concepts and cold analysis. Such knowledge is mystic, affective knowledge of the heart and imagination. Here our resources are not extensively developed, and considerable work needs to be done. Fortunately, there is a growing recognition of the direct importance of the arts and literature as tools of enablement for the discerning community. It is in this area that case studies and parables can give human breadth and depth to more discursive principles and definitions.

Group Process Tools

To handle the complex group it has gathered, beneficence needs adequate group process. Adequate process will facilitate a fullness of reflection that (1) is focused but not rigidly constricting; (2) is coextensive with the length and breadth of the problem, not ignoring essential areas, not coming to premature closure; (3) attends to persons as well as issues; (4) ensures input from all and monopoly of none; (5) allows for self-examination and interpersonal communication; (6) promotes open challenge and confrontation; and (7) includes intellection, intuition, affect, and imagination. Front-end planning of meetings cannot guarantee these characteristics but it can go far in enabling them.

Moving from Individual to Societal Realm: Two Examples

Now I want to consider two example that illustrate the U.S. tendency to assume and resolve issues as if they were issues of individual ethics and how differently the issues are discussed and resolved when we locate them on the institutional level.

Example One: Case Consultation—An Issue of Institutional, Not Individual, Ethics

First let us look at the question of case consultation as a function of ethics committees. In an article, "A Paradigm Shift for Case Consultation," a colleague and I have argued in substance—though not in these terms—that the common practice of ethics committees is to treat case consultations as a series of difficult individual cases. In effect, we are treating the problem as one with its center of gravity on the level of individual ethics. Our suggestion is that we should move our gaze to the institutional level of ethical reality and define the problem as one of institutional ethics.[24]

If we see the cases that come to the Institutional Ethics Committee as symptoms of institutional ethical dysfunction, we will diagnose the institution's problem and change the organizational systems and structures, rather than focusing on a case-by-case resolution. Our argument is developed in two theses.

Thesis One: Case consultation by an ethics committee should be recognized as an institutional embarrassment to be eliminated as soon as possible and replaced by institutional change—consistent, effective patterns of case conferencing by staff as a routine part of patient care. The chronic problem is an organizational deficit—the absence of adequate discussion of

patient care by the community of key stakeholders in the case. Because the worst effects of this chronic deficit have finally come to our attention, the "ethics case consultation," a stopgap intervention, has been invented. Using Howard Brody's metaphor of ethics-as-conversation, we would argue that because appropriate conversations were not being held by the right people, at the right times, and in the right places, the ethics case consultation was invented to ensure that at least some conversations, with some of the right persons, were being held somewhere. Given this persistent institutional deficit, the "ethics case consultation" does provide some symptomatic relief, but leaves the fundamental ethical problem—on the institutional level—unresolved. So we find ourselves in the ironic but not uncommon situation in which amelioration in terms of individual ethics becomes a disservice in terms of institutional ethics.

We propose an approach that promises more widespread and abiding results because it addresses the problem on the level of institutional ethics. Most simply put, it involves changing institutional systems and structures, as well as staff understandings and behaviors, so that the primary care community (patient, loved ones, and the clinical professionals involved in giving care) discuss the ethical dimensions of cases effectively, consistently, and adequately in the setting of care. This means institutionalizing the consistent and effective use of case conferences at the unit level.

To achieve this, a number of elements will be needed: (1) an institution will need to develop a consensus across key groups of professionals, from trustees to technicians, that case conferencing is an essential element of excellence in patient care; (2) an institution will need to identify the elements of a case conference and when such a conference would be needed; (3) an institution will need systems and structures to support this practice, including policies, procedures, integration into the quality assurance process, orientation, credentialing, and so on; (4) an institution will need to provide education so that key publics share a common fund of knowledge, including familiarity with (a) the cases that have shaped the current ethical and legal understanding of our culture, (b) the boundaries set by legislative and administrative bodies, and positions taken by major religions, cultural groups, institutions, and professional societies, and (c) basic concepts, definitions, and principles of the current discussion (e.g., autonomy, informed consent, competence, etc.); (5) an institution will also be helped by a methodology or protocol for conferencing. This overall methodology will attend to three phases of the case conference including preparation, conduct of the conference, and follow-up.

Example Two: Reducing Medical Errors
Lucian Leape has been a national leader in addressing the grave ethical issue of reducing medical errors. He asked, "Why has healthcare been so lax at error reduction?"[25] Leape's answer, translated into three-realm ethics language is this: *We have made the mistake of treating error reduction as if it were an issue of individual ethics, when, in fact, it is an issue of organizational ethics.* He says, "[W]e have been locked into an ineffective paradigm. That paradigm, which is rarely questioned, is that mistakes can be avoided if everyone is trained not

Foundation of normative ethics	Three realms of beneficence, hard choices	Ethical Goal	Principal mechanisms of respect	Ethical magnitude and complexity	U.S. cultural emphasis/ tools of public discourse	U.S. bioethics emphasis/ tools of analysis
Law of human dignity: Moral goodness is realized and measured in proportion to lived respect for human dignity	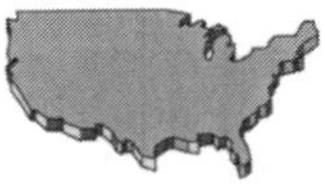 Societal	**Common good:** Society in which essential institutions thrive as balanced whole & provide social vigor & environment for flourishing of good organizations and individuals.	Essential institutions, systems, and structures of society.	▮ (large)	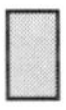 ▫ (small)	▫ (small)
Law of hard choices: Lived respect for human dignity is always realized in the condition of limits and involves hard choices— beneficence, value trade-offs, resolution of conflicting duties.	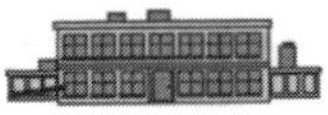 Organizational	**Organizational good:** Organization in which essential systems promote organization's flourishing, common good & environment for individuals to flourish.	Essential institutions, systems, and structures of organization.	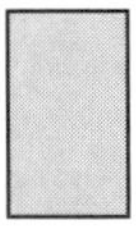 ▫ (medium)	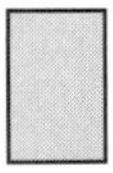 ▫ (medium)	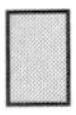 ▫ (small)
	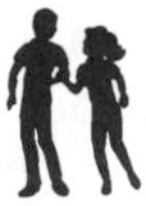 Individual	**Individual good:** Flourishing of individual through internal/external respect for dignity of self/others/ organizations/ society.	Actions of individual flowing from habits of the mind and heart.	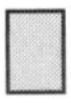 ▫ (small)	▮ (large)	▮ (large)

Figure 16.3 ❖ The graphic captures some of the major elements discussed in this chapter.

to make them and punished when they do. Some have referred to this as the 'train and blame' approach."

Organizational ethics looks first and foremost to systems and structures, while individual ethics concentrates on individual intention, attention, and performance. He sees health care's concern for errors focused on persons, not processes. "Mortality and morbidity conferences, incident reports, risk management activities, and quality assurance committees abound. But ... these activities focus on incidents and individuals."[26] Leape urges significant changes on the organizational level. We need to move from a culture of blame to one of learning and continuous improvement. This involves systems of rhetoric, self-identity, reporting, planning, incentives, evaluation, and analysis.

But Leape also recognizes the societal realm and its importance for organizational improvement, "Finally, healthcare has to deal with the culture of blame outside its walls. It is not only health professionals who are judgmental—it is a characteristic of our society. ... But the larger 'message,' that errors are systems problems not people problems needs to be spread throughout the land—to regulators, to the media, and to the public."[26]

In terms of the three-realm model, Leape urges us to move from treating errors as if they were primarily issues of individual ethics to seeing them primarily as issues of organizational ethics. This requires seeing the elements of societal ethics that require attention for our organizational efforts to thoroughly succeed.

✧ SUMMARY

I have proposed the beginnings of a partial and complementary paradigm of ethics. This paradigm begins with the experience of the law of human dignity and its demand for respect—analogous to the demand of gravity for respect. But even our fullest-hearted response is always realized in the condition of finitude. The foundational issue of ethics is therefore, where and how am I called to honor and serve human dignity because I cannot serve it all? It is important

to see such hard choices/beneficence as falling into three realms—beneficence of individuals, of organizations, and of society. These two key building blocks—the nature of beneficence and its three-tiered realization—provide the foundation for building an approach to ethics more appropriate for emerging problems.

References

1. Murray JC: We Hold These Truths. Sheed and Ward, Kansas City, MO, 1961.
2. Thompson DF: Ethics in Congress: From Individual to Institutional Corruption. The Brookings Institution, Washington, DC, 1995.
3. Lamm R: Redrawing the ethics map. Hastings Cent Rep 29(2):28–29, 2002.
4. Rasmussen L: Earth Community Earth Ethics. Orbis Books, Maryknoll, New York, 1996.
5. Cahill L: Biotech and justice: Catching up with the real world. Hastings Cent Rep 33(4):34–44, 2003.
6. Miller W: Lincoln's Virtues: An Ethical Biography. Vintage Books, New York, 2003.
7. United States Catholic Conference: Economic Justice for All. United States Catholic Conference, Washington, DC, 1986.
8. Beauchamp TL, and Childress JF: Principles of Biomedical Ethics, ed 4. Oxford University Press, New York, 1994.
9. McCormick R: Ambiguity and Moral Choice, 1973 Pere Marquette Theology Lecture. Paper presented at: Kennedy Center for Bioethics, 1973, Georgetown University, Washington, DC.
10. Schuller B: Die Begrundung Sittlicher Urteile. ed 2. Patmos Verlag, Dusseldorf, Germany, 1980.
11. Pellegrino ED, and Thomasma DC: For the Patient's Good: The Restoration of Beneficence in Health Care. Oxford University Press, New York, 1988.
12. Childress JF: Just war theories: The bases, interrelations, priorities, and functions of their criteria. Theological Stud 39(3):427–445, 1978.
13. Curran C: Toward An American Catholic Moral Theology. Notre Dame University Press, Notre Dame, 1987.
14. Schuller B: Typen der Begriindung Sittlicher Normen. Concilium 648–654, 1976.
15. Stark W: The Sociology of Knowledge, London, 1958, 54. In Stevens R (ed): In Sickness and in Wealth, American Hospitals in the Twentieth Century. Basic Books, New York, 1989.
16. Gustafson J: Moral discourse about medicine: A variety of forms. J Med Philos 15:125–142, 1990.
17. Annas GS: Life, liberty and death. Health Manage Q 12(1):5–8, 1990.
18. Jennings B, et al: The public duty of the professions. Hastings Cent Rep 17(1):1–20, 1987.
19. Hardin G: The tragedy of the commons. Science 162:1243–1248, 1968.
20. Meyer M, and Nelson L: Respecting what we destroy: Reflections on human embryo research. Hastings Cent Rep 31(1):16–23, 2001.

21. Fox R, and Swazey J: Medical Morality Is Not Bioethics—Medical Ethics in China and the United States. Essays in Medical Sociology. Transaction Books, New Brunswick, 1988, pp 645–671.

22. Glaser JW: The community of concern: An ethical discernment process should include and empower all people relevant to the decision. Health Prog March/April 83(2):17–20, 2002.

23. Glaser J: Hospital ethics committees: One of many centers of responsibility. Theor Med 10:275–288, 1989.

24. Glaser JW, and Miller R: A paradigm shift for ethics committees and case consultation: A modest proposal. HEC Forum 5(2):83–88, 1993.

25. Leape L: Can we reduce medical errors? Ethical Curr 51:1–2, 1997.

26. Leape L: Error in medicine. JAMA 272(23):1851–1857, 1994.

A Model for Ethical Decision Making to Inform the Ethics Education of Future Health Care Professionals

KAREN G. GERVAIS, PHD

Abstract

In this article the author offers a process model of ethical decision making specifying the conditions a health care professional must meet in order to make ethically informed decisions in response to ethical challenges to professional responsibility. Three types of preparation are essential, namely background knowledge, case analysis, and self-assessment. The purpose of providing this model is to serve the deeper purpose of providing a template for the identification of deficiencies in ethics education as it is currently approached, for the design of an adequate ethics education process, and for guiding the development of specialized pedagogical tools.

Ethics is a field of knowledge, yet one is hard-pressed to find an adequate model for the ethics education of future health care professionals (IICPs), a model that will support ethically informed decision making and a high standard of professional responsibility. Textbooks for the various health care professions lack such a model, and it is probably safe to say that relatively few faculty have been trained specifically to shape ethical problem-solving capacities in those they are so committed to preparing for careers exhibiting high standards of professional responsibility.

In this chapter I offer a process model for making ethically informed decisions as a health care professional. The purpose of providing this model is to enable me to articulate our educational responsibilities as ethics educators. In short, I use the model to identify the educational elements we must "teach to" in order to prepare our students to be ethically aware and competent decision makers in response to professional challenges.

I admit some reluctance in suggesting that a sound ethics education in accordance with this model will lead to ethically competent decisions. So, in fact, I am not claiming that. We cannot educate people to be ethical, but we can educate them to adhere to a disciplined process in order to arrive at ethically informed decisions, and it is the latter that I seek to support through the model I offer.

My process model specifies the conditions a HCP must meet in order to make ethically informed decisions in response to ethical challenges to professional responsibility. If it is a successful model, it will serve my additional and deeper purpose, to provide a template for the identification of deficiencies in ethics education as it is currently approached, for the design of an adequate ethics education process, and for guiding the development of educational tools.

✧ TRADITIONAL BIOETHICS APPROACHES

Bioethics has traditionally focused on the individual clinical encounter and decisions concerning clinical alternatives. It has failed to analyze the societal and institutional features that are in fact the origin of many ethical issues in the clinical setting, and has offered an ethical framework fruitful only in relation to such individualized clinical encounters. To redress the deficiencies of the ethics education model implicit in previous bioethics work, I attempt an enlarged model, one that considers the institutional and societal embeddedness of the HCP to be essential aspects of an adequate ethical analysis. The embeddedness of the HCP in societal, institutional, and professional arrangements and relationships is a veritably unlimited source of challenges to professional responsibility. The process model I offer is informed by the excellent work of Jack Glaser, another contributor to this volume.[1]

✧ THE PROCESS MODEL

Figure 17.1 provides a general overview of the model. It consists of three types of preparation for making an ethical decision—background knowledge, case analysis, and self-assessment. Each of these major process elements is complex, consisting of sub-elements. In the more detailed version of the model (Fig. 17.2), the complexities of many of the sub-elements are spelled out.

The three broad input categories leading to an ethical decision (background knowledge, case analysis, and self-assessment) are three crucial elements in the reflective process in which HCPs must engage to respond to challenges to professional responsibility. I define such challenges broadly as threats to their fiduciary or advocacy role.

Let us examine the components of the process model in detail.

Step 1: Background Knowledge

Societal and Health System Characteristics

The first claim implicit in the model is that the HCP must draw not only on the "facts" of the immediate clinical situation, but also on the societal and health system realities that constitute the context of the case. In particular, the HCP must draw on knowledge of how the delivery and financing system bear causal connections to the ethical problem.

Moral Compass: Professional Responsibility

The foundation for all HCP practice is a code of ethics specific to each profession. An ethical code, however, is not an ethical process, and it is not aspirational. A well-designed code provides enforceable standards of minimally decent conduct. Knowledge of one's professional code is an essential feeder into a process of ethical decision making, but it does not negate the need to follow an explicit process for making ethically informed choices.

An obvious principle not immediately entailed in the traditional bioethics framework is a rich principle of advocacy that is not coextensive with the duties of beneficence and nonmaleficence. The normative cornerstone of my model of professionalism is the concept of advocacy, understood as the responsibility to articulate the wishes/interests of clients/patients, *and* to identify essential institutional and system changes. A point that I will not argue for is that the traditional clinical ethics framework (the principles of autonomy, beneficence, nonmaleficence, and justice) is inadequate as an analytical framework to address many of the ethical issues arising for HCPs in today's health care environment.

The other two aspects of the moral compass are approaches to ethical reasoning and ethical principles and application. Each of these

Overview of the Process

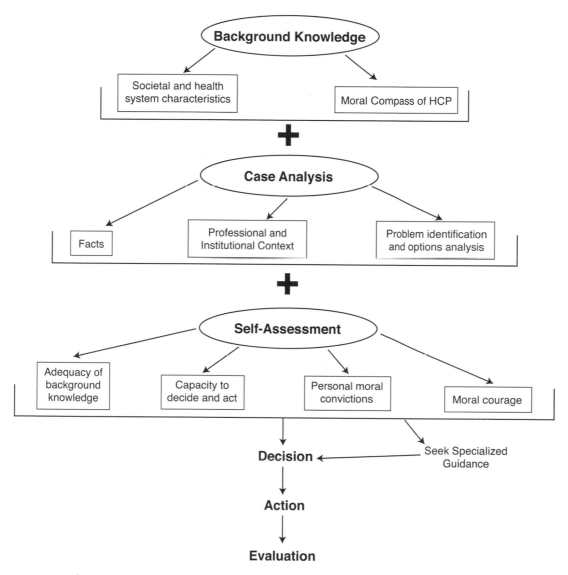

Figure 17.1 ✧ A model for ethical decision making to inform the ethics education of future health care professionals.

is an aspect of traditional approaches to ethics education, and requires no special explanation because it is not novel.

Step 2: Case Analysis

The case analysis requires a delineation of the facts of the case (also a part of the traditional ethics education model) as well as atten-

tion to further features of context—namely, the professional and institutional contexts.

Professional and Institutional Context

Further aspects of the embeddedness of the HCP include the surrounding professional arrangements and relationships, and the institutional structure and policies (both formal and

Details of Process

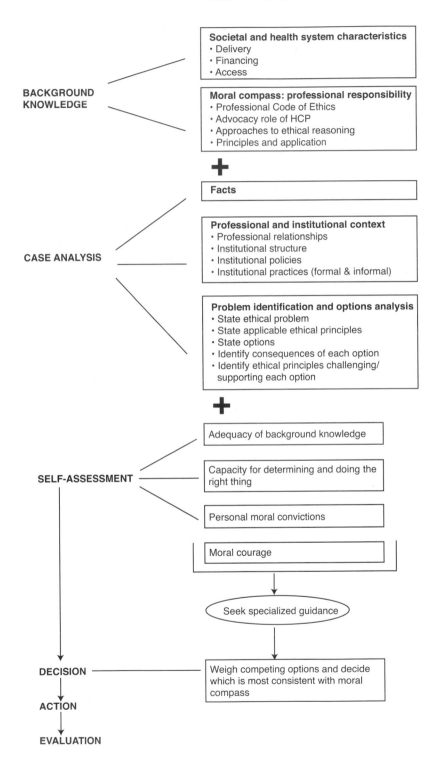

Figure 17.2 ✧ Details of the ethical decision making process are highlighted.

informal) that are often contributors to ethical problem for HCPs.

Problem Identification and Options Analysis

This element of the process model has always been a part of traditional ethics education. However, because the traditional model was insufficiently attentive to the embeddedness of the HCP, the problem identification and options analysis was thin by comparison with the thicker analysis encouraged by the model I am offering. The consideration of embeddedness, which is primarily encouraged by attention to societal and health system characteristics (part of the background analysis) and professional and institutional context (part of the case analysis), provides for this thicker analysis. It allows the HCP to identify the origin of the ethical problem and those who are in a position to address it. In some cases, this will be the HCP herself; in others, it will be a person(s) in a different role relative to the problem (e.g., an institutional administrator or a coverage decision maker). This analysis becomes critical because the HCP cannot always solve the ethical problem single-handedly. Yet the HCP may have a role in identifying the problem and advocating for change that is a critical part of the resolution of the problem.

As Jack Glaser and Ron Hamel have written,

We need to recognize the interrelationships, priorities, and interdependencies that exist between the three realms (the societal/institutional/individual)— or we make mistakes, such as thinking we can remedy significant deficits on the societal [and institutional] level[s] by the compensating behavior of individuals..."[2]

In short, the HCP needs to know where and how to exert pressure when the ethical problem originates on a level she cannot address adequately on her own.

The traditional model of ethics education has emphasized the problem identification and options analysis described in my model, and so this is not a novel aspect of my model. My central claim is that the identification and options analysis must be understood as the thick analysis I am proposing.

Step 3: Self-Assessment

This element of the model is a profoundly introspective one, and I am convinced students can be educated to engage in it in a very purposive way. Self-assessment consists of four elements, each of which I explain by conveying the question central to it.

First, the HCP must ask about the adequacy of her background knowledge. Do I fully understand my situation, the influences on it, and my professional obligations? Second, the HCP must consider her personal capacity for determining and doing the right thing. Do I have personal concerns or deficiencies concerning my capacity to do the right thing? Third, the HCP must determine whether a course of action is consistent with her personal moral convictions. Do I have moral beliefs and values that are at odds with what I am considering doing as a professional? Finally, the HCP must assess whether the situation calls for moral courage.* I know what is right, but do I have the courage to take the difficult and threatening path of advocating for this response to the ethical problem?

✦ DECISION, ACTION, EVALUATION

The final stages of the model are, as one would expect, to decide and to act, and then to conduct a retrospective evaluation of one's entire process. I have also suggested that the outcome of the self-assessment step may lead to an interim decision—a decision to seek specialized guidance, perhaps to study and reflect more deeply. The type of guidance, study, or reflection pursued would of course depend on the nature of the problem identified. If, for example, the HCP sees a conflict with her personal moral beliefs, she must stop and inquire into and analyze all of the resources available to her. Is there an institutional policy concerning conscientious objection? Does her professional

---

* Moral courage was not included in the model I presented at the conference. I am indebted to the work of Carol Davis, which led me to see that moral courage must be given a place in the model. See Chapter 20 of this volume.

code speak to this issue in any way? Or, if she is fearful but confident in her responsibility as a professional, can she identify resources available to her as she decides to act with moral courage?

If the self-assessment step does not reveal issues that require an interim step, the difficult leap of moral judgment is the next step in the process. The individual must weigh competing options and determine which is most consistent with her moral compass (a feature of the background knowledge).

✧ EDUCATION BEFITTING THE MODEL PROCESS

Assuming this process model is generally acceptable as a guide, what does it require of us as educators? Which of the items in the model have we been emphasizing in ethics education, and which do we need to take on as additional educational challenges if we are to adequately prepare future HCPs for ethically informed decision making? I suggest we embrace three major goals to enrich ethics education.

First, we must address deficiencies in the way we educate and empower future HCPs to focus on ethical challenges rooted in embed-

dedness. This means we must develop pedagogical tools that emphasize ethical challenges deriving from societal and health system characteristics (Background Knowledge) and professional and institutional context (Case Analysis).

Second, we must enrich our attention to the development of the full moral compass of the professional (Background Knowledge).

Third, we must create tools that assist in managing conflicts with personal moral beliefs, and tools that inspire moral courage (Self-Assessment).

These are tall orders for us as educators. Fortunately, it was my role to attempt to provide a model that would help us discern our need for expanded ethics educational efforts and the development of richer pedagogical tools. Hopefully, the process model I have presented will provide critical landmarks for the educational tasks that lie ahead for us.

References

1. Glaser JW: Three Realms of Ethics: Individual, Institutional, Societal, Theoretical Model and Case Studies. Rowman & Littlefield Publishers, Lanham, MD, 1994.
2. Glaser JW, and Hamel RP: Three Realms of Managed Care: Societal, Institutional, Individual: Resources for Group Reflection and Action. Rowman & Littlefield Publishers, Lanham, MD, 1997.

18

Mindfulness: Applications for Teaching and Learning in Ethics Education

GAIL M. JENSEN, PHD, PT, FAPTA

Abstract

As ethics educators we are committed to preparing students who are self-aware, reflective, and capable of understanding her or his moral responsibility as a health professional. We are all challenged in our work as we teach in professional curricula that are intensive and information-driven. Facilitating reflective habits of mind in a professional education environment is a difficult yet necessary student outcome. The purpose of this chapter is to critically examine the concept of mindfulness and its application to ethics education in the health professions. This critical examination of mindfulness includes: (a) a review of key concepts found in the literature, (b) application of these key concepts of mindfulness to clinical cases, and (c) critical self-reflection on my teaching of ethics in which I explore evidence of student learning in the area of mindfulness and pose suggestions for health professions education.

One day, at a nursing home in Connecticut, elderly residents were each given a choice of houseplants to care for and were asked to make a number of small decisions about their daily routines. A year and one half later, not only were these people more cheerful, active and alert than a similar group in the same institution who were not given these choices and responsibilities, but more of them were still alive. In fact, less than half as many of the decision-making, plant-minded residents had died as had those in the other group.[1]

The startling results of this experiment done in the 1980s led Dr. Ellen Langer and her colleagues into research on what they call "mindfulness."

Mindfulness is an ancient Buddhist practice that has to do with being in touch with our present-day lives. Mindfulness is a flexible state of conscious awareness characterized by being engaged in the present moment, noticing new things, novelty, and being sensitive to context and perspective.[1] When we approach something that we believe we know well then we tend to view it mindlessly; however, when we approach something that is novel to us we approach it mindfully.

In 1999, Dr. Ronald Epstein[2] published an article in JAMA on *mindful practice* that has caused continued discussion among medical educators about the role of mindfulness in the development of professional competence.[3,4] Epstein[2] argues that mindfulness is a natural extension of reflective practice. Furthermore, he believes that the process of critical self-reflection that is seen in exemplary or expert practice depends on the presence of mindfulness. Mindfulness means paying attention in a particular way, in the present moment and being nonjudgmental.[1] A mindful practitioner attends in a nonjudgmental way to their own physical and mental processes during ordinary, everyday tasks. This critical self-reflection enables the practitioner to fully listen to the patient, self-monitor, bring multiple sources of knowledge and deeply held values to both ordinary and complex situations.[2,5]

The concept of mindfulness appears to have many similarities with how we describe expertise. We have evidence across the health professions that expert clinicians attend to patients in a nonjudgmental way, engage in moment-to-moment self-monitoring, rely on practical wisdom gained through experience, and use their senses and awareness to acquire new information. Their ability to make clinical judgments draws from many sources of evidence, yet centers on understanding the perspective and context of the patient and family/caregiver situation.[6–9]

As an educator teaching ethics to health professions students, I struggle with the question, How do I best prepare students, who will enter the profession as novices, to have the ability and necessary moral foundation to develop expertise? Students often respond to course content in ethics and other areas of the behavioral sciences somewhat mindlessly because this content is seen in stark contrast to the intensity and perceived relevance of the basic and clinical sciences. Although there is acknowledgment that ethics is needed given the current pressures in health care, the reality of professional curricula remains. Students quickly learn the lessons of the explicit and implicit curriculum. There is strong emphasis on the "hard sciences" in which the need to memorize and digest extensive amounts of content in order to survive is seen in stark contrast with the more experiential, theoretical, and applied emphasis in the behavioral sciences.[10,11] Although many health professions educators have embraced Schon's[12] concept of reflective practice as a central component of professional competence,[5,8,13,14] there has been far less discussion and exploration of what elements may underlie critical self-reflection and mindfulness.

Dewey[15] argued that the object and reward of learning is continued capacity for growth and that students develop skills and habits of mind that will enhance their creativity and problem-solving abilities with respect to the issues they are likely to meet. The tools of ethics include developing "habits of mind" for reflection on complex, changing situations that are part of everyday practice. Facilitating reflective habits of the mind is a necessary, but difficult, challenge in a professional education environment.[16,17]

Ethics educators in occupational therapy and physical therapy, as an organized community of concern, serve a potentially critical role in facilitating necessary changes in education that lead to integration of "habits of mind" as essential elements of professional competence. The concept of mindfulness as a "habit of mind" is worthy of dialogue. The purpose of this chapter is to explore the concept and practice of mindfulness as applied to teaching and learning of ethics. First, I briefly review the literature on mindfulness and highlight the key concepts. Second, I apply these key concepts of mindfulness to clinical practice and speculate on what behaviors we might observe in mindful practice by sharing two vignettes from my students. Third, I share my own critical self-reflection on my teaching of ethics and pose suggestions for how we might teach and assess student learning in the area of mindfulness.

✧ UNDERSTANDING MINDFULNESS

The goals of mindful practice are to be more aware of one's mental processes, listen more attentively, be more flexible, recognize bias and judgments, and act with principles and compassion (Table 18.1).

Mindfulness is a practice that stems from a philosophical-religious tradition in which the underlying philosophy is pragmatic. The practice of mindfulness is based on the interdependence of action, cognition, memory, and emotion.[1,18] Mindfulness is a quality of a person or practitioner that does not place boundaries between cognitive, technical, emotional, and spiritual aspects of practice. Epstein says, "Mindful practitioners have an ability to observe the observed while observing the observer in the consulting room."[2]

Epstein suggests that mindful practice is a logical extension of reflective practice.[2] When practitioners are mindful, they are able to engage in critical self-reflection. What makes reflection critical? Brookfield would argue, "Critical reflection on experience certainly tends to lead to the uncovering or paradigmatic, structuring assumptions … For something to count as an example of critical reflection, I believe that persons concerned must engage in some sort of power analysis of the situation or context in which the learning is happening."[19] Critical self-reflection depends on the ability to monitor one's own progress, also referred to as metacognition or meta-processing.[20] The process of meta-processing begins with intrapersonal self-awareness.[20,21] This insight into self allows practitioners to see themselves as they are seen by others and helps establish satisfactory interpersonal relationships. In turn, this self-awareness helps the practitioner transcend and see connections across all areas of practice (e.g., technical, cognitive, emotional, spiritual) versus separation. Mindfulness allows the practitioner to "welcome uncertainty" and see difficult or problem patients as areas for creative problem solving versus unsolvable problems.[2,18]

Mindfulness also facilitates "connected knowing" as knowledge is not seen independently but in relationship to the one observing and using that knowledge.[22] Tacit knowledge, that knowledge that is learned through observation and critical reflection on practice, is another source of evidence for clinical judgment and decision making.[2,5] The object of mindfulness applies to any and all domains of knowledge whether explicit or tacit.[1,23]

Langer has a chapter in her book *Mindfulness* entitled, "When the light is on and nobody is home."[1] This is an example of what she refers to as mindlessness. She describes mindlessness as acting automatically according to our behavior made in the past rather than in the present. She suggests three descriptions that can help us further understand the concept of mindlessness: (1) experiencing the world when we are trapped by categories and make distinctions based on those categories, (2) automatic behavior, and (3) acting from a single perspective as if there were only one set of rules.[24] Furthermore, she believes that education has a great deal to do with fostering mindlessness when it is focused on learning the facts and getting the right answer—done without attention to the perspective or context of the situation.[18]

Table 18.1 ✧ Suggested Elements of Mindful Practice
Active observation of oneself, patient, and the problem(s)
Peripheral vision
Preattentive processing
Critical curiosity
Courage to see the world as it is rather than as one would have it be
Willingness to examine and set aside categories and prejudices
Adoption of a beginner's mind
Humility to tolerate awareness of one's areas of incompetence
Connection between the knower and the known
Compassion based on insight
Presence

Source: Epstein RM: Mindful practice. JAMA 282(9): 833–839, 1999.

What are the consequences of mindlessness in clinical practice situations? Epstein points out that when mindlessness occurs in medicine, one sees gaps between knowledge, values, and actions, "Physicians make moment-to-moment value laden decisions that entail cognitive and emotional factors.... These rapid decisions based on personal knowledge, level of skill, efficiency, and values ultimately result in actions.... Self knowledge is essential to the expression of core values in medicine such as empathy, compassion and altruism."[2]

For example, for a clinician to be empathic she must be present—understand the patient's suffering as well as be able to distinguish the patient's experience from her own. It may be a lack of self-awareness on the part of the clinician that contributes to confusion of one's own perspective with the patient's and leads to less patient-centered care.[25] In situations of uncertainty and emotional charge, mindlessness can contribute to deviations from professionalism, such as avoidance of difficult situations, externalization, or denial.[26]

Mindful Practice: What Does It Look Like?

Epstein proposes a model that outlines five levels of mindful practice.[2] Although the model has not yet been verified with research, it poses a useful tool for thinking about what we might see in clinical practice settings:

Level 0—Denial and Externalization. At the extreme level of mindlessness we would see practitioners demonstrate denial and externalization. The problem is out there with the patient. This allows the practitioner to avoid taking responsibility for the situation. "Not his problem, but the problem is centered elsewhere." A familiar scenario in rehabilitation would be the patient who is unable to engage in an exercise program or functional activity and the therapist quickly coming to the decision that it is the patient's lack of motivation that is at fault and has nothing to do with how the therapist has designed the intervention.

Level 1—Imitation: Behavior modeling. At level 1, although practitioners may not necessarily engage in reflection, they will take some responsibility for the situation and attempt to solve it by conforming to some external standard of behavior. For example, a patient is not following the procedures for his work hardening program. The therapist decides to call the case worker and make the patient aware of the proper guidelines, but does no further probing to find out what may be underlying the patient's behavior.

Level 2—Curiosity: Cognitive understanding. Here the practitioner does engage in some reflection triggered by curiosity, and makes the decision based on explicit cognitive models and focuses on the transfer of information. In doing this, personal knowledge, tacit knowledge, and emotions are ignored. Here we may see the therapist focused on sorting out the clinical signs and symptoms that are gathered through the interview and physical examination, which is central in supporting a working hypothesis for the "diagnosis." Missing from this hypothesis-oriented approach would be to fully integrate the patient's perspective (including an assessment of the patient's beliefs and values) into the diagnostic process.

Level 3—Curiosity: Emotions and attitudes. At level 3, the practitioner is open to and includes thoughts, feelings, and behaviors without judging them as good or bad. This inclusion of personal knowledge and emotions provides the practitioner with additional tools for patient-centered care. Here we would see the therapist actively seeking and gathering the thoughts and feelings of the patient but unable to integrate or act on this information as a component of the treatment intervention.

Level 4—Insight. This level includes three components of practitioner understanding—the nature of the problem, how one attempts to solve it, and the interconnectedness between the practitioner and the knowledge she has. In our example of patient refusal to participate in a rehabilitation program, a therapist at the level of insight would uncover the patient's beliefs and values to find out how they may be affecting the patient's ability to engage in the program. Then, the therapist would attempt to tailor the rehabilitation program considering the patient's belief system.

Level 5—Generalization, incorporation, and presence. At this level, the practitioner uses his or her insight to generalize, incorporate new behaviors and attitudes, overcome similar challenges in the future, express compassion, and be present. At this highest level, the therapist tailors a rehabilitation program that integrates the patient's perspective as a central component of the program. This would be done by fully being present with the patient during all interactions and gaining the patient's perspective as well as critically assessing what was successful and what could be improved. The knowledge gained from this reflection would become part of her constantly evolving clinical knowledge.

Two Case Examples of Mindfulness

How might these levels of mindfulness be applied to examples of clinical cases? Here are two contrasting clinical case examples—one representing an example of mindless practice and a second example of mindful practice. Both have been generated by doctor of physical therapy (DPT) students, one from an entry-level student and the second from an experienced therapist in the transitional DPT program. Both case vignettes are shared with permission of the students.

The Case of Sally, John, and Maria
Sally is a physical therapy student on her second 3-week clinical affiliation. She is assigned to a local county hospital that provides free health care to the community. Sally's clinical instructor, John, has been in practice for over 15 years. Maria is a 69-year-old patient who recently received a total hip replacement. She speaks no English and has no family in the area. John has been treating Maria for 1 week prior to

Sally's arrival. On this day, John briefs Sally and asks if she speaks any Spanish. John goes on to say that Maria speaks no English and he is having trouble communicating with her.

Upon Maria's arrival, Sally sits back and watches John treat her. She sees that there is no communication between the therapist and the patient. Maria's care includes manually resisted hip flexion, knee extension, and ambulating 30 feet twice with a front wheeled walker. Sally sees that Maria is bending over significantly to get out of her wheelchair and that John is extremely frustrated at how the treatment is progressing. Maria seems to be taking no active role in the therapy and treating it as a chore. After Maria leaves, Sally asks John if Maria has received any patient education as to hip protocols, transfers, or the plan of care and goals. John states that since he knows no Spanish he was unable to give the amount of education he thought was necessary. Sally asks if he thought of using a translator to which John said there were none employed by the hospital. John also states that Maria will be transferring to a local nursing home in the Latino area of town where she will get proper education.

One day a young man who spoke Spanish happened to bring Maria to the treatment room and Sally knew this was her chance. Without consulting John, she got the young man to translate the hip protocol for her. At the end of the session, Maria said she was thankful as before she had no idea what was going on and what she needed to do.

John, the clinical instructor and licensed physical therapist in this case, appears to be at mindfulness level 0, denial and externalization. He sees that the language barrier with his patient is her problem, not his. Even though he is aware of his frustration, he does nothing to address it other than ask his student if he knows Spanish. His ultimate solution is to rationalize this case in his own mind and see that the patient will get "patient education" when she returns to her community. The student writing this ethics case appears to be at level 3 as he uses his curiosity that includes his feelings and emotions about what he was observing in this clinical instructor.

In the second case, we have an experienced therapist who used this ethics case writing assignment as an opportunity to reflect back on a clinical case that he had continued to reflect on as he wondered if he had "done the right thing:"

Reflections on Blessings

I have thought long and hard about this case for quite some time. As is frequently the case in practice, we make decisions based upon our instincts and the available facts only to later reflect and question whether those decisions were truly right. Case in point, I had been called to a meeting of several important Rabbis from the Lubovich sect, one of the Hassidic Dynasties located in Brooklyn. The chief Rabbi known as The Rebbe had suffered a major stroke, and they wanted to interview me about possibly doing homecare on this case. Not being Jewish, I didn't fully appreciate the importance of The Rebbe. He was truly an international leader; many of his followers actually thought of him as the Moshiach, the savior. In fact, even though he has been dead for a long time, many of his followers still believe he will return and reveal himself as such.

Needless to say, this was an extensive interview process, which culminated in my being hired to work on this man. He was housed in his office where a hospital room had been set-up. There was always a male nurse with him and always at least two Rabbis to pray with him. I was rather intimidated by the whole scene at first, but quickly had established a good working relationship with The Rebbe and our sessions were progressing. The Rebbe was a man who was not used to having anybody say the word "no" to him. He simply got whatever he wanted, no questions asked. Therefore prior to each session, I was instructed to ask him if we could proceed with the PT session.

During the early sessions, there was considerable pressure on me to get The Rebbe walking as soon as possible so that he could lead the congregation in prayer. All went well for a few weeks until one day when he refused PT. He would occasionally do that, and I would usually wait for a while and try again. Almost always we would then proceed with the session. On this day, however, it was not to be. He refused for several days in a row, making the people in charge rather anxious.

I was not able to motivate him to participate in PT at all. It rather appeared to me that he had given up all hope and was just waiting to expire. At this point one of the Rabbis gave me some advice. He told me to ask The Rebbe for his blessing that my work with him would be a success. He reasoned that if The Rebbe gave me that blessing then he would have to consent to PT in order for the blessing to come true. This was the start of my ethical distress, although I didn't call it that at the time. I had no belief in his blessing, and he was smart and intact enough to know that. Should I lie to the patient to motivate him to agree to PT?

I had several duties at that time. First, I had a duty to my patient to provide him with sound physical therapy treatment. Part of that is the ability to motivate patients to perform when they may not be willing to do so. I also had a duty to the physician and the Rabbis who had put their faith in my ability to help them with this case. I felt a sense of duty to the whole congregation who would all gather each evening for prayer hoping that The Rebbe would lead them. On top of this, I had a duty to be honest with my patient and to respect his autonomy.

However, the guiding theory for me at that time, although I didn't know it, was an ethic of care. I had reached a point in our relationship where I truly cared for this man. I knew that his past glories would never be repeated, but if he could walk to his balcony and lead his congregation in prayer, he would benefit greatly. I knew that his fear of failure was the limiting factor, and I believed that he had let me get close enough to him to make a difference.

I approached The Rebbe and made eye contact. I quietly told him how much I wanted our work together to succeed. I asked him for his blessing that our work would be successful. He looked at me for a long hard moment, which I shall never forget, then nodded and said something in Hebrew. After a few moments we started our treatment session. Several of the Rabbis in the room were stunned. They thought I had tried to trick him into agreeing to cooperation, but when he began to participate in PT, nothing was said.

The Rebbe never refused a treatment again after that day. He progressed in his PT rather well. Shortly after the event, he did begin going to his balcony in the evenings and led the congregation in prayer. I am still held in high esteem by the people of that community for my work with their religious leader. However, I know that when he looked into my eyes he knew very well what I was trying to do, but he allowed me to get away with it. Perhaps in the final analysis he did maintain his autonomy. He could have easily ignored me or had me released from the case. The caring relationship we had built over time had paid off.

In this case, the therapist demonstrates sound evidence of mindfulness, perhaps at Epstein's highest level—presence. His critical self-reflection allowed *him to examine his own belief system and values, while still being present and nonjudgmental with his patient.*

My Reflections on Mindfulness

✧✧ As I reflect on both of these cases I ask myself, "what contributed to the students' ability to demonstrate mindfulness?" Although they used the structure of the learning experience and written clinical ethics case report as an opportunity to think back about their thinking and actions in these cases, there is evidence of mindfulness in their actions. For Sally, perhaps it was because she was initially the "observer of the observed" as she was the student watching the therapist and the patient and from a minority group herself. For the experienced therapist, it may have been that his initial handling of the case came from his tacit knowledge and intuitive decision making. Now he was using this learning experience as an opportunity to critically self-reflect on his actions using core principles from his ethics course. The case analysis provided him the structure for his reflection on his past experience. ✧

✧ MINDFULNESS: DOES IT HAVE A ROLE IN TEACHING AND LEARNING IN ETHICS?

"The greatest gift that faculty can give to students, and that they can give to themselves, is to infuse all they know with a healthy uncertainty."[1] We all know firsthand the delight with which health professions students engage in ethics when they suddenly realize that uncertainty is more prevalent than right answers. Here is a quote from one of my student's evaluations on his self-assessment: "At the beginning of this semester I was not excited about taking this course. I hated classes like this. I also was not fond of your teaching style. Your lectures were all over the place and seemed meaningless."

I believe that facilitating the development of mindfulness in our students as both a formative and summative outcome of professional competence has everything to do with teaching and learning in ethics. In fact, as I critically reflect on what we know about student learning—ethics may be the most ideal component of the professional curriculum for facilitating *true mindful learning.*

I believe that several core constructs that underlie "mindfulness" are directly related to our ultimate goal in health profession education—preparing a competent health practitioner who will engage in lifelong learning and continue to develop expertise. Epstein and Hundert define professional competence as the *habitual and judicious use of communication, knowledge, technical skills, clinical reasoning/judgment, emotions, values, and reflection in daily practice for the benefit of the individual and community being served.*[3] Furthermore, they state that competence in medicine is built on a foundation of basic clinical skills, scientific knowledge, and moral development. Essential to this building of competence is habits of mind—including several of the characteristics of mindfulness—attentiveness, critical curiosity, self-awareness, and presence.

If I look more closely at several of the terms used in discussing mindfulness, I see concepts that do not appear to be mutually exclusive but are being used in ways to bring more clarity to the concept or perhaps are being seen through a different disciplinary lens. For example, Dewey's notion of *inquiry* is a central tenet of reflection.[15] One cannot reflect or engage in inquiry unless he or she is aware of context—that is something different or problematic. *Critical self-reflection* involves thinking about one's own learning and to do that one must be mindful.[2,20,21] Brookfield emphasizes that there are three common assumptions for critical reflection: paradigmatic assumptions that structure the world into categories with the most difficult to identify being in oneself, prescriptive assumptions about what we think ought to happen in a specific situation, and casual assumptions about how the world works and how it may be changed.[27] *Transformation of learning* occurs when there has been movement and a reformulated structure of meaning.[20,21] Mentkowski and colleagues would argue that transformative learning occurs when learners have engaged in four domains of growth—development, self-reflection, reasoning, and performance.[21] In this transformative learning model, the critical elements for learners include using *metacognitive strategies* (thinking about their thinking), self-assessment of performance, and awareness of context. Doesn't this sound like mindfulness?

Inquiry into Student Learning in Ethics

I can share with some confidence evidence from my inquiry into student learning in my ethics teaching.[28] My teaching of ethics continues to evolve and be shaped through mentorship of my colleagues at the Center for Health Policy and Ethics. The past 2 years, I have continued to integrate more active learning experiences into the course and go beyond paper case analysis. I now integrate two encounters in which students must interact with standardized patients (SP). The standardized patient has a script with designated prompts to follow. The student does an interview with the standardized patient much like they would do in the clinic. Two structured levels of analysis occur following the standardized patient interaction. The first is done immediately after the student has completed the session and must respond to a series of structured questions. Each session is also videotaped so the second level of analysis is accomplished through small group review of this videotape. Here is a description of a standardized patient case experience:

> *The first SP case presents a very common dilemma for physical therapists, honoring patient autonomy when it may be in direct tension with promoting beneficence or good for the patient. One of the key elements in the case centers on the issue of patient adherence or ability to follow through with exercise programs and safety concerns. One of the challenges for therapists is being present, respecting the patient, yet listening to the concerns of the patient and family while working together toward a mutually acceptable solution. The student must be careful not to get frustrated and judge the patient. If this occurs the patient is prompted to follow the lead of the student. If however the student is present, listening to the concerns of the patient, and able to negotiate a solution the patient will follow that lead.*

Immediately following the interaction with the standardized patient, the student responds to these questions.

1. What was the **central** ethical issue you encountered?
2. At the end of the interview, why did you choose the action you did?
3. If you were the therapist in this case, what would you **do next**?
4. What still confuses you about this case?
5. What did you **learn** about **yourself** from doing this encounter? (What could you not do that perhaps you can do now?)

When I analyzed the narrative data in this initial set of student responses, I found the following: student responses and reflections centered around issues of uncertainty and self-confidence. The specific coding categories for student responses and reflections included: (1) Struggle, frustration, problem focus, personal insight; (2) Struggle, personal insight, respect for the patient, and (3) No struggle, confident, knows the solution.

Struggle, Frustration, Problem Focus, Personal Insight

The majority of student responses were in the category of the student struggle, frustration, problem focus, and personal insight. Here students acknowledge the struggle and uncertainty of the interaction with the "stranger," which is followed by their expressions of some frustration with their inability to "fix the problem" and then a reflective focus on self and need to improve their skills. Here is an example of this approach from Kate. "The problem in this case was that the patient did not want to go to a nursing home yet she could not do her ADLs. ... she was non-compliant.... I really wanted to try to provide the patient with independence and give her an ultimate last chance but it didn't work. I feel I am getting better at trying to understand the patient's needs. ... I need to look at the bigger picture."

Struggle, Personal Insight, Respect for the Patient

A smaller cohort of students (n=7) had evidence of recognizing the struggle and uncertainty of the case along with personal insight and then an ability to bring that insight together with ethical principles, as seen here with Don:

Patient autonomy was the central issue in this case. Also as a PT I did not want to do harm to the patient or the family and wanted to help them. At first, I was going off of what the family was saying was true but then it might not mean that the patient wasn't telling the truth but maybe there was a lack of communication. I had to think on my feet and I learned to give the patient the benefit of the doubt and try to think of how we could get to the underlying problem. I feel like I was able to maintain respect for the patient.

No Struggle, Confident, Knows the Solution/Judgmental

Another small cohort of students (n = 8) experienced no reported struggle, was not confused about the case at all, and the students were very confident in their ability to resolve the case based on their judgment of what needed to be done as seen here: "The patient had desires that were in direct conflict with her overall well being and health status ... I simply told the patient that we were going on with the family conference where we could hear the concerns of all involved. I learned that I can deal with an ethical issue on the fly and do that without stumbling over my words or thoughts."

Although I have spent the last 15 years priding myself on being in the role of advocate for promoting methods of facilitating reflection in my students, this inquiry into my own teaching through evidence of student learning became a critical incident for me. I will never forget that moment of my own personal insight as I realized that I had a deeper understanding of what students were actually thinking.

For the students, I believe the standardized patient interaction provides a more realistic, *authentic* learning experience that mirrors clinical reality. For physical therapy students, I believe this kind of experience enhances the *clinical credibility* of ethics. The experience also places a different emphasis on ethical case analysis that goes beyond analysis of a paper case or discussion of a media clip. Students

in the standardized patient experience are at the center of the action/interaction as part of a "lived experience." The structured debriefing questions that students responded to immediately after the interaction appear to facilitate further student reflection on the standardized patient process and provided me with insight into their reflective process.

As I continue to think about this learning experience in the context of this chapter, I see evidence of *mindful learning*. Perhaps standardized patient interactions provide an authentic performance-based learning experience more consistent with what Langer calls *sideways learning*.[18] She contrasts sideways learning with the standard top-down (traditional lecture) or bottom-up (direct experience and repeated practice) approaches that dominate most educational settings. Sideways learning revolves around facilitating a mindful state where there are the following characteristics: "1) openness to novelty, 2) alertness to distinction, 3) sensitivity to different contexts, 4) implicit, if not explicit, awareness of multiple perspectives; and 5) orientation to the present."[18]

For those students who were very confident about their ability to "fix this problem" and not confused about the case at all—there was little sense of context or perspective—only their own. For the other two groups of students, the struggle with the uncertainty led to some frustration, which in turn led to some evidence of critical self-reflection.

Remember the quote from the student who hated classes like this? Well, here is the remainder of his self-assessment. This is a young man who, in his first standardized patient interaction, was very confident and told the patient she had better exercise or go to the nursing home. I took the opportunity to reflect on his reflections of how he handled the patient interaction, providing him with a few gentle insights. This led to a dramatic observable change. He started sitting up front in class and actively participating in class. Here is what he wrote in the remainder of his self-assessment at the end of the course.

Solving ethical issues is still the hard part. My background is in science at the cellular level where I look for a certain right or wrong answer. Over the course of the semester I have learned that in many cases there is not a certain right or wrong answer and answers seem to lead to more questions. However, many times that may be the best answer.

(Then in his comments on the back of the page) … I did not see ethical problems in your examples. At this point, I was wrong about everything and I am not afraid to admit it. I have learned so much, not about the cases but about myself much of this I cannot explain in words. Your class has changed the way I look at many situations and this is for the better…

❖ CONCLUSION: ETHICS EDUCATION—AN ESSENTIAL ELEMENT OF MINDFUL LEARNING

I stated earlier in this chapter that I believe ethics education may be the most ideal component of the professional curriculum for facilitat-ing *true mindful learning.* I still believe that. Mindfulness is a graduate outcome that is an essential element of professional competence. We must however see ethics education in the larger context of clinical competence and performance. I see ethics education as a critical bridge—facilitating mindful learning through our emphasis on metacognitive strategies (habits of mind). This bridge is essential in helping students engage in their learning through authentic assessment opportunities and make connections between our traditional (normative) view of professional education as knowledge, skill, and reasoning, and the human sciences. See Figure 18.1.

We have the perfect opportunity in teaching ethics to work toward this outcome. We too, as educators, must be involved in our own critical self-reflective process and actively assess student learning in our classrooms. I will close this chapter with a quote about "a table of learning" from Lee Shulman.[29] For me this paragraph

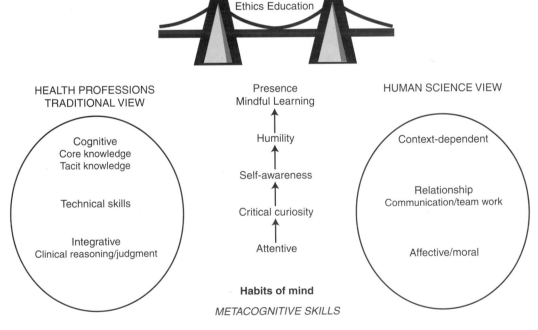

Dimensions of Professional Competence

Ethics Education

HEALTH PROFESSIONS TRADITIONAL VIEW

Cognitive
Core knowledge
Tacit knowledge

Technical skills

Integrative
Clinical reasoning/judgment

Presence
Mindful Learning

↑

Humility

↑

Self-awareness

↑

Critical curiosity

↑

Attentive

HUMAN SCIENCE VIEW

Context-dependent

Relationship
Communication/team work

Affective/moral

Habits of mind

METACOGNITIVE SKILLS

Figure 18.1 ❖ Ethics education provides a critical bridge as educators work toward facilitating habits of mind in linking our traditional view of health professions education with the human sciences. (Adapted from Epstein RM, and Hundert E: Defining and assessing professional competence. JAMA 287(2):226–235, 2002.)

embodies key elements in teaching and learning in ethics:

Learning begins with student engagement, which in turn leads to knowledge and understanding. Once someone understands, he or she becomes capable of performance or action. Critical reflection on one's practice and understanding lead to higher order thinking in the form of a capacity to exercise judgment in the face of uncertainty and to create designs in the presence of constraints and unpredictability. Ultimately, the exercise of judgment makes possible the development of commitment. In commitment, we become capable of professing our understandings and our values, our faith and our love, our skepticism and our doubts, internalizing those attributes and making them integral to our identities. These commitments, in turn, make new engagements possible—even necessary.[29]

As ethics educators in occupational therapy and physical therapy and an organized community of concern, we serve a critical role in facilitating necessary changes in health professions education. What will we do?

References

1. Langer EJ: Mindfulness. Perseus Books, Cambridge, MA, 1989.
2. Epstein RM: Mindful practice. JAMA 282(9):833–839, 1999.
3. Epstein RM, and Hundert E: Defining and assessing professional competence. JAMA 287(2):226–235, 2002.
4. Leach D: Competence is habit. JAMA 287:243–244, 2002.
5. Eraut M: Developing Professional Knowledge and Competence. Falmer Press, London, 1994.
6. Benner P: From Novice to Expert. Addison-Wesley Publishing Co Inc, Menlo Park, CA, 1984.
7. Benner P, Tanner CA, and Chelsa CA: Expertise in Nursing Practice: Caring, Clinical Judgment and Ethics. Springer Publishing Co Inc, New York, 1996.
8. Higgs J, and Tichen A: Practice Knowledge and Expertise in the Health Professions. Butterworth-Heinemann, Boston, 2001.
9. Jensen GM, et al: Expertise in Physical Therapy Practice. Butterworth-Heinemann, Boston, 1999.
10. Kopelman L: Values and virtues: How should they be taught? Acad Med 74(4):1307–1310, 1999.
11. Shepard KF, and Jensen GM: Handbook for Teaching Physical Therapists. Butterworth-Heinemann, Boston, 1997.
12. Schon DA: Educating the Reflective Practitioner: Toward a New Design for Teaching and Learning in the Professions. Jossey-Bass, San Francisco, 1987.
13. Shepard KF, and Jensen GM: Physical therapist curricula for the 1990s: Educating the reflective practitioner. Phys Ther 70(9):566–577, 1990.
14. Parham D: Toward professionalism: The reflective therapist. Am J Occup Ther 41:555–561, 1987.
15. Dewey J: Democracy and Education. Macmillan, New York, 1916.
16. Barnitt RE, and Roberts LC: Facilitating ethical reasoning in student physical therapists. J Phys Ther Educ 14(3):35–41, 2001.
17. Jensen GM, and Paschal KA: Habits of mind: Student transition toward virtuous practice. J Phys Ther Educ 14(3):42–47, 2000.
18. Langer EJ: The Power of Mindful Learning. Addison-Wesley Publishing Co Inc, Reading, MA, 1997.
19. Brookfield SD: Transformative learning as ideology critique. In Merizow J (ed): Learning as Transformation. Jossey-Bass, San Francisco, 2000.
20. Mezirow J (ed): Learning as Transformation. Jossey-Bass, San Francisco, 2000.
21. Mentkowski M, et al: Learning that Lasts: Integrating Learning, Development and Performance in College and Beyond. Jossey-Bass, San Francisco, 2000.
22. Blensky M, and Stanton A: Inequality, development and connected knowing. In Merizow J (ed): Learning as Transformation. Jossey-Bass, San Francisco, 2000.
23. Demick J: Toward a mindful psychological science: theory and application. J Soc Issues 56(1):141–159, 2000.
24. Langer EJ: Mindful learning. Curr Dir Psychol Sci 9(6):220–223, 2000.
25. Stern DT: Practicing what we preach? An analysis of the curriculum of values in medical education. Am J Med 104:569–575, 1998.
26. Feudtner C, Christakis DA, and Christakis NA: Do clinical clerks suffer ethical erosion: Student perceptions of their ethical environmental personal development. Acad Med 69:670–679, 1994.
27. Brookfield SD: Becoming a critically reflective teacher. Jossey-Bass, San Francisco, 1995.
28. Jensen GM: Exploration of critical self-reflection in the teaching of ethics: The case of physical therapy. Paper presented at: American Educational Research Association Annual Meeting, April 21, 2003, Chicago, IL.
29. Shulman L: Making differences. Change 34(6):36–44, 2002.

19

Reflections on Spirituality: Implications for Ethics Education

Linda Gabriel, PhD, OTR

Abstract

Human beings are essentially spiritual creatures because we are driven by a need to ask 'fundamental' or 'ultimate' questions.... We are driven, indeed we are defined, by a specifically human longing to find meaning and value in what we do and experience.[1]

I have only recently entered into the study of systematic reflection on and the teaching of ethics in occupational therapy. My course includes content from traditional bioethics, virtue ethics, ethics of care, and, of course, codes of ethics. The structure of the course includes frequent small group discussions designed to facilitate reflection. I keep wondering, however, if this learning will serve the students well when they encounter ethical distress and ethical dilemmas in future clinical practice. I continue to have a nagging feeling that some important affective learning element or ingredient is missing (or underrepresented) from my course. As Triezenberg and Davis stated, "So no matter how elegant our teaching, when 'push comes to shove' what really matters is that we have the will, the character to follow through with what we know is right and best."[2] This chapter provided me with the impetus to ponder this missing element. I decided that the element I wished to explore was awareness of personal spirituality and its relationship to ethical reasoning in clinical practice.

In this chapter I first provide descriptions for the terms spirituality, religiousness, religiosity, morality, and ethics. Then, I briefly examine spirituality in Western culture and medicine as the context in which the recent and increasing interest in spirituality exists. Next, an introduction to the concept of spiritual intelligence, which I believe is relevant to the discussion of a linkage between spirituality and ethics, is presented. This is followed by a brief overview of the roles of spirituality in occupational therapy practice, which also may be applicable to physical therapy practice. Difficulties with defining spirituality is reviewed and a rationale for the definition used in this paper provided. Although explicit discussion of spirituality is less prevalent in the physical therapy literature, similar concepts of ethos, empathy, moral reasoning, and moral agency are briefly reviewed. The primary purpose of this chapter is to explore the possible link between spiritual self awareness and the teaching and learning of ethics. I propose that providing students with the opportunity to increase their own spiritual awareness could be an important and powerful component of teaching ethics to occupational therapy and physical therapy students. Finally, I share some preliminary ideas about how this could be accomplished.

✧ DEFINITION OF TERMS REGARDING SPIRITUALITY

My intent in offering the following definitions is to provide clarity for this chapter. This chapter describes spirituality as a universal life force that provides an individual with a sense of meaning, value, and connectedness to self, to other people, and to a larger meaning or purpose in life.[3,4] Individuals may take one of three approaches to express spirituality: religious, sacred, or secular. A religious approach to answering spiritual questions involves the use of a theistic framework. A sacred approach rejects the theistic framework but uses belief in a higher power or ultimate truth to guide the search for answers to spiritual questions. A secular approach to spiritual questions uses alternative perspectives, such as humanism, existentialism, or reverence for nature.[5]

Religiosity is described as a "search for identity, belonging, and meaning through participation with an identifiable group of people that is organized around a spiritual goal."[5] "A religious approach to spiritual questions is based on a theistic framework often within an organized doctrine that sets out answers or teachings in response to spiritual questions."[5]

Morality: "Morality, then, is concerned with relations between people and how, ultimately, they can best live in peace and harmony."[6] It makes up the guidelines that preserve the very fabric of a society.[6]

Ethics: "Ethics is systematic reflection on morality: 'systematic' because it is a discipline that uses special methods and approaches to examine moral situations and 'reflection' because it consciously calls into question assumptions about existing components of moralities that fall into the category of habits, customs, or traditions."[6]

Spirituality in Western Culture

There appears to be a resurgence of interest in matters relating to spirituality.[1,7–11] According to Zohar and Marshall, many people in the Western cultures are spiritually undernourished, suggesting that this spiritual poverty results, in part, from the rise of individualism and rationalism that accompanied the 17th century scientific revolution.[1]

Currently, increased interest in spirituality is evident in the practice of medicine.[8,12,13] Kalb reported that according to a Newsweek poll, 72% of Americans would welcome an opportunity to talk with their physician about their faith, 84% think that praying for the sick improves their chances for recovery, and only 28% think religion and medicine should be separate.[8] The Newsweek article also noted that more than 70 of the United States' 125 medical schools offer specific courses in spirituality or incorporate the content throughout the curriculum.[8] Post, Puchalski, and Larson state that "patient expressions of spirituality should be screened for and respected by physicians."[12] Koenig urges physicians to take a spiritual history as part of a comprehensive medical evaluation.[13] During the spiritual history, the physician should listen and provide presence and support, but not attempt to demonstrate expertise in religious matters.

If the field of medicine is focusing this degree of attention on spirituality, can occupational therapists and physical therapists afford not to become more involved in it?

Spiritual Intelligence

Zohar and Marshall describe spiritual intelligence (SQ) as: "… the intelligence with which we address and solve problems of meaning and value, the intelligence with which we can place our actions and our lives in a wider, richer, meaning-giving context, the intelligence with which we can assess that one course of action or one life-path is more meaningful than another. SQ is the necessary foundation for the effective functioning of both IQ and EQ. It is our ultimate intelligence."[1]

In this passage, EQ refers to emotional intelligence, which provides the awareness of our own and others' feelings and the ability to feel emotions, such as empathy, compassion, and motivation. These authors also make a clear distinction between SQ and religion: "SQ has no necessary connection to religion. For some people, SQ may find a mode of expression through formal religion, but being religious does not guarantee high SQ. Many humanists and atheists have very high SQ; many actively and vociferously religious people have very low SQ."[1]

According to Zohar and Marshall, human beings are fundamentally spiritual beings because we are driven "by a specifically human longing to find meaning and value in what we do and experience."[1] They further argue that spiritual intelligence gives us our moral sense and it "facilitates a dialogue between reason and emotion, between mind and body."[1] The connections suggested between meaning and experience, and between mind and body, to my mind, bear a striking resemblance to the essence of occupation as used in occupational therapy.

✧ SPIRITUALITY AS RELATED TO THE PRACTICE OF OCCUPATIONAL THERAPY

Concern for the spiritual nature of human beings has been part of occupational therapy since the profession's founding, sometimes in the foreground of practice and other times relegated to the background.[14] That the spiritual nature of human beings be brought to the foreground is now voiced by many in the profession.[3-5,7,11,14-30] Peloquin underscores the need and importance of bringing spirituality front and center by writing that if occupational therapists "profess that the perspectives, values, needs, and strengths of individuals will direct their interventions, they must address the spiritual dimensions of those perspectives and values, needs and strengths."[14]

The work of many authors and organizations became highly visible in 1997. During that year both the *American Journal of Occupational Therapy* and the *Canadian Journal of Occupational Therapy* published special issues focused on spirituality. In addition, the Canadian Model of Occupational Performance was revised and placed spirituality at the core of its model.[31] Also in 1997, the *British Journal of Occupational Therapy* published a series of letters submitted from 1979 to 1996 that focused on spirituality and occupational therapy.[3] The Canadian Association of Occupational Therapists (CAOT) has defined spirituality as: "A pervasive life force, manifestation of a higher self, source of will and self-determination, and a sense of meaning, purpose and connectedness that people experience in the context of their environment" and states that "spirituality resides in persons, is shaped by the environment, and gives meaning to occupations."[4] This definition was intended to be broadly inclusive of diverse spiritual perspectives with a secular view of spirituality; one that separated it from religiosity.[4,31]

In 2002, the American Occupational Therapy Association published a new Practice Framework, which includes the spiritual context of a person's life as one of seven aspects of contexts for practice. Context "refers to a variety of interrelated conditions within and surrounding the client that influences performance."[32] Spiritual is defined as "The fundamental orientation of a person's life; that which inspires and motivates that individual."[32] As an example, the AOTA Practice Framework lists "essence of the person, greater or higher purpose, meaning, substance."[32] According to Peloquin, occupation, the core of our therapy, animates the human spirit and spirituality brings meaning to our occupations.[18] According to Christiansen, "If occupational therapy is to be complete and genuine in its consideration of humans as occupational beings, it must acknowledge spirituality as an important dimension of everyday life."[23]

A related concept, spiritual health, is defined by Hasselkus as "an optimal state of balance in life between the spiritual essence of one's inner being and the worldly connections of one's outer self."[3] She cites Bellingham and colleagues as identifying connectedness as the key element to spiritual health—connectedness to oneself, connectedness to other people, and connectedness to a larger meaning or purpose in life.[3] Egan and DeLaat write about spiritual health as being connected in three spheres.[25] The first sphere is connectedness with one's self by remaining intimately in touch with one's own feelings and exploring one's own values. Connectedness with others is the second sphere where "individuals are encouraged to assess their physical, emotional and intellectual connections with others" and to make time, space, and feelings available for others.[25] The third sphere is connectedness with the rest of creation (and they include one's creator). Egan and DeLaat suggest that creativity is also important in this sphere.[25] Urbanowski and Vargo also describe three levels of meaning related to spirituality, but these are more secular and described as having to do with the individual, the family, and the community.[15]

Swarbrick and Burkhardt describe the development of interventions directed at spiritual health in clients.[17] They define spiritual health as including, but not limited to, "faith, values, beliefs, and attitudes which are intangible components that impart vitality and meaning to life events."[17] They believe that most entry-level practitioners do not have the skills to provide interventions for spiritual health because most entry-level educational programs lack content about spiritual health. They urge the profession to continue to engage in exploring "the spiritual domain of health and the achievement of a sense of well-being through scientific inquiry and analysis of qualitative data describing clinical experiences and actual life case stories."[17]

What about physical therapy? Due to the recent interest in spirituality as part of occupational therapy practice, there are far more publications examining this construct explicitly in the occupational therapy literature than in the physical therapy literature. There are authors, however, who write about the importance of self awareness to moral agency, which I suggest could be considered aspects of personal spirituality.[2,33] In describing the process of empathy, Davis notes that the second stage of empathy (crossover) requires self awareness and a secure sense of self.[33] Triezenberg and Davis describe moral behavior as requiring moral sensitivity (ability to identify and interpret a situation containing moral content), moral reasoning (process of considering all the angles of a situation and deciding what the most right action would be), and moral character (ability to act on moral decisions).[2] In discussing moral character, these authors stress that to be effective moral agents one must understand one's core values and personal metabeliefs and ask oneself questions such as "What has ultimate meaning for me and why?"[2]

✧ DIFFICULTIES IN DEFINING SPIRITUALITY

A variety of authors in occupational therapy literature from Canada, the United States, and Great Britain have struggled to define spirituality and lamented the variability and the lack of clarity and consistency among definitions of spirituality in relation to occupational therapy.[5,7,14,15,20,24,27,28,30] Part of this uncertainty

may be the result of differing opinions about just what spirituality means.

Unruh, Versnel, and Kerr performed a broad and systematic examination of definitions of spirituality in the health literature.[5] Definitions were sorted into what became seven categories. The first of these categories included "Relationship to God, spiritual being, higher power, a reality greater than the self." A distinction was made between spirituality and religiosity within this category:

The spirituality definition proposed by Hill et al. (1998) is noteworthy in this category because it reflects the outcome of a consensus panel deliberation (a panel primarily of psychologists, sociologists, and medical specialists). Spirituality was defined as an individual search for the sacred with sacredness defined as a "socially influenced perception of either some divine being, or some sense of ultimate truth or reality" (Hill et al., 1998, p. 20). The panel contrasted religiosity with spirituality by defining religiosity as a "search for identity, belonging, and meaning through participation with an identifiable group of people that is organized around a spiritual goal."[5]

The second category was "Not of the self." The definitions in this category emphasized the spirit. These definitions implied a relationship with a higher power but were less explicit than the first category. "Transcendence or connectedness unrelated to a belief in a higher being" described the third category, and the fourth category was "Existential, not of the material world." The fifth category centered on definitions that suggested "The way in which a person constructs meaning and purpose is her or his spirituality."[5] Category six focused on the "life force of the person, integrating aspect of the person" and the final category was titled "summative" and included definitions that attempted to combine multiple features of spirituality.

Unruh, Versnel, and Kerr go on to discuss three general approaches (religious, sacred, and secular) to addressing spiritual questions:

A religious approach to spiritual questions is based on a theistic framework often within an organized doctrine that sets out answers or teachings in response to spiritual questions. A sacred approach implies that aspects of a theistic framework are rejected but belief in a higher being or ultimate truth may be retained in some way and may guide the search for answers to other spiritual questions. In contrast, a secular approach to the same spiritual questions involves a rejection of theistic and sacred frameworks with a preference for alternative perspectives such as humanism, existentialism, evolution and so on.[5]

Based upon reviewing this literature, certain questions arise. Is a consensus among therapists necessary regarding the definition of spirituality? Are there variations of the term spirituality that can coexist? At this point in my reading, I would agree with Peloquin (2003) who notes that "attempts at reconciling diverse definitions have led most to see spirituality as multifaceted."[14] Just as meaning is defined by the individual, it would seem that spirituality is also defined at the personal level. I believe it is possible and necessary to have a definition of spirituality that includes several variations, and the variation that is employed at any one point in time depends on the individual and his/her context. This precludes a unitary and specific definition of spirituality. Perhaps this approach is preferable as long as all therapists understand the breadth and depth of the term, and there is consensus about those variations of spirituality that can inform practice and allow scholars to investigate its impact. I propose for this chapter that spirituality be described as a universal life force that provides an individual with a sense of meaning, value, and connectedness to her/himself, to other people, and to a larger meaning or purpose in life.[3,4] Individuals may take one of three general approaches to express spirituality; religious, sacred, or secular.[5]

If we are to fully understand spirituality as it guides our interactions with others, we must first understand and nurture spirituality in ourselves. Connectedness to self was emphasized earlier in this paper as the most fundamental part of spiritual health.[3,15,25] Consider the following passage (particularly the fourth bulleted item) from *Spirituality in Enabling Occupation: A Learner-Centered Workbook* published by the CAOT Publications:

Attending to spirituality in the Occupational Performance Process draws one into active listening, and enriches the development of a relationship with an individual client, a group, or the representatives of an agency or organization. This relationship is based on dialogue which opens the door for the client to articulate ideas about meaning and purpose. The process includes:

- ✦ Assessment procedures which honor subjective input
- ✦ Client-centered goal formation and documentation
- ✦ The occupational therapist as advocate with and for the client
- ✦ The occupational therapist's awareness of his/her own spirituality
- ✦ Validation of the client's spirit[4]

In Box 19.1 I share part of a story from Remen, an author whose two books have had a profound effect on my spiritual growth and my ability to articulate my spiritual beliefs.[34] This passage is about personal integrity, but I think it can have a parallel meaning with one's awareness of spirituality as well.

Spirituality and Teaching Ethics

Given this discussion of spirituality, how do we begin to integrate it into education of students in occupational and physical therapy? I believe two foundations from ethics education will better prepare therapists to integrate spirituality into practice.

Triezenberg and Davis make a strong case for the deliberate and carefully planned teaching of moral reasoning to physical therapy students.[2] They describe some of the research of J.R. Rest on moral reasoning as a developmental process that requires instruction, reflection, and experience. Triezenberg and Davis also challenge faculty to examine their attitudes and behaviors and to model the professional values they want their students to acquire.[2]

The need to teach moral reasoning to occupational therapy students is also voiced by Kanny and Kyler.[35] They also cite work by Rest and state: "Action generally outweighs rhetoric, and acting in what one perceives to be the "right" manner involves more than knowing rules or a code of ethics or being able to reason through a decision. Acting in the right manner

---

Box 19.1

Integrity is an ongoing process, a dynamic happening over time that requires our ongoing attention. A medical colleague describing his own experience of staying true to himself told me that he thinks of his life as an orchestra. Reclaiming his integrity reminds him of the moment before the concert when the concertmaster asks the oboist to sound an A. "At first there is chaos and noise as all the parts of the orchestra try to align themselves with that note. But as each instrument moves closer and closer to it, the noise diminishes and when they all finally sound it together, there is a moment of rest, of homecoming.

"That is how it feels to me," he told me. "I am always tuning my orchestra. Some- where deep inside there is a sound that is mine alone, and I struggle daily to hear it and tune my life to it. Sometimes there are people and situations that help me to hear my note more clearly; other times, people and situations make it harder for me to hear. A lot depends on my commitment to listen- ing and my intention to stay coherent with this note. It is only when my life is tuned to my note that I can play life's mysterious and holy music without tainting it with my own discordance, my own bitterness, resentment, agendas, and fears."

Deep inside, our integrity sings to us whether we are listening or not. It is a note that only we can hear. Eventually, when life makes us ready to listen, it will help us to find our way home.[34]

---

requires not only recognizing an ethical issue and deciding what is right, but also, more importantly, having the motivation and forti- tude to act on what one believes to be right."[35]

Andre points out that moral behavior involves more than applying ethical rules to conflicts—one must first recognize that a con- flict exists.[36] She makes the case that clearer moral vision requires time and training in reflection. She writes, "Reflection is crucial to moral vision. Reflection consists, partly, in see- ing (into) oneself: it involves paying attention to nagging doubts, finding words for convic- tions, articulating feelings; it requires time and quiet. Reflection is less orderly and less discur- sive than reasoning."[36] I suggest that "seeing into oneself" should also involve reflection on one's spirituality.

As a foundation for spirituality, the second aspect of teaching ethics I want to highlight is the possibility of using virtue ethics. As some other authors in this book have noted, whereas ethics grounded in principles emphasizes duty and/or action, virtue ethics emphasizes the agent (person) who performs actions. Some define moral virtue as a disposition to act in a manner that is consistent with moral principles and ideals. "Virtue ethics is primarily about per- sonal character and moral habit, rather than a particular action ... One becomes just and tem- perate by doing just and temperate things."[37]

In their introduction to virtue theory in medicine, Pellegrino and Thomasma write:

Medicine is a moral community because it is at heart a moral enterprise and its members are bound together by a common moral purpose. If this is so, they must be guided by some shared source of moral- ity ... For centuries, this source was the character of the physician and, in keeping with the moral philoso- phy of the times, virtue ethics provided the concep- tual foundation for professional ethics. In modern times, for reasons we will outline briefly, virtue has been supplanted by principle- and rule-based ethics.[38]

Pellegrino argues that clinical medicine is centered on the personal encounter between physician or healer and patient.[39] Healing acts are centered on caring and alleviating pain and suffering, as well as curing. He notes, "Cure may be futile but care is never futile."[39] He goes on to write, "The optimal end of healing is the good of the whole person—physical, emotional, and spiritual."[39] The good of the whole person includes four components: the medical good, the patient's perception of the good, the good for humans, and spiritual good. He writes, "The highest level of good which must be served in the clinical encounter is the good of the patient as a spiritual being…"[39] Should this not also be the case of occupational therapy and physical therapy? And if we are to achieve this highest good of the patient as a spiritual being, would it not be important to understand the ways in which spirituality is manifested in others and in ourselves?

✧ THE CONNECTION BETWEEN PERSONAL SPIRITUALITY AND LEARNING ETHICS

I believe therapists will be better equipped to wrestle with ethical and moral dilemmas if they have a strong sense of who they are as spiritual beings. And I believe that focused attention should be given to spiritual health of students as well as faculty in entry-level curricula. Such attention should exist across the curricula based on the assumption that all clinical encounters have the potential to contain spiritual elements and that spiritual growth develops over time and with practice. In addition, I would argue that there should be focused spiritual learning experiences in the context of ethics content. It will be important to convey that working on spiritual well-being or health does not mean we are implying that one's spirit is sick or needs treatment. Rather just as cognitive, emotional, and physical growth occurs across a lifetime, so too there is spiritual growth across a lifetime (especially in adulthood). Like with psychological issues, if personal spiritual

issues exist, the student or faculty may wish to seek professional assistance or engage the services of a spiritual advisor or member of the clergy.

A review of ethics textbooks, however, reveals little or no content relative to spirituality. Haddad noted that the discussion of the relationship of spiritual beliefs to ethical decisions has not often occurred outside of theological circles. Gula believes there is an explicit connection between spirituality and ethics, although he notes, "the relation of spirituality and ethics in healthcare has not yet received much attention."[40] "My contention is that our spirituality is the wellspring of moral living. Ethics without spirituality is rootless; spirituality without ethics is disembodied."[40] He further writes:

The heart links spirituality and ethics. The language of principles and consequences that makes up our public ethical discourse is the product of cognitive reflection. Such reflection can be far removed from where our heart lies as the true expression of who we are and what we stand for. Clearer indicators of the heart come through expressions of feelings, intuitions, and somatic reactions. Ethics has for too long neglected these prereflective sources as being reliable guides to moral truth. But our spiritual tradition of discernment has relied on them as pathways for discovering what fits as true for the one making the decision. … The spiritual connects with the ethical at the point of what counts most for us in living."[40]

Zohar and Marshall make a case for using our spiritual intelligence (SQ) to forge a new ethics. In discussing Heisenberg's Uncertainty Principle, they write:

Einstein and Heisenberg helped to bring about a fundamental change in our relationship to truth and ethics. The old way was top-down, an attempt to replace the lost certainties of our biological past with reference to an externally imposed set of truths. But both Heisenberg and Einstein are saying that it all depends in some crucial way upon us. Truth depends upon our point of view, upon the questions that we choose to ask. This is a bottom-up truth, which in some fundamental sense comes from within. It is, I contend, ultimately a truth that we can access only with our spiritual intelligence.[1]

Furthermore, spiritual intelligence lights our way through what mystics have called the "eye of the heart," which can also be a metaphor for intuition. "The spiritually stunted self cannot give us an ethics based on spiritual intelligence, or on the eye of the heart. It has no deep source from which to draw its wisdom or intuition."[1]

Although I do not believe that a bottom-up approach to ethics, drawing on internal spiritual wisdom, can replace codes of ethics and other rule-based approaches, I do believe spirituality should become more central in the learning of ethical reasoning and increase the likelihood of ethical behaviors. This is not a radical departure from virtue ethics or from the early vision of occupational therapy. Peloquin reflects on the early visions of the profession, quoting from the autobiography of an occupational therapist published in 1946, *The Healing Heart* by Carlova and Ruggles, "It is not enough to give a patient something to do with his hands. You must reach for the heart as well as the hands. It's the heart that really does the healing."[41] And Triezenberg and Davis write, "In the words of Willard Gaylin, 'the only way in which knowledge may truly inform conduct is through those emotions that support the good will, the good heart, and the conscience of the individual.'"[2]

✧ IMPLICATIONS AND RESOURCES FOR EDUCATION IN ETHICS RELATED TO SPIRITUALITY

How would one teach spiritual self-awareness? Can it be taught in a college setting? What would it look like? Similar questions have been asked about empathy and moral reasoning and may provide some direction. Davis believes that professional socialization experiences and role modeling can facilitate the occurrence of empathy, even though empathy itself cannot be directly taught in the traditional sense.[33] Likewise anxiety, self-doubt, and low self-esteem can focus one's attention inward, which makes it difficult for empathy to occur. Experiences and interactions may need, there-fore, to be designed that reduce anxiety and self-doubt and increase self-esteem in students.

Triezenberg and Davis urge educators to realize that "the ability to make moral judgments is a characteristic that appears to change with time and experience."[2] They go on to say, "Dramatic and extensive changes occur in young adulthood (the 20s and 30s) in the basic problem solving strategies used to deal with ethical issues...changes in moral judgment are likely to take place during the course of professional education and that the extent of these changes can be affected through directed education."[2]

A Curriculum on Spirituality for Health Professionals

Sierpina and Boisaubin received a Templeton Award to develop a curriculum in spirituality for medical and nursing students at the University of Texas Medical Branch, Galveston.[42] A summary of the course content and listings of references and resources are contained in their article and is also available online at http://atc.utmb.edu/altmed/spirituality.htm. Their course was about the relevance of spirituality to the practice of medicine and nursing, rather than to the development of personal spirituality in students as related to ethical reasoning; however, the latter is implied and could be given greater emphasis. The objectives of the process for course development were to: (a) provide evidence about the known association between spirituality and health, (b) provide information and role models on how spirituality can be used in practice, (c) develop cases for small group discussions to stimulate spiritual thinking, (d) offer clinical formats for taking a spiritual history, and (e) provide a syllabus of materials for education and reference.[42]

The course was taught in both large group sessions and small group discussion. Small groups used case vignettes, role-playing, and panel discussions. The course philosophy held that "Spirituality includes, but is more comprehensive than, religion."[42] Learning also occurred as students shared their personal faith traditions. It was emphasized that telling about one's own religion should not be an attempt to sell that belief system to others. Any attempt to change another student's beliefs was prohibited. There were seven course objectives (learner outcomes). One of these was for students to learn several methods of taking a spiritual history. Although outcome data were not reported, the authors reported that "Spirituality can be introduced and taught in an integrated fashion in both schools of medicine and nursing."[42] They also noted that almost all of the students reported that the topic of spirituality was relevant to the practice of medicine and nursing.

Taking a Spiritual History

Learning how to take and to give a spiritual history would be a good place to start in the process of applying spirituality to ethics education. Several models were reviewed and will be briefly summarized. The HOPE approach to spiritual assessment includes questions in the following categories:

> H: *sources of hope, meaning, comfort, strength, peace, love, and connection*
> O: *organized religion*
> P: *personal spirituality and practices*
> E: *effects on medical care*[43]

Another model, developed by Puchalski, uses the acronym FICA. Spiritual questions are organized into four categories; Faith, what is Important in your life, whether you are part of a spiritual or religious Community, and how you want a health care provider to Address these issues in your health care.[44] A third model, summarized by Sierpina and Boisaubin and based on Maugans, uses the acronym SPIRIT to organize questions: Spiritual belief system, Personal spirituality, Integration with spiritual community, Ritualized practices and restrictions, Implications for medical care, and Terminal events planning.[42]

Questionnaires on Spiritual History

I believe it would be worthwhile to explore these spiritual history questionnaires, and extend the search for additional methods of producing a spiritual history (for example, writing a spiritual autobiography), for possible adaptation for use with college students or professionals to examine their own spiritual identities.

The *Spiritual Well-Being Scale* was obtained and reviewed for consideration as a tool for use with students.[45] It consists of 10 questions designed to be a self assessment of religious well-being and 10 questions designed to be a self assessment of existential well-being. The response to each question is rated on a 6-point Likert scale. Most concepts have both a positive and a negative form of the same question, such as "I feel good about my future" and "I feel unsettled about my future" or "I feel that life is a positive experience" and "I feel that life is full of conflict and unhappiness." Because of the limited scope of the questions, and the closed nature of the answers, I do not feel this scale would contribute to the type of educational experiences I am suggesting for college students or professionals.

Another self assessment, titled *Spirituality Assessment*, has good potential as a possible method for exploring personal spirituality. It was retrieved from www.courage2change.net/spiritassess.htm and identifies the author as Marty Crouch, and is freeware. The assessment begins with the following introduction: "This self assessment was developed to encourage the deepening of spiritual practice. Spirituality is different from religion. Spirituality is one's experience of self as essentially spirit, as a spiritual being with a body. In contrast, religion is an institution developed to assist people in experiencing spirituality. Many people experience the spirituality and religion together, and many do not. Some people are spiritually wounded by their experience with religion."

There are 12 statements that the reader would reflect on and answer in terms of never, rarely, sometimes, often, usually. Under each statement are examples. The 12 statements are:

I practice self care.
I tell the truth to myself and others.
I practice mindfulness.
I allow myself to experience the emotional-pain of the human condition.

I am open to learning.

I experience oneness, rather than separation.

I generously share my abundance of time, talent, and money.

I am grateful.

I participate in spiritual community on an ongoing basis.

I chop wood and carry water. Example: I enjoy what I do, even the simple things that I do.

I am aware of my life-mission.

My history is not my destiny.

Although there are ratings associated with each statement, it appears that there is no attempt to interpret scores. Rather the intent appears simply to increase awareness of where one is compared to where one wants to be, and to track growth over time.

A Workbook on Spirituality

Perhaps the most relevant and exciting resource for considering personal spirituality in the context of learning about ethics is the workbook recently published by the Canadian Association of Occupational Therapists, *Spirituality in Enabling Occupation: A Learner-Centered Workbook.* "The workbook leads occupational therapists to explore both personal and social dimensions of spirituality."[4] The workbook contains six modules and each module contains several reflective exercises. Each exercise lists guiding questions, learning resources, and learning activities. Some modules contain a vignette. Module 1 centers on personal interest in spirituality and contains two exercises, a spiritual autobiography and a professional autobiography. Module 2 centers on the context for considering spirituality and exercises explore concepts such as centeredness, connectedness, and exploring different shapes of spirituality in a secular society. Modules 3 and 4 examine how spirituality is embedded and included in concepts of enabling occupation, module 5 looks at organization of services, and module 6 asks, "How do I know when I am considering spirituality?" A number of the exercises assume that the participant has clinical experience and could be modified to apply to students.

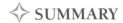

✧ SUMMARY

In summary, I propose that exploring personal spirituality be a part of the educational program for occupational therapy and physical therapy students. Further I suggest that this content be tied to ethics content or ethics courses for the purpose of facilitating moral reasoning, moral agency, and moral courage in future practitioners. This content could also apply throughout occupational therapy curricula as personal meaning of occupation is explored and the relevance of spirituality to occupational therapy intervention is addressed. Content could be applied to both occupational and physical therapy curricula as it relates to empathy and awareness in therapist/client interactions. On a personal level, I plan to spend the next 1 to 2 years exploring more sources of information, identifying collaborators and resource individuals, compiling content and activities, using focus groups of faculty and students as reviewers, and pilot-testing activities with faculty and with students. It will be important that any faculty member who is teaching in this area has completed the self assessment reflection and activities prior to working with students. Consideration will also be given to designing a study that would judge outcomes of learning/growing. Ultimately, a longitudinal study would be really exciting! On a general level, I invite any other interested faculty to use, or expand on, the ideas and resources presented in this chapter. And, should that occur, please share your experiences with me and others. "We can no longer simply hope that our students will become mature professionals with compassion and empathy for patients. We must create experiences to develop these attributes, and we must take responsibility for modeling these behaviors and reflecting on them with students, to raise their consciousness about the nature of a mature healing presence."[33]

References

1. Zohar D, and Marshall I: SQ Spiritual Intelligence. Bloomsbury Publishing, New York, 2000.
2. Triezenberg HL, and Davis CM: Beyond the code of ethics: Educating physical therapists for their role as moral agents. J Phys Ther Educ 14(3):48–58, 2000.

3. Hasselkus BR: The Meaning of Everyday Occupation. Slack Inc, Thorofare, NJ, 2002.

4. Townsand E, et al: Spirituality in Enabling Occupation: A Learner-Centered Workbook. Canadian Association of Occupational Therapists, Ottawa, 1999.

5. Unruh AM, Versnel J, and Kerr N: Spirituality unplugged: A review of commonalities and contentions, and a resolution. Can J Occup Ther 69:5–19, 2002.

6. Purtilo R: Ethical Dimensions in the Health Professions. ed 3. WB Saunders Company, Philadelphia, 1999.

7. Kroeker PT: Spirituality and occupational therapy in a secular culture. Can J Occup Ther 64:122–126, 1997.

8. Kalb C: Faith and healing. Newsweek November 10, 2003, 44–56.

9. Murphy C: Soothing solitude. Omaha World Herald. October 11, 2003, E1-E2.

10. Peloquin SM: The depersonalization of patients: A profile gleaned from narratives. Am J Occup Ther 47:830–837, 1993.

11. Rosenfield MS: Spiritual agent modalities for occupational therapy practice. OT Prac January:17–21, 2000.

12. Post SG, Puchalski CM, and Larson DB. Physicians and patient spirituality: Professional boundaries, competency, and ethics. Ann Int Med 132:578–583, 2000.

13. Koenig HG: Spiritual assessment in medical practice. Am Fam Phys 63:30–33, 2001.

14. Peloquin SM: Spirituality: Meanings related to occupational therapy. In Crepeau EB, Cohn ES, and Schell BAB (eds): Willard and Spakman's Occupational Therapy. JB Lippincott Co, Philadelphia, 2003.

15. Urbanowski R, and Vargo J: Spirituality, daily practice, and the occupational performance model. Can J Occup Ther 61:88–94, 1994.

16. Toomey MA: The art of observation: Reflecting on a spiritual moment. Can J Occup Ther 66:107–109, 1999.

17. Swarbrick P, and Burkhardt A: Spiritual health: Implications for the occupational therapy process. AOTA Ment Health SIS Q 23(2):1–3, 2000.

18. Peloquin SM: The spiritual death of occupation: Making worlds and making lives. Am J Occup Ther 51:167–168, 1997.

19. Kirsh B: A narrative approach to addressing spirituality in occupational therapy: Exploring personal meaning and purpose. Can J Occup Ther 63:55–61, 1996.

20. Howard BS, and Howard JR: Occupation as spiritual activity. Am J Occup Ther 51:181–185, 1997.

21. Frank G, et al: Jewish spirituality through actions in time: Daily occupations of young orthodox Jewish couples in Los Angeles. Am J Occup Ther 51:199–206, 1997.

22. Collins M: Occupational therapy and spirituality: Reflecting on quality of experience in therapeutic interventions. Br J Occup Ther 61:280–284, 1998.

23. Christiansen C: Acknowledging a spiritual dimension in occupational therapy practice. Am J Occup Ther 51:169–172, 1997.

24. Egan M, and DeLaat M: The implicit spirituality of occupational therapy practice. Can J Occup Ther 64:115–121, 1997.

25. Egan M, and DeLaat M: Considering spirituality in occupational therapy practice. Can J Occup Ther 61:95–101, 1994.

26. Engquist DE, et al: Occupational therapists' beliefs and practices with regard to spirituality and therapy. Am J Occup Ther 51:173–180, 1997.

27. Hammell KW: Intrinsicality: Reconsidering spirituality, meaning(s), and mandates. Can J Occup Ther 68:186–194, 2001.

28. Hume C: Spirituality: A part of total care? Br J Occup Ther 62:367–370, 1999.

29. Low JF: Religious orientation and pain management. Am J Occup Ther 51:215–219, 1997.

30. McColl MA: Muriel Driver Memorial Lecture: spirit, occupation and disability. Can J Occup Ther 67:217–228, 2000.

31. Sumsion T: Overview of client-centered practice. In Sumsion T (ed): Client-centered Practice in Occupational Therapy: A Guide to Implementation. Churchill-Livingstone Inc, Edinburgh, UK, 1999, pp 1–14.

32. American Occupational Therapy Association: Occupational therapy practice framework: Domain and process. Am J Occup Ther 56:609–639, 2002.

33. Davis CM: What is empathy, and can empathy be taught? Phys Ther 70:32–36, 1990.

34. Remen RN: My Grandfather's Blessings. Stories of Strength, Refuge, and Belonging. Riverhead Books, New York, 2000.

35. Kanny EM, and Kyler PL: Are faculty prepared to address ethical issues in education? Am J Occup Ther 53(1):72–74, 1999.

36. Andre J: Learning to see: Moral growth during medical training. J Med Ethics 18:148–152, 1992.

37. Edge RS, and Groves JR: Ethics of Health Care: A Guide for Clinical Practice, ed 2. Delmar Publishers, Albany NY, 1999.

38. Pellegrino ED, and Thomasma DC: The Virtues in Medical Practice. Oxford University Press, New York, 1993.

39. Pellegrino ED: The internal morality of clinical medicine: A paradigm for the ethics of the helping and healing professions. J Med Philos 26(6):559–579, 2001.

40. Gula R: Spirituality and ethics in healthcare: The two do not inhabit separate spheres, but are connected. Health Prog July-August:17–19, 2000.

41. Peloquin SM: Reclaiming the vision of reaching for heart as well as hands. Am J Occup Ther 56:517–526, 2002.

42. Sierpina VS, and Boisaubin E: Can you teach medical and nursing students about spirituality? Comp Health Pract Rev 6:147–155, 2001.

43. Anandarajah G, and Hight E: Spirituality and medical practice: Using the HOPE questions as a practice tool for spiritual assessment. Am Fam Phys 63:81–88, 2001.

44. Puchalski CM, and Romer AL: Taking a spiritual history allows clinicians to understand patients more fully. J Pall Med 3:129–137, 2000.

45. Ellison CW, and Paloutzian RF: Spiritual Well-Being Scale. Life Advance, Inc., Nyack, NY, 1982.

20

Educating Adult Health Professionals for Moral Action: In Search of Moral Courage

CAROL M. DAVIS, EDD, MS, PT, FAPTA

Abstract

Meaningful behavior modifications that result in instinctive patterns in people are made most forcefully in the first few years of life, during the human period of prolonged dependence, requiring caring adults. Altering automatic predispositions toward self-interest or indifference in adults is possible, but difficult, and requires the encouragement of both reason and emotion from skilled teachers. How do we develop our moral consciousness and conscience as adults? This chapter first reviews the components of moral action (i.e., thought, emotion and social interaction), and then distinguishes between two common emotions, sympathy and empathy, and links them to altruistic behavior. Moral sensitivity and judgment are then contrasted with moral courage and action. A review of the literature on influencing the moral behavior of children and adolescents follows and finally, suggestions are made, again from the literature, about how to best educate and inspire adults to moral courage, particularly adult physical and occupational therapy students, clinicians, and faculty.

✧ THE CURRENT HEALTH CARE SYSTEM—THE ETHICS OF PROFIT AND BUSINESS

Patients are no longer the center of attention in this current health care "industry." With the Balanced Budget Act of 1997, managed care, cost containment from the Health Care Finance Administration, and the increased emphasis on efficiency, billing, "collectibles," and economic control of costs from insurance companies, we find ourselves practicing in an economic driven, dehumanized jungle of impersonal care. Health care has shape-shifted to business, and profit and business ethics prevail. With that comes an erosion of the appropriate professional moral climate from service to self-interest in all of its forms: greed, fraud as a way of getting what's owed from the government and third-party payers, pleasing powers seen and unseen in order to keep our positions and get paid, expedience, pragmatism, and as Purtilo suggests, the opposite of moral courage: indifference and apathy.[1]

My students have come to me from the clinics with stories featuring each of these forms of self-interest, and I have witnessed many myself in my patient care practice and in my research on how physical therapists think when they resolve ethical dilemmas. What is needed is what most, if not all professionals involved, would advocate—a return to true patient-centered care and service, and a de-emphasis of economics over personalized attention. What is needed is true empathy and sympathy, or the "enlightened" Golden Rule of Edmund Pellegrino: Give the other person the same opportunity that you would want given to you to tell you what it is that they want and need.[2] How do we get from where we are to there? This chapter attempts to shed light on part of this complex problem.

❖ EMPATHY, SYMPATHY, AND ALTRUISM

In 1973, my father was diagnosed with a virulent throat and laryngeal cancer. Over the next 2 years he willingly participated in a clinical trial at a cancer center 6 hours from our home in Pennsylvania. On many of my visits, I was astonished at how poorly he was being cared for by some of the physicians and nursing staff. I wondered, "Surely these people do not recognize the negative impact that their behavior is having on my father, or they would not do what they do. They did not become health professionals to treat people with this kind of indifference and negativity." My stewing about this urged me back to graduate school with the burning question, "What are the roots of compassion? How can we educate health professionals so that they resist stress and recognize the impact that their negative behavior might have on patients and their families?" I recognized that my quest must have something to do with empathy, but I resisted the current (at that time, mid-1970s) flavor of empathy that was being taught and written about: the misinterpretation of Carl Rogers' work in the counseling literature that turned empathy into a skill that one could master and be "graded on" for level of accuracy of repeating back what the person just said. My scholarly efforts were rewarded in the work of Edith Stein, a phenomenology student of Husserl, active in the existential movement in Germany and France in the 1930s.[3] From my work in phenomenology, I settled on the following distinction between sympathy (from the work of Max Schleler[4]) and empathy: whereas sympathy is "fellow-feeling," or a close alignment in thought with another, empathy is a more complex process. Empathy is given *non-primordially*, or after the fact, much like memory (one cannot "empathize" because it happens to you and you realize it after the fact), and it takes place in three rapidly overlapping stages—a mental lining up of thought and awareness (self transposal or perspective-taking) followed by an emotional identification or "crossing over" into the lived experience of the other, followed by getting oneself "back" from the crossing over and a resultant feeling of "fellow feeling" or sympathy, accompanied by a sense of deep understanding and shared emotion.

This definition is accepted in the phenomenological literature, and indeed, formed the foundation of my dissertation research on "A Phenomenological Description of Empathy as it Occurs Within Physical Therapists for their Patients."[5] I collected many cases that illustrate the lived experience of the "crossing over" of empathy in physical therapists with their patients. Most importantly, when they experienced this empathy, they described a true caring relationship with their patients, and were quite moved to act in highly altruistic ways, with true caring beyond that of a rule-based beneficence orientation. Beneficence tells us to do what is right and good for our patients, but does not admonish us to care or act in any way beyond our contractual responsibilities as health care providers. Benevolence, rather than beneficence, implies doing good out of genuine care and concern. Thus, empathy seemed to inspire altruistic action, selfless regard and concern for another, a true caring for patients and a desire to do what is right and good for them as a result of this connection as a result of the moment of crossing over.

But what is more relevant to this work is that not only does the counseling literature reject this fuller explication of empathy—that is, it equates empathy to self transposal or the first of the three stages alone (putting yourself in the place of the other), so too, the moral education literature seems to have adopted this watered down version of empathy with an emphasis on empathy as perspective taking. Ironically, empathy was introduced most emphatically in the moral development literature in response to the inadequacies of the theory that intellect alone can spur one to moral action. Emotion, in the form of empathy, was thought to be essential, along with cognition, in moral decision making and action.

✧ THOUGHT, EMOTION, AND SOCIAL INTERACTION— COMPONENTS OF MORAL ACTION

Contemporary moral education authors and researchers contend that moral thoughts must be accompanied by emotions to lead to moral actions, a point emphasized by several other authors in this book. The emphasis on moral thought alone, from authors such as Piaget, Rawls, and Kohlberg, all the while ignoring emotion, stimulated the research and writing of Hoffman and others.[6] Finally, adding social interaction to cognition and emotion we find the works of Damon, *The Moral Child*[7]; Kurtines and Gewirtz, *Moral Development Through Social Interaction*[8]; and Eisenberg, *Altruistic Cognition, Emotions and Behavior*,[9] among others. The current view of stimulating appropriate moral action in children and adolescents requires experiences that feature not just intellectual moral awareness and judgment, but the emotional aspects of empathy and sympathy as a way of stimulating a fuller awareness of the effect of one's behavior on another person. As John Gibbs puts it, "The attenuation of egocentrism means in positive terms the accurate understanding and consideration of others' viewpoints, needs, rights, feelings and so on."[10] The "affective" point is that such consideration tends to elicit empathic feeling for those others.

Moral Sensitivity and Judgment Versus Moral Courage and Action

James Rest defines **moral sensitivity** as the ability to understand how the actions of one individual may affect others. **Moral judgment** is the ability to analyze a situation and make a good moral decision.[11] Neither of these abilities necessarily infers action, only cognition. Rest goes on to identify **moral character** as the moral attributes and courage needed to act on moral

decisions. Students need to be taught how to identify and resolve ethical dilemmas, but no matter how thorough and refined our education process, a huge gap exists between knowing what is good and right and doing it. Again in Rest's words, moral character is "having the strength of your convictions, having courage, persisting, overcoming distractions and obstacles, having implementing skills, having ego strength."[12] This is quite different from doing what one thinks is right in order to obey the rules, avoid punishment, or please others. These are self-serving reasons for acting, and do not reflect moral courage, in spite of the possible beneficence of the action. One can make a case for enlightened or justified self-interest: acting to protect oneself from a violent patient, or choosing to act in the interests of one's children over one's professional responsibilities are two examples often given. When one acts in this form of self-interest, safety seems to prevail as the key factor, either one's own or one's dependents' safety, rather than greed or expedience or laziness.

To discern moral courage, one needs to look deeper than the action itself, into the motives and intention. The negative, self-serving actions that are listed above stem mainly from fear, whereas moral courage and true altruism flow from a generous and caring heart. Consciousness raising activities for example, exercises that help one to identify deep-seated prejudice, can stimulate moral awareness in adults, but only true caring about others can stimulate one to moral action from moral courage. In the words of Eugene Gaylin from the Hastings Center:[13]

>...the power of knowledge to inform behavior will be greatly influenced by whether the knowledge is sown on the soil of a good conscience. The bad news is that good conscience is set in the first few years of life; the good news is that in the areas from which bioethics emerges—that is, the question of moral dilemmas—knowledge is a powerful tool. And the reasoning of sophisticated philosophers is a source of great help. Bioethics must continue to confront the real world of the passions acted out in the public spaces of the sickroom and the private places of the heart.[13]

Purtilo suggests that readiness for purposive moral action can be facilitated by four main activities: (1) Anchor students in the moral foundations of the health professions; (2) Teach students to gain the full grasp of facts in a situation; (3) Encourage creative responses that foster good practice generally and moral courage specifically, that is, imaginative problem solving accessing key resources and information; and (4) Name and affirm moral courage whenever it is found.[1]

Influencing the Moral Behavior of Children and Adolescents

Damon maintains that the research shows that "childrens' morality is a product of affective, cognitive, and social forces that converge to create a growing moral awareness."[7] The child begins with some natural emotional reactions to social events; these are supported, refined, and enhanced through social experience. In the course of this social experience, the child actively participates in relations with peers and adults, always observing and interpreting the resulting interactions. "From this web of participation, observation, and interpretation, the child develops enduring moral values."[7] Consider how much more dynamic and interactive that description is than what some believe, that children simply learn and perpetuate the rules of the house, or their church, mosque, or synagogue.

For adults to contribute positively to a child's moral development, parents and teachers must operate within an awareness of the child's holistic developmental needs. Adults must practice what Damon calls "respectful engagement" with the child, and moral education must be a cooperative, productively engaging activity, "where the child's own initiatives and reactions must be respected."[7] Children are not their best when left alone.

Children must "learn to direct their moral emotions towards effective social action … learn to modulate their emotional reactions … and above all learn to channel their emotional responses into streams of moral motivation that impel productive action."[7]

Damon and Eisenberg both caution that children can get carried away with empathic responses, and in their emotional intensity, they lack the ability to inhibit certain behaviors like anger.[7,9] Once this occurs, personal distress takes over and actions form not from altruistic reasons, but from self-interest due to "over-arousal." Eisenberg maintains that sympathy, which she defines as a feeling of sorrow or concern, is far more useful in developing altruistic moral action in children than is empathy (putting yourself in the place of the other) due to the potential aversive reaction to the apprehension of another's state.[14] One more point here: All those who research and write about the moral development of children point out the importance of effective parenting and mentoring from adults. In addition to respectful engagement, Damon advocates "authoritative parenting" in which children are confronted with the consequences of bad behavior.[7] Although there are various theories regarding the most effective way to inspire positive development in children and adolescents, most researchers are united in their belief about the characteristics of poor parenting—self centered, immature, delayed responses that result from harsh and arbitrary power-assertive punishment, void of any reasoning or invitation for the child to take the other's perspective. For example, "Stop your crying or I will give you something to cry about."[15] Damon says, "the coercive harshness of these parents reflects their own egocentric needs rather than objective assessments of the child's behavior."[7]

Martin Hoffman calls proper discipline "inductive discipline" and maintains that it must be matched to the developmental level of the child.[16] For example, at first, "If you keep pushing him, he'll fall down and cry." Years later followed by, "Don't yell at him. He was just trying to help you." And later, "He feels bad because he was proud of his tower and you knocked it down."

In working with adolescents and juvenile delinquents, John Gibbs stresses both inductive discipline and providing a cognitive role-playing opportunity, and also cultivating empathy by directing the child's attention to the distressed victim.[15] Positive, "caring" groups using the techniques of positive peer culture and related group approaches serve as the mechanism for guided group discussions of moral problem situations. "[T]hrough the give-and-take challenges and induction-like probes of these discussions, self-centered thinking is attenuated and more mature moral judgment is stimulated."[15] Thinking about others before acting is stressed. Cognitive distortions are aggressively confronted, even more so now due to a culture that emphasizes the morality of expedience, excuses, and rationalization. Blaming others and sloppy self-centered thinking are challenged as thinking errors and adolescents under Gibbs care are taught to correct them. "Considering the 'look out for number one' distortions poisoning our entire society, even non-delinquent kids may not evidence a more fair and caring behavior unless cognitive distortions are corrected."[15] A cognitive distortion is an error in thinking. An example would be the thought that a person who is so stupid as to keep their keys in their car while they run into the store deserves to have the car stolen. The person stealing the car is thus exonerated of guilt by a cognitive distortion.

To summarize, current literature advocates developmentally appropriate active engagement with children and adolescents to facilitate fair and caring behavior, emphasizing (a) accurate thinking, (b) empathic or sympathetic feeling and (c) social interaction as the main foci. What does the literature suggest for adults?

Influencing the Moral Behavior of Adults

Damon and Colby studied morally exemplary adults in in-depth case studies to discern key characteristics.[17] Their criteria for moral exemplars included (a) a sustained commitment to definable moral principles, (b) a consistent tendency to act in accordance with these principles, (c) a demonstrated willingness to affirm (rather than deny or misrepresent) one's acts and to express overtly the principles that constitute one's moral rationale for such acts, (d) a demonstrated willingness to risk personal well-being for the sake of one's moral principles, (e) a capacity for creating and projecting a moral vision, including particularly the ability to generate innovative solutions to moral problems, (f) a talent for inspiring others to moral action, and (g) a dedicated responsiveness to the needs of others.

As you can see, these criteria are indicative

not only of moral sensitivity and judgment, but also of moral character and courage. Both interviews with living people and the biographies of those no longer living served as data sources for their research. They report that their results confirm the importance of the "goal theory model of social influence."[17] In this model, moral development is brought about through the gradual transformation of one's goals by way of social influence, or the inducement of others, in interaction, to adopt new, more satisfying goals. "Over an extended period of time, an entire social perspective can be transferred through this route."[17] The authors use Andrei Sakharov as a case example:

Until the age of 36, Sakharov was a pillar of the Soviet establishment. He was considered both a patriot and a brilliant scientist of unique stature: He was the inventor of the Soviet H-bomb and the youngest person ever to be elected to the Soviet Academy of Sciences.... He enjoyed unparalleled comfort and privilege as a Soviet citizen of the highest order. Beginning in 1957... Sakharov became involved in activities that were permanently to alter his role in Soviet society. These activities, which can only be considered extraordinary from a moral point of view, became progressively challenging to the Soviet order over the next three decades.[17]

The authors chronicle a series of events over 30 years that show a growing maturity in Sakharov's moral development. His moral concerns and his subsequent actions constantly "broadened in scope and implication throughout his adult life." Social influence was determined by the authors to play a major part. "First, it is clear that Sakharov's active engagement in the civil rights cause occurred only after he had established frequent communication with a group deeply concerned about this matter."[17] Prior to this, his moral energies were devoted to issues like nuclear testing and scientific integrity that were directly connected with his own experience and expertise. Sakharov was drawn into this circle of dissidents as his concerns matched some of theirs. Over time, as his colleagues shared their information and insights with him, he was "... introduced to a broader set of issues and was asked to extend his activism accordingly...Collaborative activity induced in the learner a new and broader set of goals." Only later, and under the pressure of repeated urgings and compelling observations, did Sakharov himself take direct public action. So again we see the initial match of goals and procedures, followed by the trying out of the new procedures, followed finally by the adoption of broader goals.[17]

These case study results are important to the treatment of this question in a couple of ways. Moral growth can seem to take place later in life. And second, given a strong moral core, people can and do choose to move forward rather than withdraw from a moral challenge. Just as with developing the moral abilities of children, engagement with others is the key. Sakharov brought his own moral component to the mix, and allowed himself to be open to the influence of a rationale that compelled him to expand his views about right and wrong, best and better, and in the end, he moved out of moral awareness and judgment to moral courage and action.

Sakharov valued truth and justice, and found he could not retreat from the challenges he encountered, no matter what the risk to his life. His colleagues provided him with what the moral development researchers call "positive scaffolding" and he was able to build a new set of moral goals more consistent with his own central value core. The Soviet system did not offer this same positive pull, and in the end, he lost all contact with them and became an "enemy of the people." In 1980, he was exiled from Moscow to Gorky. "He said, 'There is a need to create ideals, even though one can't see a route by which to achieve them; because if there are no ideals there can be no hope, and then one is completely in the dark, in a hopeless, blind alley.' "[17] In his Nobel Prize address (delivered by his second wife, Elena Bonner) Sakharov stated, "We must make good the demands of reason and create a life worthy of ourselves and of the goals we so dimly perceive."[17]

Isn't this a noble cause for us to take up today, as the ways out of our current economic driven health care system seem dark and confusing and inaccessible to us? But the goals we so dimly perceive are becoming more apparent as the situation worsens.

How Do Physical Therapists Think When Making Moral Decisions?

In 1992, my students and I conducted qualitative research on how physical therapists think when they are confronted with moral dilemmas. Thirteen physical therapists, men and women, ranging in age from 29 to 59 years old and representing from 3 to 30 years of experience in acute care, outpatient care, sports physical therapy, home care, rehabilitation, administration, and university teaching were asked, "Tell me about a time when you seemed 'stopped' from moving forward in your clinical work. A problem arose that seemed to bewilder you and you weren't quite sure what to do." Of course, what this question stimulated was the memory of a moral dilemma without having to use the term as such. Taped interviews were transcribed and analyzed by four independent people with consultation from a nurse phenomenologist and physical therapist phenomenologist, and then my students and I identified recurring themes. The results indicated that half used a teleological utilitarian thinking approach (usually "to do what is best for my patient"), and half weighed principles before acting. Each therapist interviewed revealed that he or she cared very much about the patients they spoke of, and, what was quite surprising to us was that, rather than consult the Physical Therapy Code of Ethics or even a colleague, each used an inner discernment to decide what was the best thing to do, and this inner values source stemmed from values taught at home when they were children.

Wise from the College of St. Scholastica recently completed a dissertation entitled, "How Practicing Physical Therapists Identify and Resolve Ethical Dilemmas."[18] She also interviewed 10 physical therapists and came up with a model to describe their process: Identify the problem, weigh the contextual factors involved, gather and share information (including discussion with colleagues and consulting the APTA Code of Ethics), problem solve, decide and act and then, finally, reflect. Her subjects also "determined ... right or wrong, good or bad, dependent upon the values and morals instilled in earlier life."[18] And she too was struck by how present an "ethics of care" was, over a more rational, duty-oriented thinking. In her words:

> ... ethics of care places merits on the emotional reasons for acting and behaving in an ethical manner. By focusing on the relationship between two people, the one-caring and the one cared for, how humans conduct their lives from an ethical standpoint goes beyond duty and consequences. It involves the connection with another human being in order to make the best and most of the situation. The ethics of care requires the one-caring to set aside personal preferences in order to address the specific situational needs of the one cared for....It can be argued that healthcare providers always consider caring and the patient/practitioner relationship when making decisions. However the ethical decision making models...presented in textbooks and professional literature [do] not include this aspect. The fact [that] this research indicates a direct human connection in the weighing of factors involved grounds this important aspect of the decision making process.
>
> ...findings of this study point to the importance of the resources, but the decisions reached are assisted by asking others what they might do or what they might have done if faced with a similar situation....the desire to benefit and care for the patient...outweighed the sense of confidentiality.[18]

Wise's work directs us to look more closely at the emotional and the social interaction or relationship aspects of moral action.

Noddings, best known for her scholarship in the ethics of care, describes caring as "an ethical relationship between individuals that involves receptivity, engrossment, and reciprocity."[19] When she talks about engrossment, she says, "Caring involves stepping out of one's own personal frame of reference into the other's. When we care, we consider the other's point of view, his objective needs, and what he expects of us....We act not to achieve for ourselves a commendation but to protect or enhance the welfare of the one cared-for."[19] This phrase "stepping out" seems to me to point more toward Edith Stein's "crossing over" part of empathy in contrast to perspective taking or putting one's self in the place of the other.

Romanello, a physical therapist, and her colleague wrote an interesting piece entitled "The 'Ethic of Care' in Physical Therapy Practice and Education: Challenges and Opportunities,"[20] in which she reinforces a case made earlier, that an ethic of caring goes beyond simple beneficence or benevolence:

> But benevolence falls short of an ethic of care that allows health care practitioners 'to truly and consistently connect with, be with, and attend to and do for their patients.' A relational ethic of care is a critical component of physical therapy that compels practitioners to construct this relationship with patients as subjects, rather than objects of the healing encounter. Benevolence is an important virtue, but it is not a sufficient ethic to guide practitioners in today's work climates. The ethic of care goes beyond benevolence to build a relationship based on the needs and goals that arise out of the physical therapist-patient relationship.[20]

The authors suggest that educators stress the distinction between one's ethical duty to not harm a patient and one's deeper role in the relational ethic of care. Although the authors do not use the terms, basically they make a recommendation for moving beyond educating for moral sensitivity and judgment to action based on an ethic of care. The importance of developing the skill of listening and paying attention and the relevance of individual patient-centered care is stressed. Journaling or reflective writing and the storytelling of case studies shared by therapists with students will assist in identifying the dilemmas of practice, at the same time emphasizing that the caring relationship must always be at the heart of all that we do in rehabilitation. This demands time and energy that the current health care climate is not willing to give easily. But the patient-practitioner relationship is primary and we must "expect to deal with risks that produce conflict and guilt." Experience alone will not foster an ethic of care. Educators must teach directly about this moral philosophy, and point it out in case studies and in clinical practice. "How to consider a patient's wants, needs, concerns, and values can be interwoven with the teaching of evaluation and therapeutic exercise skills so students learn to combine an ethic of care with their scientific knowledge in order to put the patient's interests before their own."[19]

Teaching Physical and Occupational Therapists for Their Role as Moral Agents

The literature is not without books and articles suggesting the best ways to go about teaching ethics to various health professionals, not just physical therapists or occupational therapists. The Winter 2000 issue of the *Journal of Physical Therapy Education* edited by Dr. Elizabeth Mostrom has several articles directed to the ethics education for this group, particularly articles by Jensen and Paschal ("Habits of Mind: Student Transition Toward Virtuous Practice"), Triezenberg and Davis ("Beyond the Code of Ethics: Educating Physical Therapists for Their Role as Moral Agents"), Barnitt and Roberts ("Facilitating Ethical Reasoning in Student Physical Therapists"), Purtilo ("Moral Courage in Times of Change: Visions for the Future"), and the article by Romanello and Knight-Abowitz on the ethic of care mentioned above ("The 'Ethic of Care' in Physical Therapy Practice and Education: Challenges and Opportunities").[21] All suggest creative educational opportunities and learning experiences that emphasize going beyond moral awareness and judgment and developing moral action. All emphasize the importance of going beyond instruction in bioethics. But after reviewing the literature for this paper, I would like to emphasize certain aspects of this literature as being most important for the times we find ourselves in now at the beginning of the 21st century.

Hillman, in his book, *The Force of Character and the Lasting Life*, says this:[22]

*I am here following a tradition that begins with Socrates, who considered ignorance, especially ignorance of the soul, to be evil, and dedication to enlightenment to be the primary calling in human beings. The tradition insists that a "good" character requires a psychological education, which is nothing more than the dispelling of ignorance. It is a work in the shadows. Socrates and Freud labored in the same cave. I differ from them inasmuch as their path of insight is analytical, mine imaginative. You do not **know** yourself; you discover yourself. You catch a glimpse, recognize a characteristic response, a preference. You see the consistency of your image despite the ups and downs of mood. **And you need others to wake you up if you're to find your face**. (emphasis mine) Self-knowledge appears and disappears as insights in the play of life. Since a differentiated intelligence about one's character takes a lifetime, education of character cannot be accomplished in the younger years.[22]*

It seems as if we can extract a few more important clues from the literature that will serve to extend the excellent writings to date on how to educate for moral agency in the health professions. It is not that these clues have not been mentioned, but I believe that they need a different emphasis.

✧ TEACHING FOR MORAL AGENCY IN ADULT HEALTH PROFESSIONALS

The key is to pull students up from the self-interest positions of Kohlberg's stages one to four (avoiding punishment, reciprocity, social correctness, and rule-based rationales) to level five, in which the importance of the value of the other person is the key consideration for moral action.

Robert Nash is an educator revered by health professionals for his emphasis on the importance of narrative and stories that link us to the everyday context of moral decision making.[23] Because we have some data showing that, when making ethical decisions, physical therapists tend to emphasize the importance of an ethic of care over rule-based problem solving, and also that they tend to place highest emphasis on values instilled in them at a young age, I believe that Nash's emphasis on the importance of stories that capture one's moral autobiography, as well as stories that serve as case examples from practice illustrating the primacy of patient care-giver relationship, are powerful learning experiences for adult health professionals. In addition, Nash's work on one's "first moral language," or the bringing to awareness of important background beliefs that support students' understanding of moral truths taught to them at an early age, is an excellent way to take advantage of the tendency to use inner discernment of personal values as the final step in deciding what to do in ethical situations. Finally, Nash emphasizes the importance of using intuition as a primary resource in resolving dilemmas, even at the risk of seeming too emotional or anti-intellectual.[23] Nash says:

Do not be afraid to consult your intuitive stirrings and your feelings as you work your way through your dilemma. Intuitive flashes of insight and emotional stirrings can often be powerful guides to moral deliberation, if you learn to trust them—even though you also need to treat them with caution. I once submitted an article to a leading journal in higher education on the productive role that intuitions and feelings can play in helping us to arrive at ethical decisions which are reality-based and multi-layered. The critical feedback to the editor from the prepublication reviewers was acerbic, in spite of which the article was eventually accepted and published.

✦ *'This is a very dangerous article. Reject it. It is anti-intellectual.'*

✦ *'Is the author saying that ethical decision-making is all about subjectivity and merely letting our feelings be our guide? I've heard it all now. Throw reason to the winds; just get in touch with your feelings. The answer will automatically come. The writer must be kidding.'*

✦ *[And perhaps most biting of all:] 'The author must be a devotee of Oprah Winfrey, getting in touch with his inner bliss. He should know that there is no place for New-Age, emotional wallowing in higher administration.'[23]*

Nash goes on to say, "Of course, as I continually point out in my teaching, the best approach to ethical decision-making is one that fully integrates feeling, intuition, reason, logic, facts, context, socialization, and professional norms and codes."[23]

Important Elements in Teaching Adults Moral Agency

In sum, the literature emphasizes that, when working with adult occupational and physical therapists to influence moral action, the following are important elements to include:

Recognition of values that were instilled early in life, and comparing them to the values inherent in their health profession for consistency and relevance.

Meaningful interaction with individuals and groups that share moral concerns and who are likely to extend one's moral thought into moral action.

Teaching the foundations of medical ethics for moral sensitivity and moral judgment.

Teaching and modeling the ethics of care, "an ethical relationship between individuals that involves receptivity, engrossment and reciprocity."[19] "Teach students the importance of building relationships with patients based on the needs and goals that arise out of the patient-therapist relationship."[20] Patient-practitioner relationship is primary.

Point out examples of moral courage and ethics of care in case examples and in clinical activity.[1]

Activities that will reinforce these elements are activities already recommended in many of the articles mentioned previously. I feel that particular emphasis should be placed, on the teaching of those interactive processes that further empathy and sympathy: active listening skills, neurolinguistic psychology, assertiveness training, and conflict resolution skills are examples.[24–26] In addition, stories of one's own moral history should be encouraged and analyzed by students and faculty. Relevance to modern-day patient care should be emphasized. As mentioned before, the importance of reflection is critical to this activity, and students often have to be directed to reflect. Journaling is one way to encourage this activity.

Case studies and patient stories emphasizing moral dilemmas and situations should be analyzed. Finally, as Jensen and Haddad suggested in a moral education workshop at the 2003 American Physical Therapy Association Combined Sections meeting, the use of trained actors playing patients with moral dilemmas is invaluable in asking students to think and act morally on the spot.[27] These interactions can be videotaped, and the "patients" are to give direct feedback to the students at the conclusion of the role-play, and later the student and a faculty member inspect the videotape for further learning. More on this pedagogy is described by Haddad in Chapter 27 of this book.[28]

✦ CONCLUSION

Paraphrasing the words of James Hillman, "We need others to wake us up if we are to find our face."[22] Finding our face, or our character, or our foundation for moral action includes an interactive process that acts to pull us up above Kohlberg's first four stages, and into Gilligan's horizontal emphasis Noddings' ethic of care.[19,29] Teaching the four common values of the health professions (beneficence, nonmaleficence, autonomy, and justice) and their three rules (fidelity, confidentiality, and veracity) is important, and teaching the ability to identify and resolve dilemmas is important as well. But we err when we stop here. We must go further to engage students in the elements listed above, and further enlist the aid of clinical faculty in the environment of patient care. We must commit not just to influencing our students to act with moral courage, we must **inspire** them to it. This is the key element that cannot be taught. It must be modeled. We need to be moral exemplars ourselves, and locate others in the community to work with our students to inspire them to action, and then perhaps meaningful change can begin to take place on a grander scale.

References

1. Purtilo R: Moral courage in times of change: visions for the future. J Phys Ther Educ 14(3):4–6, 2000.
2. Pellegrino ED: What is a profession? J Allied Health August:168–176, 1983.
3. Stein E: On the Problem of Empathy. Translated by W. Stein. Martinus Nijhoff, The Hague, 1970 (Original work published in 1930).
4. Schleler M: The Nature of Sympathy. Archer Books, Hamden, CT, 1970.
5. Davis CM: A Phenomenological Description of Empathy as it Occurs Within Physical Therapists for Their Patients. Boston University School of Education, Boston, 1982.
6. Hoffman M: Empathy and Moral Development. Cambridge University Press, Cambridge, MA, 2000.
7. Damon W: The Moral Child. The Free Press, New York, 1988.
8. Kurtines WM, and Gewirtz JL: Moral Development Through Social Interaction. John Wiley and Sons, New York, 1987.
9. Eisenberg N: Altruistic Cognition, Emotions and Behavior. Erlbaum, Hillsdale, NJ, 1986.
10. Gibbs J: Social processes in delinquency. In Kurtines WM, and Gewirtz JL (eds): Moral Development Through Social Interaction. John Wiley and Sons, New York, 1987, p 312.
11. Rest JR: Moral Development: Advances in Theory and Research. Praeger, New York, 1986.
12. Bebeau MJ, Rest JR, and Narvaez D: Beyond the promise: A perspective on moral education. Educ Researcher 28(4):22, 1999.
13. Gaylin E: Knowing the good and doing good. Hastings Cent Rep May-June:36–41, 1994.
14. Eisenberg N: The Development of empathy-related responding. March 3, 2003, University of Miami.
15. Gibbs JC: Fairness and empathy as the foundation for universal moral education. Comenius jrg Netherlands 14:12–23, 1994.
16. Hoffman ML: Moral development in adolescence. In Adelson J (ed): Handbook of Adolescent Psychology. Wiley-Interscience, New York, 1980, p 295.
17. Damon W, and Colby A: Social influence and moral change. In Kurtines WM, and Gewirtz JL (eds): Moral Development Through Social Interaction. John Wiley and Sons, New York, 1987.
18. Wise D: How Practicing Physical Therapists Identify and Resolve Ethical Dilemmas, Capella University, 2000.
19. Noddings N: Caring: A Feminine Approach to Ethics and Moral Education. University of California Press, Berkley, CA, 1984.
20. Romanella M, and Knight-Abowitz K: The "Ethic of Care" in physical therapy practice and education: Challenges and opportunities. J Phys Ther Educ 14(3):20–25, 2000.
21. Mostrom E. Guest Editorial: Moral and ethical development in physical therapy practice and education: Crossing the threshold. J Phys Ther Educ 14(3):2–4, 2000.
22. Hillman J: The Force of Character and the Lasting Life. Random House, New York, 1999.
23. Nash RJ: "Real World" Ethics—Frameworks for Educators and Human Service Professionals. ed 2. Teachers College Press, New York, 2002.
24. Davis CM: What is empathy, and can empathy be taught? Phys Ther 70:32–36, 1990.
25. Davis CM: Patient/Practitioner Interaction—An Experimental Manual for Developing the Art of Heath Care. ed 3. Slack Inc, Thorofare, NJ, 1988.
26. Purtilo R, and Haddad A: Health Professional and Patient Interaction. ed 6. WB Saunders Company, Philadelphia, 2002.
27. Jensen GM, Haddad A, and Purtilo R: The impact of critical self-reflection on student professional development: Applying a model of scholarship of teaching and learning. Paper presented at: American Physical Therapy Association Combined Sections Meeting; February 14, 2003; Tampa, FL.
28. Haddad A: Teaching for enduring understandings. In Purtilo R, Jensen GM, and Royeen CB, (eds): Educating for Moral Action: A Sourcebook for Health and Rehabilitation Ethics. FA Davis Co, 2005.
29. Gilligan C: In a Different Voice. Harvard University Press, Cambridge, MA, 1983.

21

Environment, Professional Identity, and the Roles of the Ethics Educator: An Agenda for Development of the Professional Ethics Curriculum

LAURA LEE (DOLLY) SWISHER, PHD, MDIV, PT

Abstract

Changes in the health care system during the last two decades of the 20th century produced significant challenges to notions of professionalism and professional ethics. These challenges illustrate the need to locate the ethics curriculum within appropriate educational, organizational, professional, and educational environmental systems. At the same time, the curriculum must be rooted in a strong professional identity. The purpose of this chapter is to outline an agenda for occupational therapy and physical therapy ethics education that attends to both professional identity and environmental influences. In pursuit of this goal, I propose five suggestions for the advancement of ethics education in occupational therapy and physical therapy:

Development of the ethics curriculum requires an appreciation of its social and environmental context.

The content of the ethics curriculum must address the multidimensional nature of moral behavior through didactic material directed toward moral sensitivity, moral judgment, moral motivation, and moral courage/implementation.

The most appropriate emphasis for teaching and evaluation of moral judgment is intermediate concepts (such as, confidentiality, patient autonomy, conflict of interest) rather than the more abstract level of developmental theories or more concrete professional codes of ethics.[1]

Professional role and the moral obligations of professionalism should be the emphasis of the moral motivation curriculum.

Further development of the ethics curriculum requires ongoing research and scholarship focusing on professional identity in relationship to its environmental context.

Each of these proposals suggests a related role for the ethics educator: organizational construction worker, curriculum architect, everyday philosopher, midwife, and scholar.

When I began to write this paper, I started with a simple idea: physical therapy and occupational therapy ethics education should not occur in isolation from the health care system that students were being trained to enter. The concept that I proposed to develop was that the curriculum and the educator should be seen as a part of the health care system. However, as I reflected on these ideas, it became increasingly clear to me that the term "system" is not a good fit with current health care services. A system is a whole whose parts interrelate and that is not a good description of the current fragmented health care system. I came to believe that the postmodern organizational metaphor of "collage" is more representative of the present state of affairs.[2] In contrast to the postmodern collage, the metaphor proposed by Hatch for the classical perspective (1900s) was the machine, and that of the modern period (1950s) was the organism or "living system."[2]

As the collage metaphor implies, our experience with the health care system is frequently fragmented, with each of us seeing a slightly different part of the whole, and whose parts may stand in juxtaposition. Health care policies often pull in opposite directions. Precisely because of this fragmented experience, it seemed more appropriate to think of the health care *environment* than the health care *system*.

Changes in health care during the last two decades of the 20 century produced significant challenges to notions of professionalism and professional ethics. Indeed, one can argue that managed care has created a professional identity crisis among health care professionals and that this crisis extends to the realm of professional ethics. For example, Morreim has described managed care as a "balancing act" in which physicians must balance the interests of the patient with societal goods and self-interest in an environment of "fiscal scarcity."[3] This represents a distinct departure from traditional notions of fidelity that obligate the professional to be guided at all times by the welfare of the individual patient. Health care professionals before the advent of managed care may not have fully realized that professionalism and professional ethics are socially constructed concepts embedded in and influenced by their social context.

The professional "identity crisis" generated by managed care has spawned discussion among health care professionals about the nature of professionalism, especially among physicians. A 1996 study of 1011 family physicians found that they believed that managed care had negative impacts on relationships with patients, ability to carry out ethical obligations, and the quality of care.[4] Medical journal publications ask how to revitalize professionalism,[5] what does being a professional mean in these times,[6] how can physicians restore their clinical autonomy,[7] have physicians been deprofessionalized,[8] and how should educators train physicians in professionalism?[9]

A smaller number of publications in occupational or physical therapy suggest that therapists have confronted similar issues about their professional role.[10-18] A survey of 56 occupational therapists in an academic rehabilitation environment found that 43% of the 103 ethical issues identified were related to reimbursement.[10] Within physical therapy, Purtilo and Giffin delineated ethical concerns of managed care, and Emery described the impact of reimbursement changes on the types of ethical issues encountered in clinical education.[15-18]

Taking the lessons of managed care to heart, I contend that professional ethics education must be grounded in a fully developed notion of professionalism in relationship to the social, professional, and health care environments. The fact that marked changes in the health care system can produce such a crisis points to the need to locate the ethics curriculum within appropriate educational, organizational, professional, and educational environments. An environmental perspective on ethics education incorporates an understanding that professionalism and professional ethics are dynamic social constructs that evolve within the environment of individual organizations, the profession, health care systems, and the larger social environment.

✧ DEVELOPING AN ETHICS CURRICULUM FOR THE NEW MILLENNIUM

In this chapter, I outline a theoretical framework for appropriate content of the physical therapy ethics curriculum in the new millennium and delineate implications of environmental systems theory for curriculum development. The purpose of this chapter is to present an agenda for physical therapy ethics that attends to both professional identity and environmental influences. This theoretical framework may also apply in occupational therapy. In pursuit of this goal, I have four suggestions for the advancement of ethics education in physical therapy:

1. Development of the ethics curriculum requires an appreciation of its social and environmental context.

2. The content of the ethics curriculum must address the multidimensional nature of moral behavior through didactic material directed toward moral sensitivity, moral judgment, moral motivation, and moral courage/implementation.

3. The most appropriate emphasis for teaching and evaluation of moral judgment is intermediate concepts (such as, confidentiality, patient autonomy, conflict of interest) rather than the more abstract level of developmental theories or more concrete professional codes of ethics.[1]

4. Professional role and the moral obligations of professionalism should be the emphasis of the moral motivation curriculum.

Further development of the ethics curriculum requires ongoing research and scholarship focusing on professional identity in relationship to its environmental context.

Each of these recommendations suggests a related role for the ethics educator: organizational construction worker, curriculum architect, everyday philosopher, midwife, and scholar.

An analysis of ethics knowledge in physical therapy suggests that physical therapy has neither fully developed nor fully articulated its professional ethic.[19] Similarly, Foye and associates allude to the relative paucity of ethics research in occupational therapy, with only one empirical study of ethical issues between 1984 and 2002.[10] Accordingly, dialogue with relevant environmental systems must include research into the professional role, the unique nature of the dilemmas encountered by physical therapists and occupational therapists, ethical concepts that guide decisions, and appropriate methods to evaluate the moral behavior of therapists. Ongoing reform of the ethics curriculum is, therefore, tied to research grounded in moral dialogue between faculty, clinicians, patients/clients, representative organizations, students, and faculty.

Environmental Context of Professional Ethics Education: Organizational Construction Workers

As educators we learn a great deal from the content and process of students' learning. It has been a humbling experience for me to observe that a student who can easily resolve an ethical case dilemma in the classroom may not recognize that same situation as an ethical issue in the clinical environment, a "disparity" similar to the concern expressed by Hack.[20] At the same time, I should add that it has been equally rewarding when students take on the responsibility for sensitizing their clinical instructors to overlooked ethical aspects of clinical problems. However, it is more often the case that students come to view the time spent in the ethics part of the curriculum as an "academic ivory tower" experience somewhat removed from the realities of the clinic. Occupational and physical therapy ethics educators develop an appreciation for the power that the statement, "This is how we do it in this clinic" may hold for the student and novice therapist. The fact that this phrase uttered in 5 seconds can negate hours of moral discourse in the classroom reinforces the power of environmental context.

From the modernist organizational theoretical perspective, the environment is an objective "entity" external to one's own distinct organizational boundaries and comprises certain elements and sectors.[2] In the modernist view, environments control organizations and organizations respond to the environment (Fig. 21.1).

The external notion of organizational environment subtly frees us of responsibility for our environment, except for attempts at "boundary spanning" to ensure our own organizational survival. In contrast to this passive and reactive view of the organizational and environmental interaction, more recent organizational theories (symbolic, interactive, and postmodern) postulate that the environment is a social construction in whose creation we actively participate. Clinical educators have long recognized that the clinical environment in which students practice skills introduced in the academic context is crit-

ical. In spite of the importance of clinical education, most clinical educators would concede that they feel little control over clinical sites, clinical educators, or the organizational environments where clinical education takes place.

The potential of the clinical environment to serve as a laboratory to mold ethical character, identify ethical issues, and refine moral judgment has not yet been fully developed. Faculty who teach professional ethics in occupational therapy and physical therapy programs cannot concentrate solely on the "ethics curriculum," educating students about the environment. Instead, we must see ourselves as and become change agents within the clinical and organizational environments in which students will practice. To accomplish this mission requires us to visualize ourselves working together in constructing a shared environment characterized less by distinct boundaries than partnerships and dialogue with the numerous groups and stakeholders that contribute to an ethical environment for education (Fig. 21.2).

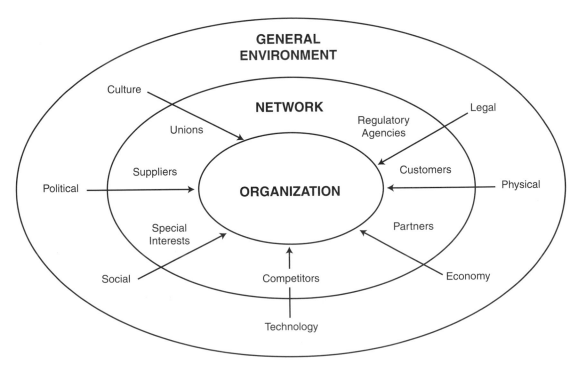

Adapted from Hatch.[2] By permission of Oxford University Press.

Figure 21.1   ✧   Modernist view of organization and environment.

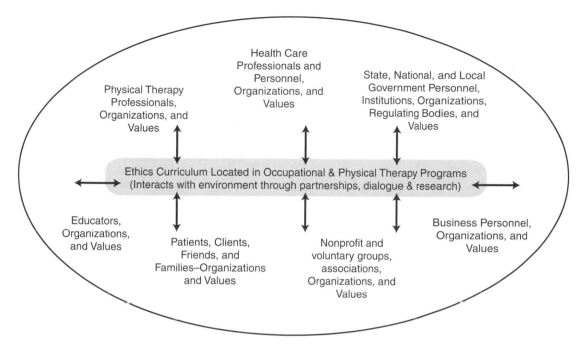

Figure 21.2   ✧   Context of ethics education in occupational and physical therapy.

As Hatch notes, "...[O]nce we recognize our role as construction workers who build organizational reality, we can free ourselves from situations we do not like and create something else."[2]

The Educator as Architect: Curricular Content for Multidimensional Ethical Behavior

Recall the example of the student who can easily resolve an ethics case presented in class but fails to even recognize the same issue as an ethical problem in the field. We have already explored the idea that this failure might be due in part to the influence of the external environment. Another reason for the student's difficulty may be that these actions (deciding and recognizing) represent different ethical processes. Rest and associates[21,22] proposed that ethical behavior involves four component psychological processes: moral sensitivity, moral judgment, moral motivation, and moral courage (Table 21.1). It is important to note that these are overlapping psychological processes rather than sequential steps. A person who is skilled in recognizing ethical problems may not have commensurate skills in moral judgment. Likewise, someone may make excellent decisions (moral judgment) and have few implementation skills (moral courage).

To illustrate the differences between two of these component processes, consider the following example. Muriel Bebeau[23] relates that she often works with dentists who have run afoul of the dental ethics process. In one case, two dentists who were partners seemed to have complementary ethical abilities. Evaluation showed that one had decreased moral judgment abilities and the other decreased moral sensitivity. While one assumes that this could work out differently, in this case the result was that one partner would get into an ethical situation without thinking about it (moral sensitivity) and the other partner could not make an appropriate decision to resolve the problem (moral judgment). An important distinction for educators is that these overlapping processes are not identical to the separate educational domains of cognition, behavior, and affect.[21] From Rest's perspective, the idea of separate domains for moral cognition, behavior, and affect is contradictory to the overlapping nature of the moral processes.

Table 21.1 ✧ Four-Component Scaffold for Ethics Curriculum Content

COMPONENT	MORAL SENSITIVITY	MORAL JUDGMENT OR REASONING	MORAL MOTIVATION OR COMMITMENT	MORAL COURAGE AND IMPLEMENTATION
Process Based on Rest[21] pp 23–25.	Interpreting situations—requires empathy, taking the perspective of others, recognizing ethical issues, projecting consequences, developing a plan.	Making decisions about right and wrong	"Prioritizing ethical values in relation to other values"[21]	Implementation of moral decisions, persevering against adversity
Educational Content	Personal and professional values Communication skills Discrimination Enculturation/Socialization Differences based on race, class, gender, religion, sexual orientation, and culture. Health care system, organizational dynamics and ethical implications	Professional documents—Code of Ethics and Guide for Professional Conduct Ethical theories and frameworks Intermediate ethical concepts Applying ethical concepts to specific cases Law and ethics State Practice Act Government regulations	Meaning of professionalism Identifying personal values—individual, religious, cultural, organizational Professional values and obligations Balancing personal and professional obligations	Communication Assertiveness Conflict-Resolution Negotiation skills Organizational and social action Virtue Integrity Whistle blowing Unethical colleagues
Sample of Educational Activities	Professional code Case studies Personal values history Relating to different backgrounds and experiences Role playing Standardized patients Audio and videotapes Portfolio or journals	Professional code Case studies Ethical decision making models Readings Standardized patients Audio and videotapes Portfolio or journals	Professional code Personal ethical and value history Values clarification Ethics and Values Coat of Arms Exercise Organizational analysis Case studies Portfolio or journals	Exemplars Exposure to courageous role-models through readings, panels Problem solving Case studies Examination of failure of moral courage
Evaluation Tools	Practical exam with standardized patients Evaluation of portfolio or journals Self-assessment	Defining Issues Test (Rest) Moral Judgment Interview Test of intermediate concepts Practical exam with standardized patients Scored case analysis	PROI-PT[60] Professional role essay Practical exam with standardized patients Evaluation of portfolio or journals Objective exam	Practical exam with standardized patients Evaluation of portfolio or journals

Source: Rest JR: Background: Theory and Research. In Rest JR, and Narvaez D (eds): Moral Development in the Professions: Psychology and Applied Ethics. Lawrence Erlbaum Associates, Publishers, Hillsdale, NJ, 1994, pp 1–26 and Bebeau MJ: Influencing the moral dimensions of dental practice. In Rest JR, and Narvaez D (eds): Moral Development in the Professions: Psychology and Applied Ethics. Lawrence Erlbaum Associates, Publishers; Hillsdale, NJ, 1994, pp 121–146. Adapted with permission.

Given the multidimensional nature of ethical behavior, the content of the physical therapy curriculum must at least include each of the component psychological processes. Table 21.1 provides a schematic representation of possible curriculum content organized by each component of the four ethical processes outlined by Rest. For a further elaboration of the possible use of the four-component model in physical therapy education, see Triezenberg and Davis,[24] and for dental education, see Bebeau.[25] For delineation of approaches to the occupational therapy curriculum, see Haddad,[26] and DeMars, Fleming, and Benham.[27]

In spite of the usefulness of the four-component model as a basic foundation for the occupational and physical therapy ethics curriculum, we should also recognize its limitations. The theoretical framework of the four-component model is at best a "bare-bones" psychological theory of moral behavior that demonstrates the limitation of confusing moral behavior with simple moral judgments. A more adequate theory might also recognize the numerous influences on these four components including context, personal abilities, and individual coping strategies. Building on the work of Haan, Bredemeier and Shields developed a 12-component theory of moral behavior that includes some of these considerations.[28–30] Reacting against Kohlberg's emphasis on moral cognition at the expense of social interaction, Haan had conceptualized moral behavior as a social interaction in which the individual utilizes "ego processes" to solve moral problems. She defined "ego processes" as "characteristic ways of solving problems that come to be durable aspects of their personality...Ego processes describe the way people *interact* with situations, determined by both situations and personal preference."[29] By incorporating the insights of Haan, the 12-component model provides insight into the nature of internal and external influences that may come to bear on the 4 major component processes of moral behavior.

An expanded model for moral behavior may also indicate the manner in which managed care has been so successful in shifting the ethical landscape of the health care environment. Contextually, managed care altered the moral atmosphere, realigned power structures, and shifted organizational priorities. At the same time, the change in environment created challenges for individuals' ego processing; that is, situational moral problem solving through social interaction by therapists.

Designing an ethics curriculum to address the influences and components of moral behavior suggests a second role for the ethics educator: architect. The end-result may be simple or complex but the resulting curriculum must be comprehensive and capable of preparing the student for the prevailing environmental stresses.

Teaching Moral Decision Making: The Ethics Educator as Everyday Philosopher

Although the ethics curriculum must address all four components of ethical behavior, a primary goal of the professional curriculum must be to prepare graduates to make sound ethical judgments. As educators, we spend significant amounts of time developing students' abilities to make sound ethical judgments. An important question in teaching moral judgment is the amount of philosophy that students need to know in order to make sound ethical judgments. Just as students must understand the foundational sciences of anatomy and biomechanics to make judgments about human movement disorders, students require a basic appreciation of the major philosophical underpinnings of ethical decision making. Should they read Kant, Mill, and Aristotle?

Bebeau and Thoma argue persuasively that teaching moral judgment should focus on "intermediate principles," those principles that are not as abstract as moral developmental schema but more abstract than the conduct rules of the Code of Ethics.[1] Bebeau and Thoma focus on the three major developmental schema of moral judgment (personal interest, maintaining norms, postconventional) proposed by Kohlberg and refined by Rest and colleagues.[22,31,32] Beauchamp and Childress take a similar approach to describing the level of abstraction of ethical concepts; deontological concepts are quite abstract but codes of ethics are relatively concrete.[33] If we combine the developmental perspective of Bebeau and Thoma with the philosophical perspective of Beauchamp and Childress, the hierarchy of ethical guidance from most abstract to most specific would look something like Figure 21.3. As indicated by Figure 21.3, each level influences the others, and each level is affected by the environment. From this perspective, moral judgment proceeds both inductively and deductively.[1,22,33]

The educational significance of level of abstraction is twofold. First, the most abstract ethical guidelines offer little or no direct assistance in making decisions for the student in a professional program. Cognitive developmental stages or schemas are not consciously available to the subject to guide decisions. Instead, as Bebeau and Thoma describe, stages or schemas act as a kind of "default" background for making ethical decisions.[1] The individual does not say, "As a maintaining norms thinker I value rules and laws and this means that the correct action is X." Similarly, with the exception of trained philosophers, few people will say, "since I am a deontologist, I must choose action B." Second, neither abstract philosophical principles nor developmental stages lend themselves to establishment of norms for the measurement of student educational achievement.

Instruments to measure moral judgment, such as the *Defining Issues Test* (DIT) of Rest and the *Moral Judgment Interview* (MJI) of Kohlberg are capable of measuring long-term shifts in moral judgment and can demonstrate effects from educational interventions.[22,31,32,34,35] However, as Bebeau and Thoma argue, measures targeted at intermediate concepts may provide a better indication of educa-

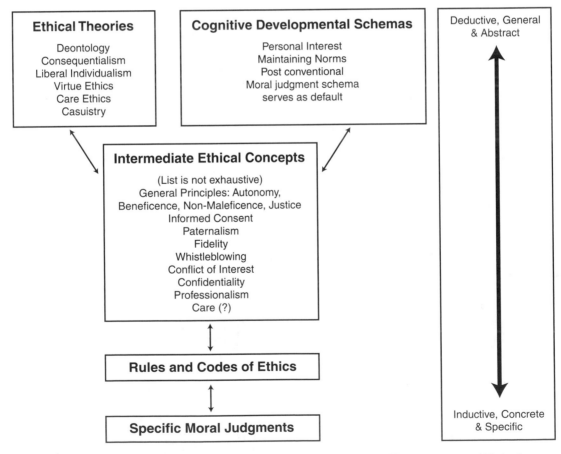

Based on concepts presented by Beauchamp and Childress[33], Rest et al.[22], and Bebeau and Thoma[1]

Figure 21.3 ✧ Levels of abstraction in ethical theories, principles, and rules.

tional interventions than developmental measures.[1] It may be that developmental measures such as the DIT and MJI are not sensitive enough to detect smaller changes resulting from a course of instruction among most subjects, or perhaps application of intermediate concepts taps into a different aspect of moral judgment.

We still know little about the moral reasoning of physical or occupational therapists. Sisola has found a significant correlation between performance on clinical education affiliation and moral reasoning among physical therapy students.[36] In occupational therapy, Greene found that a service-learning experience did not improve moral reasoning among occupational therapy students.[37] In a study of British occupational and physical therapists, Barnitt and Partridge's research revealed that the two groups encountered similar ethical problems and context, but used different reasoning processes.[38] While physical therapists used a diagnostic or procedural approach within the biomedical model, occupational therapists used a narrative approach within an illness or disability model.[38] Further research in this area would be valuable for educators in designing the moral judgment portion of the ethics curriculum.

A major challenge in teaching intermediate ethics concepts occurs in the selection of the most important concepts for focus. Although there are numerous intermediate ethical concepts in the medical literature, it is often the case that these concepts do not "translate" to the physical or occupational therapy context. Consider the example of informed consent. From a philosophical point of view, the elements of informed consent might be considered to be identical for all health care providers.[33] For this reason, physical and occupational therapy ethics instructors feel comfortable in teaching the basic elements involved in obtaining informed consent. However, it can be difficult to adapt the basic principles of informed consent to the day-to-day work environment of therapy.

Beauchamp and Childress are emphatic in stating that informed consent in medicine should not be reduced to "shared decision-making," although they concede that "[t]his proposal is plausible when consent involves ongoing exchanges of information between patients and health care providers...."[33] They contrast this type of informed consent to the type of informed consent involved in giving consent for a specific intervention. The nuances within Beauchamp and Childress' discussion of informed consent indicate that environment and role profoundly influence how occupational and physical therapists experience ethical concepts.[33] Occupational and physical therapists encounter informed consent in different circumstances and with different legal or organizational responsibilities than physicians. Perhaps, informed consent for intervention by occupational and physical therapists is more like shared decision making in most patient/client management situations. These observations about informed consent point to the need for therapists to reflect upon and discuss their own experiences with intermediate concepts rather than importing ethical concepts as they have been developed in medicine or even nursing. Recent debates about informed consent in the physical therapy literature confirm that physical therapists have not yet reached consensus about how one should obtain informed consent and what should be disclosed to the patient.[39,40]

Two particular ethical concepts that require attention are the ethics of care and professionalism. A study of peer-reviewed ethics publications in physical therapy between 1970 and 2000[19] uncovered only one article using the care framework.[41] Since that time, Romanello and Knight-Abowitz have published an article that explored the use of an ethic of care in physical therapy education.[42] A cursory review of occupational therapy literature also suggests that there are relatively few articles from the care perspective.[43,44] The ethic of care has, of course, played a prominent role in nursing ethics and in feminist ethics. It is possible that the ethics of care could contribute greatly to occupational and physical therapy ethics. Much more work remains, however, in order to delineate how an ethic of care would guide moral practice in both fields.

One unresolved issue is whether care functions as an intermediate principle or a theoretical framework. As an ethical framework, the care paradigm is to some degree incompatible with other theoretical paradigms because they start from different central moral assumptions. From an educational standpoint, care provides a powerful critique of dominant Western rational ethical paradigms. In my experience, it is more difficult to teach students to "think within" the care paradigm because this way of thinking is so new and because there are few good examples of ethical analysis from the care perspective in the educational literature and texts for therapists. Further development of care ethics in occupational and physical therapy could make a significant contribution to our body of knowledge.

In 1978, Purtilo observed that those in the allied health professions encountered unique ethical dilemmas due to the nature of their work and that these unique dilemmas require moral problem solving skills.[45] Currently, we take for granted that physical and occupational therapists have the ability and authority to make ethical decisions. Purtilo's observations, however, were at that time very radical because most presumed that only the work of physicians required moral judgment. Twenty-five years later, we still have a significant amount of work to do to fully assume the moral role implied by Purtilo's observations. A vital component of this work includes defining our unique dilemmas and relevant intermediate concepts as we encounter them in the health care environment as physical therapists and occupational therapists.[10,46–49]

Identification of the most important intermediate ethical concepts for occupational and physical therapists, crafting appropriate scenarios, and reaching consensus on action choices require that we engage in the scholarship implied by Purtilo's early work, working toward the goals described by Bebeau and Thoma. Full delineation of intermediate ethical concepts in occupational and physical therapy would provide a strong foundation for the moral judgment portion of the ethics curriculum.

A final note about the importance of intermediate concepts in professional ethics education relates to the theme of this chapter. A focus on intermediate concepts embraces the concept of environmentally embedded professional identity. As revealed by Figure 21.3 and by the work of Beauchamp and Childress, it is not the case that either abstract theories or more specific rules have absolute primacy in moral judgment.[33] Instead, we hammer out professional ethical judgments by reasoning both inductively and deductively. Specific situations inform our understanding of theories and principles; principles shape our interpretation of situation and context.

Professionalism and Identity as the Focus of Moral Motivation: The Ethics Educator as Midwife

In the previous section, I explored the idea that professionalism could serve as an important intermediate concept in the curriculum directed toward moral judgment. However, professionalism and professional role are also foundational to the portion of the curriculum dedicated to moral motivation. In professional ethics, professional role and identity provide strong motivators to put ethical and professional values above others (moral motivation) and to persevere against barriers (moral courage).

Educators face serious challenges in teaching professional role because there has been relatively little scholarship about how physical and occupational therapists view their professional role. Our tendency has been to appeal to the early sociological functionalist literature that defines professions in terms of traits, such as professional autonomy, responsibility, accountability, body of knowledge, service orientation, and code of ethics.[50–52] Studies in both physical and occupational therapy have examined individual therapists' commitment to sociologically defined attributes, such as sense of calling, belief in self-regulation, commitment to the professional organization, public service, perceived status, and sense of autonomy.[53–55]

Physical therapy has been especially focused on professional autonomy as the mark of the professional.[56] This dated and static notion of professionalism represents a normative concept of our professional role without realistic reference to our responsibilities in an environmental context and without significant reflection upon our profession from a historical perspective. I am not suggesting that we totally abandon the insights of the "trait" approach to the professions, but we must define what these concepts mean for occupational therapists and physical therapists. Extensive literature has developed in medicine attempting to redefine professionalism in response to the challenges of the current health care environment. Further development of the ethics curriculum requires ongoing research and scholarship focusing on professional identity in relationship to the environmental context and to the self-understanding of occupational and physical therapists in dialogue with patients and clients.

At the opposite end from the cognitive developmental portion of the professionalism curriculum is the concern for "generic abilities."[57] This approach proposes that professionalism entails 10 behaviors: commitment to learning, interpersonal skills, communication skills, effective use of time and resources, use of constructive feedback, problem solving, professionalism, responsibility, critical thinking, and stress management. An instrument based on these generic abilities involves ongoing self-assessment of these behaviors. The best use of generic abilities provides a powerful tool for both students and instructors to reflect on skills, take responsibility for growth in professional behaviors, and quantify their evaluations. Generic abilities, however, may not be entirely synonymous with "professionalism" as a guide for ethical behavior.

A recent study by Jette and Portney attempted to establish construct validity of the generic abilities instrument.[58] Factor analysis of the resulting ratings confirmed 7 rather than 10 professional behaviors: professionalism, critical thinking, professional development, personal balance, working relationships, communication management, and interpersonal skills. Notably, the behaviors for professionalism accounted for only 48% of the variance in scores and there was no significant difference in professionalism between students based on amount of clinical education. As the authors suggest, this may indicate the "need to further explore the constructs of professional behavior in physical therapy."[58] A further implication of the study is that the instrument may not be sensitive enough to detect changes in professional behaviors. In spite of these limitations, the generic abilities instrument is one of the few instruments with known psychometric properties available for measuring elements of professionalism other than moral judgment in physical therapy.

Bebeau, Born, and Ozar[59] developed the *Professional Role Orientation Inventory* (PROI) to evaluate how professionals in dentistry conceptualize a professional role along four dimensions: autonomy, responsibility, authority, and agency. For the purposes of the instrument, autonomy was defined as the "extent to which an individual feels freedom and independence in his/her role," and responsibility was the "breadth of an individual's commitment to others."[59] Authority was defined as the "degree to which a person sees the self as knowledgeable, a good judge of outcomes, respected, and deferred to for expertise."[59] Agency referred to the professional's "sense of control and power in his/her life as a practicing professional."[59] The authors of the PROI based these four dimensions of professionalism on the philosophical literature describing professional obligations. The PROI was successful in differentiating experts in ethics from practicing dentists and first-year dental students from fourth-year students. Bebeau has successfully used this instrument in the educational setting to provide feedback to students on their changing professional role concept.

In a separate study, I adapted the PROI for use with physical therapists (PROI-PT).[60] After eliminating some items and switching the associated dimension of others, the reliability of the individual scales improved from alpha scores of 0.35–0.70 to a range of 0.50–0.70. Although I recognize that current reliability may limit the ability to draw conclusions, one interesting feature of the results of this study of 478 physical therapists was that physical therapists scored significantly lower on autonomy than dentists. With further revision and appropriate adaptation for occupational therapy, this instrument could perhaps provide valuable information about the evolving professional role concept of occupational and physical therapy students.

Within the component of moral motivation, the ethics educator may serve as midwife in the development of the student's professional role concept. Individual professionals construct an internalized professional role concept that brings together ideas from the profession, society, and the inner self. This individual notion of professional role provides not only a conceptual road map of professional obligation, but also emotional resources to fulfill those commitments. As suggested by the metaphor of midwife, the ethics educator does not "give" the student a professional role concept but assists the student in bringing it to life.

Securing the Future: The Ethics Educator as Scholar

The need for scholarship in ethics and professional role has been a recurring theme in this chapter. Responsibility for research into professional ethics as a basis for education in physical therapy should be viewed as a high priority as occupational and physical therapists seek more autonomous roles because this area of scholarship has been relatively neglected in the past. Occupational and physical therapist educators must, therefore, also assume the role of scholar and researcher. The following topics should have some priority in this undertaking:

+ Intermediate ethical concepts
+ Professionalism and professional role identity
+ Outcomes of educational interventions
+ Environmental context

Given the theme of this chapter, it is appropriate to address the professional environment for occupational therapy and physical therapy scholarship in the area of ethics. One would assume that evidence-based practice (EBP) would welcome scholarship about ethical practice and the professional role of rehabilitation professionals. However, the dominant model of EBP by Sackett, Straus, Richardson, Rosenberg, and Haynes delineates a very narrow definition of evidence.[61] Most disturbing is the value placed on the randomized controlled trial, an inappropriate design for studying most questions about ethics or professional role.

In spite of these concerns, the evidence-based practice movement raises an important question for those doing scholarship in this area: What constitutes good evidence in ethics?

Although it is clear that we cannot endorse a narrow model of evidence that shuns value considerations, we must develop some consensus on the proper grounds for evaluating social science and humanistic research. Working in our role as "organizational construction workers," ethics educators should advocate for a model of evidence-based practice that embraces the full spectrum of questions about occupational and physical therapy practice, and this will require moral courage.

In a previous section, I discussed Bebeau and Thoma's suggestion to develop instruments to evaluate students' use of intermediate concepts to evaluate moral judgment.[1] They proposed that the four-component model could serve as a framework for the development of instruments to evaluate the outcomes of each component of morality in the ethics curriculum. Although we can never accurately measure all of the outcomes of the ethics curriculum, scholarship in this area would provide a basis to measure much more than we currently measure. Appropriate research would also provide the ability to compare student performance to that of practicing occupational and physical therapists.

The practice of physical therapy and occupational therapy occurs in a complex environment of individuals and organizations, with differing notions of professionalism and ethics. Some have suggested that professionalism is best conceived as a reflection of an implicit contract with society. From this perspective, appropriate notions of professionalism require an understanding of the legitimate expectations of patients/clients. However, we know little about patients'/clients' view of the appropriate role of occupational and physical therapists or their perceptions about ethical dilemmas.[19] Research about ethics and professional role in physical and occupational therapy requires partnership and dialogue with patient groups, other health care providers, and other stakeholder groups in the environment.

✦ CONCLUSIONS

This chapter has proposed that ethics education in occupational therapy and physical therapy requires an understanding of both professional identity and environmental context. I put forth five major propositions for curricular inclusion. These propositions require that ethics educators must also assume the roles of organizational construction worker, curriculum architect, everyday philosopher, midwife, and scholar.

Managed care has highlighted the importance of environment and our responsibility to participate in shaping the environment. In the role of organizational construction workers, ethic educators must engage in dialogue and partnerships to improve the ethical environment of health care. In dialogue and through partnerships, however, we must listen to the concerns of practicing therapists, patients/clients, government officials, and advocacy groups. By partnering and listening, we gain an understanding of the environment that students will enter, enabling us as curriculum architects to develop appropriate educational experiences using a multidimensional model of moral behavior. As architects of the ethics curriculum, the four-component model can be a useful tool for organizing curricular content and intermediate ethical constructs provide the appropriate focus for the moral judgment portion of the curriculum.

In addition to understanding the environment, occupational and physical therapy students must also have a strong sense of professional identity. Professional identity serves as a strong rudder with which professionals navigate the sometimes turbulent ethical waters of managed care. This chapter has proposed that professional identity or professionalism should be the focus of that part of the ethics curriculum dedicated to moral motivation and that ethics educators may serve as midwives for students in creating a professional role identity. A full understanding of professional identity requires that ethics educators participate in research to investigate professionalism, ethics, and appropriate outcomes measures. Research of this nature demands that we partner with those within the environment, taking us back to the role of organizational construction workers. Completing this circle illustrates the multiple roles ethics educators must assume.

References

1. Bebeau MJ, and Thoma SJ: "Intermediate" concepts and the connection to moral education. Educ Psychol Rev 11(4):343–360, 1999.
2. Hatch MJ: Organization Theory: Modern, Symbolic, and Postmodern Perspectives. Oxford University Press, New York, 1997.
3. Morreim EH: Balancing Act: The New Medical Ethics of Medicine's New Economics. Georgetown University Press, Washington, DC, 1995.
4. Feldman D, Novack DH, and Gracely E: Effects of managed care on physician-patient relationships, quality of care, and the ethical practice of medicine. Arch Intern Med 158:1626–1632, 1998.
5. Cruess RL, Cruess SR, and Johnston SE: Renewing professionalism: An opportunity for medicine. Acad Med 74:878–884, 1999.
6. Castellani B, and Wear D: Physician views on practicing professionalism in the corporate age. Qual Health Res 10:490–506, 2002.
7. Morreim EH: Professionalism and clinical autonomy in the practice of medicine. Mt Sinai J Med 69:370–377, 2002.
8. Reed RR, and Evans D: The deprofessionalization of medicine: Causes, effects and responses. JAMA 258:3279–3182, 1987.
9. Siegler M: Training doctors for professionalism: Some lessons learned from teaching clinical medical ethics. Mt Sinai J Med 69:404–409, 2003.
10. Foye SJ, et al: Ethical issues in rehabilitation: A qualitative analysis of dilemmas identified by occupational therapists. Top Stroke Rehab 9(3):89–101, 2002.
11. Walker KF: Adjustments to managed health care: Pushing against it, going with it, and making the best of it. Am J Occup Ther 55(2):129–137, 2001.
12. Brayman SJ: Managing the occupational environment of managed care. Am J Occup Ther 50(6):442–446, 1996.
13. Howard BS: How high do we jump? The effect of reimbursement on occupational therapy. Am J Occup Ther 45(10):875–881, 1991.
14. VanLeit B: Managed mental health care: Reflections in a time of turmoil. Am J Occup Ther 50(6):428–434, 1996.
15. Purtilo R: Interdisciplinary health care teams and health care reform. J Law Med Ethics 22:121–126, 1994.
16. Purtilo R: Managed care: Ethical issues for the rehabilitation professions. Trends Health Care, Law Ethics. Winter/Spring,10(1–2):105–118, 1995.
17. Giffin A: Coping with the prospective payment system (PPS): Ethical issues in rehabilitation. Issues on Aging 23(1):2–8, 2000.
18. Emery MJ: The impact of the prospective payment system: Perceived changes in the nature of practice and clinical education. Phys Ther 73:11–25, 1993.
19. Swisher LL: A retrospective analysis of ethics knowledge in physical therapy (1970–2000). Phys Ther 82(7):692–706, 2002.
20. Hack LM: Disparity in practice: Healing the breech. In Purtilo R, Jensen GM, and Royeen CB (eds): Educating for Moral Action: A Sourcebook for Health and Rehabilitation Ethics. FA Davis Co, Philadelphia, 2005.
21. Rest JR: Background: Theory and Research. In Rest JR, and Narvaez D (eds): Moral Development in the

Professions: Psychology and Applied Ethics. Lawrence Erlbaum Associates, Publishers, Hillsdale, NJ, 1994, pp 1–26.

22. Rest JR, et al: Postconventional Moral Thinking: A Neo-Kohlbergian Approach. Lawrence Erlbaum Associates, Mahwah, NJ, 1999.

23. Bebeau MJ: Teaching Professional Ethics. Ethics in Practice and the Professions. Paper presented at Association for Practical and Professional Ethics, August 3–7, 1997, Missoula, MT.

24. Triezenberg HL, and Davis CM: Beyond the code of ethics: Educating physical therapists for their role as moral agents. J Phys Ther Educ 14(3):48–58, 2000.

25. Bebeau MJ: Influencing the moral dimensions of dental practice. In Rest JR, and Narvaez D (eds): Moral Development in the Professions: Psychology and Applied Ethics. Lawrence Erlbaum Associates, Publishers; Hillsdale, NJ, 1994, pp 121–146.

26. Haddad A: Teaching ethical analysis in occupational therapy. Am J Occup Ther 42(5):300–3304, 1988.

27. DeMars PA, Fleming JD, and Benham PA: Ethics across the occupational therapy curriculum. Am J Occup Ther 45(9):782–787, 1991.

28. Haan N: Two moralities in action contexts: Relationships to thought, ego regulation, and development. J Pers Soc Psychol 1978;36(3):286–230, 1978.

29. Haan N, Aerts E, and Cooper BAB: On Moral Grounds: The Search for Practical Morality. New York University Press, New York, 1985.

30. Bredemeier BJ, and Shields DLL: Applied ethics and moral reasoning in sport. In Rest JR, and Narvaez D (eds): Moral Development in the Professions: Psychology and Applied Ethics. Lawrence Erlbaum Associates, Publishers, Hillsdale, NJ, 1994, pp 173–187.

31. Kohlberg L: Stage and sequence: The cognitive-developmental approach to socialization. In Goslin D (ed): Handbook of Socialization Theory and Research. Rand McNally, Chicago, 1969.

32. Kohlberg L: Moral stages and moralization: The cognitive-developmental approach. In Lickona T (ed): Moral Development and Behavior. Holt, Rinehart and Winston, New York, 1976.

33. Beauchamp TL, and Childress JF: Principles of Biomedical Ethics, ed 4. Oxford University Press, New York, 1994.

34. Rest JR: Development in Judging Moral Issues. University of Minnesota Press, Minneapolis, MN, 1979.

35. Rest JR: Guide to the Defining Issues Test, Version 1.3. Center for the Study of Ethical Development, Minneapolis, MN, 1993.

36. Sisola SW: Moral reasoning as a predictor of clinical practice: The development of physical therapy students across the professional curriculum. J Phys Ther Educ 14(3):26–34, 2000.

37. Greene D: The use of service learning in client environments to enhance ethical reasoning in students. Am J Occup Ther 51(10):844–852, 1997.

38. Barnitt R, and Partridge C: Ethical reasoning in physical therapy and occupational therapy. Physiother Res Int 2(3):178–192, 1997.

39. Scott RW: Spinal manipulation and patient informed consent in orthopaedic physical therapy. Orthop Phys Ther Pract 13:9–11, 2001.

40. Tygiel PP: Letter to the editor. Ortho Phys Ther Pract 14:24–28, 2002.

41. Mattingly SS: The mother-fetal dyad and the ethics of care. Phys Occup Ther Pediatr 16(1–2):5–13, 1996.

42. Romanello M, and Knight-Abowitz K: The "Ethic of Care" in physical therapy practice and education: Challenges and opportunities. J Phys Ther Educ 14(3):20–25, 2000.

43. Brown K, and Gabriel L: Ethical perspectives on school-based practice: Care, rights, justice, and compromise. Occup Ther Health Care 9(2–3):3–15, 1995.

44. Brown K, and Gillespie D: Recovering relationships: A feminist analysis of recovery models. Am J Occup Ther 46(11):1001–1005, 1992.

45. Purtilo R: Ethics teaching in allied health fields. Hastings Cent Rep 8(2):14–16, 1978.

46. Guccione AA: Ethical issues in physical therapy practice: A survey of physical therapists in New England. Phys Ther 60:1264–1272, 1980.

47. Triezenberg HL: The identification of ethical issues in physical therapy practice. Phys Ther 76:1097–1107, 1996.

48. Hansen RA, Kamp L, and Reitz S: Two practitioners' analyses of occupational therapy practice dilemmas. Am J Occup Ther 42(5):312–319, 1988.

49. Crabtree JL, and Caron-Parker LM: Long-term care of the aged: Ethical dilemmas and solutions. Am J Occup Ther 45(7):607–612, 1991.

50. Carr-Saunders AM: Professionalization in historical perspective. In Vollmer HM, and Mills DL (eds): Professionalization. Prentice-Hall, Englewood Cliffs, NJ, 1966.

51. Dingwall R, and Lewis P (eds): The Sociology of the Professions: Lawyers, Doctors, and Others. St. Martin's Press, New York, 1983.

52. Etzioni A (ed): The Semi-Professions and Their Organization: Teachers, Nurses, Social Workers. Free Press, New York, 1969.

53. Bell BD, and Bell JK: Professionalism as a multidimensional perspective. Am J Occup Ther 26(8):391–398, 1972.

54. Silva DM, Clark SD, and Raymond G: California physician's professional image of therapists. Phys Ther 61(8):1152–1157, 1981.

55. Dunkel RH: Survey of attitudes of Arkansas physicians and physical therapists toward the professional capacity of the physical therapist. Phys Ther 54(6):584–587, 1974.

56. Rothstein JM: Autonomy or professionalism? Phys Ther 83:206–207, 2003.

57. May WW, et al: Model for ability-based assessment in physical therapy education. J Phys Ther Educ 9(1):3–6, 1995.

58. Jette DU, and Portney LG: Construct validation of a model for professional behavior in physical therapist students. Phys Ther 83:432–443, 2003.

59. Bebeau MJ, Born DO, and Ozar DT: The development of a professional role orientation inventory. J Am Coll Dent 60(2):27–33, 1993.

60. Swisher LL, Beckstead JW, and Bebeau MJ: Factor analysis as a tool for survey analysis using a professional role orientation inventory as an example. Phys Ther 84(9):784–99, 2004.

61. Sackett DL, et al (eds): Evidence-Based Medicine: How to Practice and Teach EBM. ed 2. Churchill Livingstone Inc, New York, 2000.

22

Integrating Theories and Practices of Adult Teaching and Learning: Implications for Ethics Education

SUSAN W. SISOLA, PHD, PT

Abstract

The need for ethics education in professional health care programs is clear and convincing. Students enter these programs, however, with varying levels of capacity and motivation for moral and ethical development, and some have not yet achieved the levels of cognitive, relational, and self-reflective skills necessary for the development of ethical competence. Although students generally recognize limitations to their clinical knowledge and technical skills and they are motivated to learn, some students see little need for understanding and mastery of the skills necessary for ethical competence. Faculty attitudes can also be barriers that diminish the effectiveness of ethics education in professional health care programs. Some faculty report feeling uncomfortable teaching in "softer" areas of the curriculum, and report not to know "how" to teach ethics. Theories and methods for teaching and learning out of the adult education literature offer unique and useful perspectives in ethics education. This paper addresses selected barriers among both students and teachers that present challenges to developing and implementing ethics education, and underscore the need for modes of teaching and learning that differ markedly from the traditional didactic approach in health care education. Two interrelated perspectives of adult learning, Mezirow's theory of Transformative Learning, and King and Kitchner's Reflective Judgment Model, as well as Brookfield's writing on critical reflection, offer direction and support for overall curricular design, and for specific educational strategies in ethics education. Selected educational strategies that follow these perspectives of teaching and learning are included, to promote further exploration and discussion.

✧ INTRODUCTION

In the final analysis, the challenge of college, for students and faculty members alike, is empowering individuals to know that the world is far more complex than it first appears, and that they must make interpretive arguments and decisions—judgments that entail real consequences for which they must take responsibility and from which they may not flee by disclaiming expertise.

The Challenge of Connected Learning, Association of American Colleges[1]

The need for ethics education in professional health care programs, including the development of attitudes and behaviors supporting ethical competence, is clear and convincing. In the current health care environment, issues relating to cost controls, an increasingly diverse patient population, and limited access to health care result in frequent and complex ethical challenges for physical therapists.[2] Understanding and developing specific educational strategies to bring about the necessary attitudes, behaviors, and skills sufficient to meet these professional expectations for ethical practice has yet to be fully explored. The health professions are now heeding the early calls of Purtilo and others, for ethics education to be an integral and prominent component of physical and occupational therapy education.[3] With the involvement of a widening circle of educators, researchers, and clinicians, new and promising curricular models are being proposed and implemented.

Theories and strategies for teaching and learning out of the adult education literature offer unique and useful perspectives on the development of curricular initiatives in ethics. In addition, these authors provide valuable insight into why some of our efforts in ethics education have, at times, been less than successful. This chapter describes selected attributes and attitudinal barriers among both students and teachers that present challenges to the development and implementation of ethics curricula. These barriers underscore the need for models of teaching and learning that differ markedly from the traditional didactic modes of education currently employed in many occupational and physical therapy programs. Two interrelated perspectives of adult learning, Mezirow's theory of Transformative Learning, and King and Kitchner's Reflective Judgment Model, as well as Brookfield's writing on critical reflection for teachers and learners, offer direction and support for overall curricular design, and for specific educational strategies in ethics.

✧ STUDENT ISSUES IN ETHICS EDUCATION

Students enter physical and occupational therapy programs with varying levels of capacity for further development in the ethical components of clinical practice. In a study using Rest's Defining Issues Test (DIT)[4] as a measure of moral reasoning for students entering physical therapy programs, Sisola[5] reports the mean

DIT score indicating the relative importance subjects gave to items representing principled moral thinking (p-score) was 47.05, consistent with that for incoming students in medicine (50.2), nursing (46.3), and dentistry (47.6). Meanwhile, the range of DIT scores for the physical therapy students (21.7 to 75.0) reflects significant variability in their capacities for moral reasoning, extending from that of junior high students (DIT average 20.0), to that of graduate students in philosophy (DIT average 60.0 to 75.0).[5] These data support the anecdotal comments of physical therapy faculty involved in ethics education, reporting that while some students appear well prepared and motivated to expand their existing abilities for recognizing and resolving ethical dilemmas, other students appear to struggle and even resist this component of the curriculum. Rest responded to the question, "What difference does a moral judgment score make?" suggesting that a DIT p-score below 50 means that the student is unable to conceptualize ethical problems in terms of balancing the interests of affected parties.[4] "For low scoring students, discussions of intermediate-level concepts such as informed consent, paternalistic deception, and confidentiality, do not find lodging in ... basic cognitive structure, but rather seem like superfluous solutions for problems neither foreseen nor recognized. For these students, ... principled solutions to ethical problems must be learned one at a time (as special *overrides*), largely by rote, since their default schemas do not provide a general perspective for anticipating principled solutions."[4]

In addition to cognitive readiness to engage in ethics education, students enter professional programs with varying degrees of motivation for genuine engagement with the ethics curriculum. The reality of the competitive academic experience common to many students seeking entry into graduate health care programs reinforces an egocentric perspective, driven by the need to succeed over others. Triezenberg and Davis describe patterns early in life and in the undergraduate experience of physical therapy students that predisposes them toward self-interested patterns of thought and action.[6] Tannen suggests that this competitiveness among students is generally reflective of

American culture, leading us to think adversarily in terms of winning and losing, or in proving ourselves to be smart or worthy.[7] Tannen describes ours as an "argument culture," where we are conditioned to approach situations requiring resolution as a fight between opposing sides.[7] With this mind-set, individuals see two sides to every issue, and readily choose the "right" side while negatively labeling the other side. The focus is on winning, rather than working toward an understanding of other perspectives and the possibilities of common ground. Tannen suggests that helping students move away from this argument culture is a necessary step in developing skills in empathetic listening and informed constructive discourse.[7]

Students entering occupational and physical therapy, as well as other health care programs, must be assumed to be good people who desire positive outcomes for those whom they will see as patients/clients.[2] Despite these good intentions, some students appear to have not yet achieved levels of cognitive, relational, and self-reflective skills necessary for subsequent development of ethical competence at the professional level. In addition, unlike the attitude of students toward other components of the didactic curriculum, where they recognize the limits of their knowledge and skills and are motivated to learn, some students see little need for education and mastery of the ethics curriculum.[8] Student comments to the author reflecting this perspective include:

✦ "Talking about ethics isn't as important as my clinical learning and skills."

✦ "I care about patients—isn't that enough? I wouldn't ever do anything that would harm anybody."

✦ "What I need to know about ethics I already learned before I got to PT school—you learn that stuff at home, when you are a kid."

✦ "I already took an ethics class in undergrad; it was kind of interesting, but we never got down to the real answers to anything."

These students may, in fact, have the capacity for logical thought, have strong technical skills and generally good intentions, but they appear vulnerable to finding themselves overwhelmed when confronted with the complexities of real-world ethical problems, or they may simply fail to recognize the presence and implications of critical ethical issues.[4]

✧ CURRICULAR AND FACULTY ISSUES IN ETHICS EDUCATION

Curricular issues can also create barriers that diminish the effectiveness of ethics education in professional health care programs. Powerful message are sent to students regarding what is and what is not taught. Shepard and Jensen call attention to the "null curriculum," the content or skills not taught.[9] When a topic area is not prominent, or is not reinforced throughout the curriculum, the message sent to students is "this isn't particularly important in practice." Although accreditation requirements for professional health care programs mandate ethical content in the curriculum, failure to reinforce ethics throughout the curriculum relegates ethics to an "add-on" or optional status. Providing opportunities for students to recognize and address ethical issues in the context of clinical practice, and as part of ongoing clinical decision making, is further reinforced when modeled by the core program faculty.

Faculty attitudes and beliefs can also create barriers for effective ethics education. The following comments reflect these perspectives in the author's discussions with physical therapy faculty regarding teaching ethics:

✦ "I feel more confident teaching in the basic science or clinical components of the curriculum; I'm not as comfortable in the softer (ethics) areas of the curriculum."

✦ "I don't think that we know how to teach ethics, and I'm not sure that we're very successful in terms of what students learn about recognizing and resolving ethical dilemmas. It makes me feel like I'm not a very good teacher."

✦ "I'm committed to student development in ethics—it's essential for good clinical practice—but I get frustrated when there's no support from the rest of the faculty. The other faculty see ethics as my job."

◆ "I doubt that we can effectively teach ethics in school—certainly not at the graduate level. Isn't learning about ethics supposed to happen in undergrad, or at home, long before they get to us? Our job is to teach the clinical stuff."

These views reflect conflicted faculty attitudes and beliefs about the role of ethical competence in practice, and a lack of consensus on the value of ethics in the physical therapy curriculum. Similarly, Kanny and Kyler discuss concerns regarding faculty preparation for teaching ethics to occupational therapy students.[10] Faculty concerns about a lack of understanding and experience with effective educational strategies for teaching ethical content and skills can also lead to a lack of confidence on the part of faculty. Brookfield describes what he calls the faculty "imposter syndrome," where college instructors frequently feel incompetent: "If I'm not careful I will be found out to be teaching under false pretenses."[11] Armed primarily with confidence in one's area of clinical expertise but little formal training in the art and skill of teaching can leave professional health care faculty feeling insecure in their role as educators. This attitude can be especially prevalent in academic institutions where mentoring of faculty in their role as teachers is rare, and it is generally assumed that the content or discipline expertise of the teacher is sufficient to ensure that students will learn. These feelings of impostership can be heightened whenever faculty venture into new content areas or they attempt alternative methods of instruction. Brookfield suggests, "…the further we travel from our habitual practices, the more we run the risk of looking incompetent."[11] Sellheim, in her research on faculty beliefs about teaching, reports that physical therapy faculty, like that in other disciplines, describe their teaching methods as being based primarily on what they themselves experienced as students.[12] Cross describes faculty as victims of their own past.[13] "Many of the bone-weary teachers teach as they were taught. There is nothing in their preparation and training to break the cycle of teaching as telling. All too often information flows from the notes of the professor into the notebook of students without passing through the minds of either."[13]

Barr and Tagg describe these traditional teaching methods as teacher-centered, where knowledge is primarily delivered in definable segments, as lectures by the instructor who is considered to be the expert.[14] Knowledge, in this model is assumed to transfer from the teacher-expert to the students, whose role is that of passive receivers of knowledge. This mode of teaching and learning has been demonstrated by Pratt and others to push students toward rote memorization and other superficial modes of learning, with minimal long-term retention of knowledge or skills.[15] Sellheim reports that even when the physical therapy faculty participating in her study expressed an awareness of more learner-centered modes of instruction, where students are more actively engaged in the learning process, the faculty reported being fearful of trying new teaching methods, especially if doing things differently meant covering less content or losing what was perceived as "core" content.[12] The faculty's "implicit beliefs about teaching, such as the teacher must tell students the content in order for the students to learn it" prevents them from implementing more student-centered methods of teaching.[12] Sellheim reports that few mechanisms were in place to assist the faculty in her study toward increased development and confidence in using instructional methodologies that result in deeper learning and higher-order thinking.[12,16] The result of this faculty reluctance to explore alternative teaching methods is a firmer grasp on more traditional, but potentially less effective teaching strategies for ethics as well as other components of the curriculum, and fewer faculty willing to participate in teaching ethics across the curriculum.

What are the goals of the ethics curriculum, and in what ways do teaching and learning in ethics require different teaching strategies than those historically present in professional health care programs? Treizenberg and Davis argue that ethics should be at the "philosophical center" of the physical therapy curriculum with specific goals to improve the moral behavior of students, and to integrate these new professionals into the value system and expected behaviors of the profession.[6] Critical skills for ethical competence for physical therapists involve the development of attitudes and behaviors that reflect the values or "ethos" of the profession, an understanding of one's own values and morality, and the values and cultural context of patients, families, and colleagues.[17] Ethical competence also requires skill in critical thinking, including an attitude or disposition that determines how individuals view and manage information and beliefs. Thus, in contrast with the traditional health professional curriculum, with its primary focus on the acquisition of declarative knowledge, clinical reasoning, and technical skills, education in ethics involves developing a meaningful awareness of self as a professional, a personal commitment to patients as central to the process of healing, and attitudes supporting genuine critical reflection in ethical decision making.[6] Successful curricular strategies supporting the development of these attitudes and behaviors by occupational and physical therapy students must reflect the unique nature of these learning goals. The interrelated theoretical perspectives of *transformative learning* and *reflective judgment* and concepts of critical thinking described in the adult learning literature can be instructive in considering the development and implementation of the ethics curriculum. A description of some overlapping educational strategies that extend from these theoretical constructs follows a brief overview of these educational theories.

✧ TRANSFORMATIVE LEARNING

Transformative learning is an area of educational theory and practice first described by Mezirow.[18] The educational theorist Habermas described three domains of knowledge with related theories of learning: technical learning includes the acquisition of content including facts, concepts, problem-solving strategies or practical skills.[19] In this domain, the educator is recognized and valued as an expert, and the student sees herself or himself as gaining necessary knowledge or skills. Practical learning is concerned with understanding what others mean; this includes understanding social norms, val-

ues, and political concepts, as well as making our selves understood. Emancipatory learning is a process of freeing the individual from forces or perspectives that limit her/his options and control over their lives, forces or perspectives that have been taken for granted or seen as beyond the individual's control.[19] Transformative learning comes out of the domain of emancipatory learning where, through a process of critical self-reflection, an individual revises old or develops new assumptions, beliefs, or ways of seeing the world.[20]

The phrase "frames of reference" is used by transformative learning theorists to describe complex webs of assumptions, expectations, values, and beliefs that act as filters or screens through which we view the world and ourselves.[21] Mezirow describes two dimensions of a frame of reference.[18,22] A meaning scheme is a set of related and habitual expectations governing cause-effect and category relationships. These meaning schemes are implicit and habitual patterns for interpreting what is occurring; we expect to see the sun rise in the east, and food is to satisfy our hunger. Meaning perspectives (habits of mind) are higher-order beliefs, attitudes, value judgments, and orienting predispositions that shape our interpretation in a broader way. Mezirow describes one category of meaning perspectives as "the distinctive ways an individual interprets experience at what developmental psychologists describe as different stages of moral, ethical, and ego development and different stages of reflective judgment."[18] These frames of reference are derived from our cultural background, our prior knowledge, beliefs, and psychological makeup, and are important in providing a sense of stability, coherence, and identity in our lives. This is how we are able to make sense of the chaos around us. It is not surprising, then, that challenges to this frame of reference can be very disturbing and the initial reaction to alternative views is often highly emotional and defensive. Other viewpoints may be quickly dismissed as distorted, deceptive, or "just plain wrong." Learning within this mode is narrowly confined to adding only those ideas that are compatible to an already existing frame of reference. This perspective calls to mind the emotional resistance demonstrated by students at times, when they are challenged to explore alternative views of complex situations. The students' distress can be interpreted as their reaction to a perceived threat to an established and trusted frame of reference.

Brookfield reports that adults can be particularly tenacious in holding on to their set of beliefs or assumptions.[22] Transformative learning theorists cite research, however, suggesting that this disposition to reject challenges to an existing frame of reference can be altered, in favor of developing a more effective and dependable frame of reference.[23] This frame would be open to other viewpoints, would be critically reflective of assumptions and emotionally capable of change, and would allow the integration of past experiences. Thus, transformative learning is a reformulation of structures of meaning through a process of critical reflection and reconstruction of frames of reference. The result is not only a significant change in life perspective, but it is an actualization of that perspective. True transformative learning is said to occur when life is not merely seen from a new perspective, but is lived from that perspective.[24]

Mezirow discusses the "habits of mind" as a set of assumptions acting as filters, interpreting the meaning of one's experiences. These filters can be sociolinguistic—stemming from social norms, customs, cultural canon; epistemic, including individual learning styles or sensory preferences; they are philosophical, including one's religious doctrine or a "world view." They can be psychological, including one's self-concept, and personality traits; or aesthetic, including values, attitudes, and judgments about what is beautiful, and what is ugly. These habits of the mind, occurring quite outside of conscious awareness, shape one's interpretation of events, and lead us to act in given ways.[18] Taylor, in his critical review of research in transformative learning theory, reports that adults in a variety of settings do, indeed experience perspective transformations initiated by a disorienting dilemma and followed by a series of specific learning strategies involving critical reflection, exploration of options, and negotiation of relationships.[23] Other authors suggest that incremental introduction to alternative perspectives may also lead to transformative learning.[25]

Given this brief overview of transformative learning, what educational strategies extending from this theoretical base could be incorporated into professional health care programs to promote critical reflection as a foundation for ethics education by both teachers and students? The selected strategies that follow reflect a limited representation of the extensive literature base on the theory and methods of transformative learning, and are included here to promote further exploration and discussion, which may pertain to ethics education.

✧ PROMOTING TRANSFORMATIVE LEARNING

What is the educator's role in promoting transformative learning, and how can this process be useful in supporting student ethical development? Cranton describes three critical aspects in promoting transformative learning: fostering learner empowerment (setting the stage for critical self-reflection), stimulating transformative learning, and supporting the process.[20] While the educational strategies described here may be familiar to some occupational and physical therapy educators, it is useful, nevertheless, to place them within this theoretical framework. These transformative learning strategies can then be recognized as quite distinct from the traditional didactic educational approaches used in the majority of professional health care programs, with potential as educational approaches within the ethics thread of the curriculum. By grounding classroom approaches in a theoretical foundation, teaching strategies once considered merely "novel," can be identified and further studied as potentially valid and effective instructional approaches, capable of supporting the learning objectives of the ethics curriculum.

Fostering Learner Empowerment and Involvement

Necessary conditions for discourse and self-reflection include an environment where participants are free from coercion, and students are encouraged to fully participate. When students lack confidence or feel unsupported, they may be unwilling or unable to sufficiently overcome their fears and participate in self-reflection in a meaningful way. An important first step in fostering student empowerment is the instructor's recognition of the various forms of power he or she holds in the classroom, and exploration of how this power can be shared with students.[20]Certainly, teachers are not free to, nor should they, give up all power; grades must be awarded, schedules for courses must be maintained. Thoughtful consideration of ways to share power with students can, however, yield surprising opportunities. Among the many examples are, acknowledging that the faculty do not have all the answers, sitting with the students rather than standing in front of the room, planning activities that draw knowledge, questions, and answers from the students whenever possible, allowing students to help construct how you will do your work together, and promoting peer feedback, so faculty are not seen as the only credible evaluators of student work.[20] The educational environment promoted here is consistent with that described by Barr and Tagg as learner-centered rather than teacher-centered.[14] Students are not only encouraged, but are expected to be active in the learning experience. Teachers act as facilitators of learning, rather than as providers of knowledge.

Stimulating Critical Self-Reflection

Creating an environment conducive to learner empowerment does not ensure that students will engage in critical self-reflection. A critical role for the educator is to stimulate and encourage this reflective process, while refraining from imposing her or his own values, beliefs, and assumptions. Cranton describes the role of the teacher as a "provocateur," promoting critical self-reflection in order to stimulate "perceived discrepancies between the learner's beliefs, values or assumptions, and new knowledge, understanding and insights."[20] These discrepancies can be initiated through provocative readings, discussions with peers or faculty, and practical experience. Posing well-structured critical questions is an important step setting

the stage for student insight into their assumptions or experiential learning. These questions should create a sense of disequilibrium for the student, which Mezirow describes as a necessary "trigger" for transformative learning.

Consciousness-raising can be another effective strategy to increase self-awareness. Activities such as role-playing, simulations, and games invite students to look at familiar things from new perspectives. Care must be taken to allow those who are uncomfortable with activities such as role-plays to initially act as observers, in order to allow progress within a supportive, empowering environment.[20]

Journaling is used in many health care programs, most commonly in relation to clinical education experiences. Journals can also be a positive means for students to express thoughts and feelings relating to values and attitudes previously undetected and unexplored.[26,27] Once identified, these values, beliefs, and attitudes can be examined in relation to their influence on the student's actions. Frequently, it is the students who might benefit most from transformative learning experiences who are puzzled by the process of journaling ("what do you want me to write?"). One suggestion for encouraging more genuine reflection versus "keeping a daily log" is to ask students to divide the pages of the journal in half vertically and use one side for descriptions and observations and the other half for feelings and thoughts relating to the descriptions.[20] The goal of the self-reflective process in relation to ethical development is to provide the opportunity for the students to move beyond mere rote citation of ethical principles or an ethical code toward identification and potential revision of previously unexamined values and beliefs about ideas such as one's ethical obligation to patients and patients' rights.

Supporting Transformative Learning

An important way that educators can support students in the transformative learning process is by demonstrating this process themselves and being what Cranton describes as "authentic."[20] The more the educator identifies and relates with the experience of the students as they attempt self-reflection, the more supportive the interactions will be. Demonstrating that the educator is also a learner can reinforce the value and methods of transformative learning. An interesting aspect of critical reflection for the teacher is reflection on her or his own style and methods of teaching. "If we accept the assumption that critical self-reflection is one goal of adult education, and we accept the assumption that adult educators are also adult learners, we can move easily to the view that educator development includes opportunities for transformed perspectives on teaching."[20] The strategies for unearthing critical assumptions about teaching can reveal surprising insight into our practices in the classroom and interactions with students. Brookfield suggests a process of discovery through the teacher's autobiography as a learner as an important first step.[27] I suggest that transformative learning can be integrated with the ethics curricular thread.

✧ REFLECTIVE JUDGMENT MODEL

The Reflective Judgment Model of intellectual development as proposed by King and Kitchener focuses on how people arrive at judgments and decisions about complex and controversial problems.[28] This model draws on John Dewey's early work on reflective thinking.[29] Dewey described reflective judgment as that required in the presence of uncertain and problematic situations where formulas will not work and there is no way to prove that a proposed solution is correct.[29] Moral problems can certainly be included within this description of uncertain and problematic situations.

King and Kitchener distinguish reflective thinking from traditional critical thinking in two ways.[28] First, although the logic associated with critical thinking may address complex problems through the application of a formula or set of principles, reflective judgment includes epistemological assumptions about what can be known and how knowing occurs. Those who assume that knowledge is authority-based also assume that an authority can provide a solution for a problem—"uncertainty does not exist."[28]

Conversely, reflective judgment requires examination and evaluation of information, opinions, and possible explanations followed by the construction of plausible solutions for problem at hand. Solutions would then be open for further evaluation. Thus, true reflective judgment is not assumed to yield "absolute truth," but rather to provide a process for assessing what can be known.

The second distinction between critical thinking and reflective thinking relates to the structure of the problem, the degree to which a problem can be described completely, and the certainty that a correct solution can be identified. Logic can address well-structured problems or "puzzles," where one possibly complex but correct way of thinking is the appropriate pathway to the solution. Ill-structured problems require consideration of alternative perspectives, seeking out new evidence, and the evaluation of reliability of data and sources of information. Ill-structured problems cannot be described with any high degree of certainty. Experts may disagree about the best solution to these problems, and in the end, it may be difficult to determine when a solution has been reached. Proponents of this theoretical construct suggest that the development of reflective judgment is the outcome of the interaction between a student's conceptual skills and environmental factors that can promote or inhibit these skills. I believe that promoting students' capacity for reflective judgment is a critical component of ethics education.

The Reflective Judgment Model describes a developmental progression of reasoning skills in adulthood that the authors suggest can provide a foundation for teaching students to think and judge reflectively.[28] King and Shuford illustrate the profoundly divergent ways that college students describe and support their beliefs:[30]

Why do some students seem to ignore the factual evidence in arriving at a point of view, whereas others have a seemingly insatiable appetite for more and more information, thereby delaying or deferring judgment for long periods of time? Why do some students dismiss contradictory explanations as "merely different opinions," whereas others go to elaborate means to explain the basis for the differing perspec-

tives? Why do some students quickly make judgments about complex problems, confidently asserting the correctness of their views? Why do others resist making judgments, worrying that to do so would be an irrevocable denial of the basis of different perspectives?[30]

Drawing on other models of cognitive development, the Reflective Judgment Model uses stages to describe assumptions about knowledge and how knowledge claims affect reasoning.[28] In the "pre-reflective" stages, reasoning is characterized by assumptions that knowledge is gained through direct, personal observation or from an authority figure. In the middle set of stages, characterized as "quasi-reflective," the use of evidence is central to deliberations, but there is acknowledgment of ambiguity in gathering and interpreting evidence. At the quasi-reflective stage, students see the rationale for conflicting interpretations, but are unsure how to choose among competing alternatives.[28] Guthrie reports students in the quasi-reflective stage to be "caught up in the dilemma with no apparent means to reason their way to a solution."[30] In the fully reflective stage students express an understanding that knowledge is not given, but constructed, taking into consideration the context in which the knowledge claims are grounded. Students exhibiting fully reflective thinking can more readily evaluate knowledge claims, and use criteria to determine coherence, usefulness, and soundness of the data. These students recognize that knowledge is uncertain at times, but in the end, they can make reasonable judgments on the basis of information at hand. Students reasoning at the reflective level demonstrate complex cognitive ability, and they are able to argue on the basis of evidence. At this fully reflective stage, simplistic or dualistic positions are rejected, and students are able to critique their own thinking.[29] A review of research on the intellectual development of college students using the Reflective Judgment Model reports two-thirds of college freshmen in the pre-reflective mode.[28] Reasoning of the college seniors in these studies was typical of quasi-reflective thinking, with fully reflective thinking consistently demonstrated only among advanced graduate students. Interestingly, adult learners tended to enter college at the pre-reflective level similar to traditional age freshmen, but the adult students progressed to fully reflective levels more quickly.

Kitchner and colleagues suggest a structural similarity in the development of conceptions of moral rights and obligations, and conceptions of knowledge and justification described in the Reflective Judgment Model.[31] Consistent with the pre-reflective stages of the Reflective Judgment Model, initial concepts of morality are generally viewed as absolute and concrete (an act is good or bad). With developmental progression, the differentiation and complexity of conceptions of morality increase. In the later, more fully reflective stages, abstract concepts of morality are understood, and the ability to balance competing interests, and apply moral principles to moral judgments within the context of a complex ethical case emerges. Advising that further study is needed, these authors cite data from longitudinal studies of the Reflective Judgment Model suggesting that reflective judgment and moral reasoning are interrelated, and that developing reflective judgment will not necessarily lead to, but may be required for, more principled moral thinking. "Educators who want to promote moral development might address this goal by helping students consider issues of how they can better reason about ill-structured problems in the intellectual domain as well as in the moral domain."[28]

Promoting Reflective Judgment

How can educators promote reflective thinking about ethical problems in a way that recognizes the complexity of the issues and encourages students to speak from their own, rather than others', convictions? King and Shuford describe the important role that faculty can play in promoting this process, including recognition of individual student levels of reflective judgment, and the application of supports and challenges appropriate to the student's current level of thinking.[30] Challenges beyond the student's existing capabilities or a perceived lack of support by the educator may cause the student to withdraw from true self-reflective activity, and progress in reflective thinking is then diminished. The desired learning environment provides sufficient and appropriate challenge toward higher-order judgment in the presence of adequate support. King and Shuford suggest that students using pre-reflective assumptions (base their judgments on the "correct" view of authority figures) can be challenged to find factual evidence or reasoned positions to support their conclusions.[30] Students in the quasi-reflective stage (identify evidence for various perspectives but are unable to determine the adequacy of the data), will be challenged when asked to select and defend a particular point of view. Describing her use of the Reflective Judgment Model in an undergraduate literature course, Kroll suggests, "...when their responses are dogmatic, I foster all their doubts; when they seem mired in skepticism or paralyzed by complexity, I push them to make judgments; when their tactics are not fully reflective, I encourage their best efforts to use critical, interrogative, or evaluative thinking."[32] These authors caution that research on progression of students' reasoning demonstrates age-related ceilings on the level of reflective judgment they can use.[33] Students are generally able to produce reasoning only one to two stages beyond their typical thinking. Recognizing the reasoning levels for individual students allows the educator to develop or respond to learning experiences that can challenge but not overwhelm the learner.

Modeling reflective thinking for students through presentations of controversial problems or dilemmas within the discipline is encouraged.[28] Lynch and colleagues describe the importance of students seeing examples of what it means to "probe, question, compare, and evaluate sources of information.... and what it means to decide an issue on the basis of the soundest claims, the best evidence, and the most reliable experts."[33] Consideration of multiple perspectives is critical in demonstrating the reflective process, as well as allowing students to "try on" these various perspectives to encourage an emotional as well as an intellectual response. Students are further supported in this process when emotional responses are recognized as a legitimate and expected part of the learning process.

✧ CONCLUSION

Attitudinal barriers among both students and faculty in occupational and physical therapy programs present challenges for ethics education. In contrast with the traditional health care curriculum, with its primary focus on the acquisition of declarative knowledge, clinical reasoning, and technical skills, education in ethics involves developing a meaningful awareness of self and one's professional commitment to patients. Successful curricular strategies supporting the development of ethical competence must reflect the unique nature of these learning goals.

Theories and perspectives from the adult learning literature offer a rich and extensive base from which to explore and test distinctive methods for teaching ethics in occupational and physical therapy programs. While curricular models and teaching methods consistent with the concepts of transformational learning and reflective judgment may be viewed by some as novel or risky when compared with traditional curricular approaches, further study of these perspectives can yield important new and valid approaches supporting the transformation of students into mature and ethically competent practitioners. Critical elements to consider in the development of curricular strategies for teaching ethics include attention to a supportive environment for the pivotal process of self-reflection for students and faculty alike. In addition, it will be necessary to recognize and respond to the developmental levels of individual students. Attention to the overall curriculum framework as context for ethics education as well as specific strategies to promote ethical competence can advance the effectiveness of ethics education in occupational and physical therapy programs.

References

1. Association of American Colleges: The Challenge of Connecting Learning. Project on liberal Learning, Study-in-depth, and the Arts and Sciences Major. Association of American Colleges, Washington, DC, 1991.
2. Jensen GM, and Paschal KA: Habits of mind: Student transition toward virtuous practice. J Phys Ther Educ 14(3):42–47, 2000.

3. Purtilo RB: A time to harvest, a time to sow: Ethics for a shifting landscape. Phys Ther 80(11):1112–1119, 2000.
4. Rest JR, and Narvaez D. Moral Development in the Professions. Lawrence Erlbaum Associates, NJ, 1994.
5. Sisola SW: Moral reasoning as a predictor of clinical practice: The development of physical therapy students across the professional curriculum. J Phys Ther Educ 14(3):26–34, 2000.
6. Triezenberg HL, and Davis CM: Beyond the code of ethics: Educating physical therapists for their role as moral agents. J Phys Ther Educ 14(3):48–58, 2000.
7. Tannen D: The Argument Culture. Random House, New York, 1998.
8. Barnitt RE, and Roberts LC: Facilitating ethical reasoning in student physical therapists. J Phys Ther Educ 14(3):35–41, 2000.
9. Shepard KF, and Jensen GM: Handbook of Teaching for Physical Therapist, ed 2. Butterworth Heinemann, Boston, 2002.
10. Kanny EM, and Kyler PL: Are faculty prepared to address ethical issues in education? World Fed of Occup Ther Bull 39:7–11, 1999.
11. Brookfield SD: Becoming a Critically Reflective Teacher. Jossey-Bass, San Francisco, 1995.
12. Sellheim D: Physical Therapy Students' approaches to learning: Faculty beliefs and other educational factors that influence them. University of Minnesota, 2001.
13. Cross KP: A proposal to improve teaching or what 'taking teaching seriously' should mean. AAHE Bull 39:4–17, 1986.
14. Barr RB, and Tagg J: From teaching to learning: A new paradigm for undergraduate education. Change November/December, 1995.
15. Pratt DD: Five Perspectives on Teaching in Adult and Higher Education. Krieger Publishing Co., Malabar, FL, 1998.
16. Newble DI, and Entwistle NJ: Learning styles and approaches: Implications for medical education. Med Educ 20:162–175, 1986.
17. Stiller C: Exploring the ethos of the physical therapy profession in the United States: Social, cultural and historical influences and their relationship to education. J Phys Ther Educ 14(3):7–16, 2000.
18. Mezirow J, et al: Fostering Critical Reflection in Adulthood: A Guide to Transformative and Emancipatory Learning. Jossey-Bass, San Francisco, 1990.
19. Habermas J: The Theory of communicative Action. Vol. 1: Reason and the Rationalization of Society. (T. McCarthy trans.). Beacon Press, Boston, 1984.
20. Cranton P: Understanding and Promoting Transformative Learning. Jossey-Bass, San Francisco, 1994.
21. Mezirow J: On critical reflection. Adult Educ Q 48(3):185–194, 1998.
22. Brookfield SD: The Skillful Teacher. Jossey-Bass, San Francisco, 1990.
23. Taylor EW: Analyzing research on transformative learning theory. In Mezirow and Associates, (eds): Learning as Transformation. Jossey-Bass, San Francisco, 2000.
24. Cranton P: Professional Development as Transformative Learning. Jossey-Bass, San Francisco, 1996.
25. Mezirow and Associates, (eds): Learning as Transformation. Jossey-Bass, San Francisco, 2000.
26. Tryssenaar J: Interactive journals: An educational strategy to promote reflection. Am J Occup Ther 49(7):695–702, 1996.
27. Brookfield SD: Critically reflective practice. J Cont Educ Health Prof 18(4):197, 1998.
28. King PM, and Kitchener KS: Developing Reflective Judgment. Jossey-Bass, San Francisco, 1994.
29. Dewey J: How We Think. Regnery, Chicago, 1933.
30. King PM, and Shuford BA: A multicultural view is a more cognitively complex view. Am Behav Sci 40(2):153–154, 1996.
31. Kitchener KS, et al: Consistency and sequentiality in the development of reflective judgment: A six-year longitudinal study. J Appl Develop Psychol 10:73–95, 1989.
32. Kroll BM: Reflective inquiry in a college English class. Lib Educ 78(1):10–13, 1992.
33. Lynch CL, Kitchener KS, and King PM: Developing Reflective Judgment in the Classroom. A Manual for Faculty. U.S. Department of Education, Fund for the Improvement of Postsecondary Education. Project No. P116B00926, Washington, DC, 1994.

23
Reflections on Student Learning

ERNEST NALETTE, EDD, PT

Abstract

In this reflective, pedagogical chapter the author discusses the philosophical concepts that frame his case study approach to ethics instruction. He describes, with supporting evidence from his experience, how four overlapping concepts: concreteness, objectivity, analysis and skepticism of convention, are foundational to his teaching of ethics.

The author proposes that practitioners generally do not use an ethical language when discussing morally troubling clinical situations, thus resulting in moral silence. This moral silence is proposed as a contributing factor in a weakening focus of the purpose of helping professionals—to help patients become well again. Ethics instruction of professional students is offered as a way of ameliorating this problem by replacing the moral silence with a robust ethical language.

Over the last three decades I have been an observer of health care practitioners. As a retrospective reflection, a central observation from this time period was a slow change in language. The focus of clinical language during the first decade of my practice was patient stories. Practitioners knew their patients well and understood what was necessary to meet those patients' needs. The patient stories were told in a rich, relational language that was ethical by nature. Knowing someone's story evokes the compassion that takes concern for others toward action on the behalf of the other. During the second decade the language was one of diminishing resources and clinicians' struggles to meet patient needs. The richness of thick patient stories is diminished as practitioners have insufficient time to know their patients. Practitioners tell stories focused more on reimbursement categories than on the uniqueness of the patient. The third decade saw a maturing of a corporate language in which patient care was a means to the end of meeting the financial needs of an organization. At some point, patient stories become so thin as to no longer be relational between the patient and the practitioner. Under these circumstances the conditions that naturally support an ethical clinical language evaporate, resulting in a moral silence.

A purpose of the health professions is to help patients become well again, which is a fundamentally ethical practice disposition.[1] For an ethical purpose to live, it must be spoken of in an ethical language. Moral silence results in the loss of a profession's ethical purpose. A necessary component of refocusing our ethical professional purpose is to diminish the deafening moral silence of our practitioners. Ethics instruction to our student of health professions is a reasonable strategy for reintroducing a robust ethical language into clinical practice. In this chapter, I share personal experiences and reflections on my work of training students to speak an ethical language that refocuses practice on the needs of patients.

✧ PERSONAL NARRATIVE

I became a physical therapist in 1972, completing my professional education during the era of the Vietnam War and the civil rights movement. This era of personal activism provided what McIntyre might refer to as my "moral starting point."[2] From this starting point I presumed one acts on what one believes. During my early professional life, the majority of persons around me were remarkable individuals who were willing and able to help me advance my clinical reasoning and skills. At that time, we were focused on providing patients with necessary services and usually succeeded in improving the patient's quality of life. Over the ensuing quarter century, I practiced in a diverse clinical setting at an academic medical center, served on local ethics committees, was Advisor to the Vermont Secretary of State for physical therapist practice, and was a member of the American Physical Therapy Association (APTA) Ethics and Judicial Committee. I began teaching student physical therapists in both clinical and academic settings in the mid-1970s and have been a full-time educator since 1998.

Throughout my clinical practice experience I accumulated a multitude of troubling stories. At the time, I did not recognize these as ethical situations. They felt like problems— I saw a human being, usually a professional, treating another human being, usually as patient, in an unkind, unfair, or incompetent manner. I knew human beings were supposed to be kind and fair to other human beings based on lessons learned from my parents and my church. I knew professionals were supposed to be competent based on my professional education. Something was amiss.

I began to understand the importance of ethics in 1985, when I took my initial ethics class. Prior to this time I saw myself as a well-educated, well-trained, effective clinician. During this ethics course I realized, however, I was inept at discussing the moral aspects of my professional practice. I then realized what was amiss; patients were being treated unethically. My ethics education began to give me a language with which to discuss and act on the morally troubling stories I had accumulated from 13 years of clinical practice.

Language is used "in order to communicate thoughts and feelings [among a] group of people with a shared history or set of traditions."[3] The language of the physical therapist is powerful, especially in relation to a patient. One evening I saw the x-ray of a 17-year-old young man's severely fractured and dislocated thoracic spine indicating a severed spinal cord. Early the next morning he asked me, "Will I ever walk again?" I concur with Drane that language creates reality and the professional holds a power over that reality.[4] The response to this question from a trusted professional will create a new reality for this patient. An ongoing part of a professional's life is to contribute to the patient's reality by using language competently and compassionately with humility. Without a professional language our professional practice does not exist.

During a recent ethics class conversation a student said, "I believe most of us care about ethics in the clinic. I don't think we know how to talk about it." Over many years, students and practitioners have expressed the same thought. When we are silent about moral concerns because we do not know "how to talk about it," the ethical subtext drops from our language, resulting in moral silence. This language void is not self-sustaining but is filled with other languages. From my observations over the past three decades, the languages of efficiency, corporate regulations, and professional power have filled this ethical language void. All of these languages make important contributions to the care of patients. However, in the absence of a robust ethical language, the other languages are insufficient to support our professional purpose. During our period of moral silence, our purpose slides away from helping patients and toward profit, legal defensiveness, and professional aggrandizement. I am proposing that we need to reintroduce a robust ethical language into our classroom and our clinics if we are to fully realize our purpose of helping patients become well again.

The use of a moral language is essential to our professional practice but I do not intend any disrespect to those individuals who do not speak an ethics language. I have met, and continue to meet, individuals who do not speak an ethical language but who are of the most amazing moral character. Believing that those who do not speak an ethical language are morally lacking is the erroneous belief that a good moral character can only be achieved through the study of philosophy.[5] However, our profession will be of greater service to society when all physical therapists consistently speak an ethical-clinical language, thereby filling the moral silence and professing our purpose. As professionals profess, they "express their moral character in every public declaration of belief they make... always declaring openly, by their words and their actions, what is morally important to them."[6]

❖ FOUR BASIC CONCEPTS FOR ETHICS PEDAGOGY

It is with this particular background and philosophical disposition that I have been wondering what concepts may be most helpful to my ethics pedagogy. My intent in this chapter is to share selected clinical and academic experiences that have influenced my ethics pedagogy and to discuss four overlapping concepts that are now central to my ethics instruction for entry- and postentry-level physical therapist students. The concepts are (1) concreteness: the practical use of ethics in clinical practice, (2) objectivity: ethical standards external to one's self, (3) analysis: a systematic approach to ethical reasoning and action, and (4) skepticism of convention: a disposition of skepticism toward the status quo and a commitment to act from one's own reasoning.

On Concreteness

My early recollections of patient care include having sufficient time to listen to patients, to consult as needed with others, and read literature relating to a specific patient's problems. I have only a few memories of limited resources during these early years of practice. However, 1983 marked a radical change in clinical practice with the introduction of Diagnostic Related Groups (DRGs).

I met a new patient late one afternoon. The medical resident had written a goal of "discharge to home" in the patient's medical record. My evaluation indicated the patient required a few days of additional hospitalization to ensure a safe and functional home discharge. The next morning I asked the Resident about the timing of the discharge plans. He pulled a list out of his pocket (I later learned this was a list of DRGs with average length of stay for each DRG) and responded, "This afternoon." I said, "She will not be safe." He responded, "She's out of here! The Attending is under a lot of pressure to make this service look more efficient to the administration."

The Resident's action was wrong. He was acting in what he believed to be the best interest of his Attending Physician while disregarding the best interest of the patient; he was rejecting a necessary intervention and failing to be concerned about potential patient harm. Stating my clinical concerns was not sufficient to change the Resident's focus from serving his Attending to serving his patient. I participated in many similar stories that only seemed to accumulate more rapidly as resources necessary to care for patients became more limited within the practice setting.

A few years later, during my first ethics course, I remember thinking, "This is it. I can use ethics to make sense of these clinical problems!" Prior to this ethics class I had accumulated 13 years of clinical experience, had been responsible to thousands of patients, and had experienced a multitude of morally troubling situations. Ethics was instantaneously concrete as the content was directly applicable to actual, specific patient situations for which I was ultimately responsible. I began to realize that ethics, when integrated with my professional education, could help me more comprehensively understand my clinical experiences. I also had the sense I would be able to more effectively advocate on behalf of my patients.

There is a caution here. The language of philosophy, and therefore ethics, can become so esoteric as to be inaccessible to most students and practitioners. The irony for me as an ethics instructor, and the biggest challenge for my entry-level students, is that most of my students are learning ethics in the reverse order that I learned ethics. They are learning ethics with only a few weeks of clinical experience. They frequently ask, "What does ethics have to do with patient care?" and adopt an initial position that ethics is so abstract as to be useless. Bringing these students to a position of ethical concreteness is the initial challenge for the ethics instructor.

An objective of my ethics instruction is to foster the use of ethical language, what Nash refers to as the "moral conversation," in the classroom.[6] My hope is that this classroom talk will move into the clinical setting and reduce the moral silence. I am more successful in achieving this objective when it is made explicit that I intend to avoid two topics: the law and clinical decision making. The primary reason for avoiding cases that pivot on legal concepts is that it is not the purpose of the course. In addition, I am not an attorney and not competent in teaching the law. Of course, the law cannot be totally avoided, given the web of laws that both create and direct our practice. However, I am explicit with my students that the purpose of our time together is not to share opinions about the law. Likewise, it is helpful to avoid discussions centering on clinical decision making. These discussions are usually disagreements regarding the efficacy of intervention A versus intervention B in situation C. As with the law, clinical decision making is not the purpose of the course. However, I use these situations to make the point that the practitioner must limit their practice by staying within the bounds of their personal competency. Knowingly practicing in a broader scope places patients at risk and is avoided by ethical practitioners.

Students move toward ethical concreteness when they purposively use ethical languages and apply ethical concepts to patient situations for which they feel responsible. To facilitate this movement toward concreteness I assign pre-course reading and writing. I have assigned a variety of texts over the years [6–10] but rely most heavily on Robert Nash's *"Real World"* *Ethics*. The text includes concepts that have been very helpful in my teaching, such as background beliefs, rules/principles ethics, virtue ethics, and methods of analysis. Most students express concerns that the text(s) are difficult to read and most do not immediately see the application of concepts from the reading to their practice. Much of what I ask the students to read includes concepts that are new

to them. Given these are new concepts, students require mentored opportunities for application of these new concepts. The ethics instructor can facilitate the use of the readings during class discussions of particular situations by asking the students, "What might our author say about this topic?" Responses to this type of question have the effect of enriching the classroom by bringing the author of the text into the classroom. Another way to enrich the classroom is having students write and discuss case narratives.

As I assign pre-course readings, I also assign the writing of an experiential, patient-centered case narrative. The case narrative is drawn from the student's clinical experience of a morally troubling situation in which the student functioned as the moral agent in the case. Drawing the case from one's own experience contributes to the sense of concreteness that I seek to bring to the topic of ethics. This student-written case will be grist for the ethical analysis carried out later in the course. Some students arrive at the beginning of the course believing they do not have a sufficiently meaningful case to write for the course. This presumption is almost never true. Students presume a case needs to be dramatic to be meaningful. It is important to help students recognize that ethics is a part of each patient-therapist relationship. In each relationship I have with a patient: Am I respectful? competent? fair? compassionate? courageous? Adopting this point of view makes ethics not only a retrospective act of analysis but also a prospective disposition to view ethics as a way of being, thereby avoiding unethical behavior on an ongoing basis.

This disposition is rooted in our background beliefs. Our background beliefs are "the most fundamental assumptions that guide our perceptions about the nature of reality and what we experience as good or bad, right or wrong, important or unimportant."[6] Understanding one's background beliefs provides a solid foundation for our moral character. For most students, this will be the first time the student has been asked to access and reflect upon his or her background beliefs and even more certainly, the first time to make their deepest beliefs public. This requires practice. Background beliefs anchor one's character and need to be gently investigated. The need to understand your own point of view precedes the need, and maybe the ability, to understand someone else's point of view. Understanding another's point of view does not equal acceptance of that point of view.

After sharing the above reflections with the class, a student is asked to read her or his case to the class. Reading cases to the class serves two functions. First, the instructor has the opportunity to ask questions of the reader to assist comprehensiveness of the case. Second, the discussion helps writers of other cases improve the clarity of their case and assists them in seeing the moral relevance of a case. As soon as the instructor discerns it is feasible, the other students are encouraged to participate in seeking answers to the questions they have regarding the presented case. The intent is to extend the conversation, not to intimidate the presenters. The instructor needs to ensure this manner of questioning or risk losing the moral conversation.

I have been increasingly reliant on student-written case studies as I have observed their ability to make ethics more concrete for students in the classroom. At the same time, it is important to remember that, although these cases may "point toward reality," they are not reality.[11] The situations we discuss in the classroom usually occur in the clinical setting and the classroom is fundamentally different. Although the writer of the case is in the classroom, the other morally relevant actors in the case are not present. In addition, most of the time, the student cannot act on the case while in the classroom. Based on the setting, our purposes are different than if the conversation happened in the clinical environment. In the classroom, our purpose is understanding—it is not our means but our end. In the clinical setting, understanding is the means to an end—taking action in the patient's best interest. Emphasizing the concreteness of the narrative moves our work toward reality but does not equal reality.

Our class discussions move cases toward being factually complete, reliable, and having "conceptual clarity."[12] The instructor can frequently facilitate this process by asking ques-

tions of the author of the case study and by asking the other students, "What additional information might you want to know about this particular situation?" Students will sometimes ask to review "good cases" written by former students. Generally, these requests do not advance the students' learning and delay the hard work required to write their own cases. For a period of time in the past, I had provided previously completed cases for student review. My novice case writers tended to change some of the facts of the case by substitution and essentially replicate the example narrative's story structure. This approach created a block to the student's effort to tell a full story from her or his perspective.[13]

Each case must be written by the moral agent—the ultimate decision maker in this particular situation.[6] Student physical therapists become more concrete as they become more cognizant of the breadth and depth of their professional responsibility. In ethics, responsibility and advocacy can be addressed within the concept of moral agency. Patients need assistance in agency due to their current degree of vulnerability. Moral agency ranges across a wide spectrum of responsibility. At one end of the spectrum, our agency is weak as the practitioner actively supports the competent patient's autonomous decisions. At the opposite end of the spectrum, agency is strong as the practitioner makes decisions on behalf of the incompetent patient. Practitioner decisions across this spectrum are made in the patient's best interest. Moral agency can be well done only if the relationship with the patient is sufficient to allow the therapist to discern what would be in the patient's best interest in the particular situation.

The moral agent has direct evidence of the case. Nonmoral agents frequently rely on hearsay and cannot directly verify the "facts" of their case. Therefore, a symptom of a case written by someone other than the moral agent is factual vagueness. If the author cannot be specific about the facts of the case, she or he is usually not the moral agent and the instructor requests the student write up a different case. The instructor is being kind to the student when requesting a rewrite because the student will not be able to complete the upcoming analysis without being the moral agent. The earlier the instructor can help the student recognize he or she is not the moral agent, the better for the student.

I will pause here to comment on the obvious—the ethics instructor must teach ethically. Being ethical in the classroom includes being concerned about student privacy and safety. The student should be supported to share only what that student feels comfortable in sharing—both verbally and in writing. I continue to be shocked by some of the stories that are shared by my students, most recently sexual misconduct by a fellow student. Students vary widely in what they are able to share. Remember, this is part of a person's life; students brings their story into the conversation, and students carry it away from the conversation. Moreover, the storyteller may be at risk due to relationships within the classroom not known to the instructor. Does the classroom contain a professional competitor, a disgruntled former employee, or a supervisor? All of these relationships challenge the student's ability to effectively learn within the course. Of course, it can also provide opportunities to do some very challenging work of ethics.

During the process of writing up the case, the instructor is asking the student to look within herself. The well-written case is an individual's subjective (from inside one's self) perspective of a filtered series of "facts." The student's initial thoughts about the case are usually limited to their own background beliefs and life experiences. Being a professional includes the responsibility to have an objective (from outside one's self) perspective on one's practice. What does my Code of Ethics say about this case? What does my practice act say about professional conduct in my state? What do others think about my case? I am advocating that the moral agent actively seek and consider an objective perspective on the case. However, I am not advocating the rejection of our subjective perspective. Rather, I am saying an objective perspective should be added to our internally held perspective before we move toward making a decision about a situation for which we are responsible. When we look outside ourselves and consider others' wisdom, we broaden our knowledge and enhance the probability of making a good decision.

On Objectivity

My findings from a new patient evaluation were surprisingly better than findings from prior similar patients. I documented my findings in the patient's record. Later that day, the patient's Attending Physician pointed out that the data I entered in the medical record would not qualify the patient for the desired DRG and that I should initially document lesser patient abilities to allow the patient a longer LOS. The Attending's concluding comment was, "I expect your documentation to change. Besides, you get paid a salary, why should it make any difference to you?" I felt coerced by the physician in this situation and that he was trying to compel me to act in a way that might cause me harm.

Two public documents came to mind following this interchange—the state practice act and the American Physical Therapy Association Code of Ethics.[14] I agreed to adhere to the content of these documents when I voluntarily accepted my license to practice and I became a member of the APTA. At the time of this incident, I viewed these documents as quasi-legal documents, as lists of rules to be followed by the practitioner. I later responded to the Attending that my documentation did make a difference to me, "I can't do what you are asking me to do. If I get caught it could cost me my license and I would no longer be able to practice. I can't afford to take that chance." I was not standing on my character but standing on authoritative documents. I wasn't reflecting on who I hoped to become as a person. Rather, I wanted to remain employed and continue to receive my income. As time passed, I less frequently felt the need to refer to these documents and simply explained that I choose not to lie in the patient's medical record. Doing otherwise would harm my character and move me toward being a liar and less of a trustworthy person.

As DRGs and other cost controls became a more dominant part of the practice culture, some practitioners began moving away from knowing the patient as a unique human being with different stories and telling a story in the patient's medical record that fit the patients into one of various DRG categories. Losing the patient story results in morphing a skillful physical therapy workup into a diagnosis that did not accurately represent the patient's medical condition but resulted in an assignment of the patient to a DRG with the greatest LOS and the greatest financial benefit to the organization.

The assigned pre-course readings provide a source of objectivity for students. As an additional source of an objective perspective, students are asked to review, and bring to class, a copy of the American Physical Therapy Association Code of Ethics as well as the student's state practice act. A few students are asked to take the responsibility of monitoring our conversation from the perspective of the APTA Code or practice act. A question from one of these students or the instructor such as, "Given what has been said so far in this case, what does the code (or practice act) have to offer to your thought process?" helps anchor the case to these objective standards. As a reminder, I am asking that students add their objective reflections about the case to their subjective thoughts. Too often we seem to ask students to choose between A or B when the answer is frequently found in the space between A and B.

Asking good and timely questions is an important skill for any instructor. I used to act as though talking and directing were my central classroom functions. With experience, I am more effective when I ask a good question and then follow the students' lead. I am most effective in the classroom when I can fade into the background of the classroom conversation while the students carry on. I will not be in their conversations when they return to their clinical practice after completion of the course. The instructor owes the student the opportunity to become as autonomous an ethicist as possible within the brief time shared in our moral community. This requires a diminishing instructor role as the course progresses.

Seeking an objective perspective on a given particular situation provides an opportunity to make a fundamental point about ethics. Most of my students enter our coursework with a quasi-legalistic mind set. This is an understandable perspective given the pervasive nature of the law in our culture. Stories based on the law are omnipresent in newspapers, on radio and, most particularly, on television. This cultural influence creates a minimalist mind-set characterized by statements like, "If I don't get caught I haven't done anything wrong; I haven't broken the law." Of course, one has broken the law when one's behavior wanders outside of the behavior prescribed by the law. Getting caught refers to, not infraction of the law but enforcement of the law. Holding this perspective on how one ought to behave simply encourages one to be crafty in avoiding detection, not to behave within the boundaries that society has deemed as appropriate. Ethics, on the other hand, asks that one aspire toward human excellence, especially when no one is watching.

Another source of objective moral perspectives is established ethical principles from the published literature. All professional students ought to be facile in the use of a set of ethical principles in addition to the code. A very small number of students come to my course with a vague idea of ethical principles. I propose that students practice with the widely accepted bioethics principles popularized over the past three decades by Beauchamp and Childress[15] of nonmaleficence, beneficence, autonomy, and justice. This work serves well as a pre-course reading or the students can be provided with operational definitions of these principles. Asking that the students reflect on questions such as the following also facilitates application of these principles: How do I avoid doing harm to the patient? How do I ensure a patient is benefited from my intervention? How may I foster the patient's self-governance? How might I act to ensure the patient is treated in a fair manner? The rules/principles language is the dominant ethical language in our society. Although virtue ethics has been making a recent comeback, being facile in the language of ethical principles allows the physical therapist access to more of the ethics literature and to colleagues with whom they may want to discuss ethics.

At this point in the course, the students, as moral agents, are involved in a rich moral conversation involving a significant set of particular circumstances and perspectives. Adding a structured case analysis further enriches the moral conversation. Based on my experience, formal ethical analysis is not part of the physical therapist's daily practice and most see ethical analysis as the responsibility of an expert—an ethicist. Of course, all physical therapists need to be ethicists as ethical practice is part of their daily responsibility.

On Analysis

I first taught ethics in an academic institution within an entry-level professional issues course. The content was primarily composed of ethical theories and the APTA Code of Ethics. I did not offer thoughts on ethical analysis. The course seemed to help students be more aware of the moral aspects of clinical practice and to think ethically about selected topics. A common student response to the course was "It was enjoyable to think in a different way about a different kind of content." A couple of years later, I was invited to teach an ethics course at a different academic institution.

I am working with a group of postentry-level students ranging in age from 28 to 49 years with 5 to 21 years of clinical experience. Early in the course, a student said, "This is interesting theory but can't you help us understand how to apply these concepts to help our patients?" I realized during the ensuing discussion that using ethical analysis had become a tacit part of my clinical practice. Also, I had come to assume that if a clinician learned ethical theory that clinician would naturally apply the concepts to patient care. This application had not come to me naturally—I was instructed and mentored. The students were focused on the purpose of ethics—to think about morally relevant situations and to act on that reasoning. My pedagogy was separating theory from technique. We reorganized the course. The students agreed to write case studies (as described above) about actual situations from their clinical practices. I agreed to help them apply ethics, through these cases, to their clinical practice.

As previously mentioned, I rely on student-written narratives in my ethics instruction as an anchor to concreteness. However, I was initially fearful of using student-written case studies in teaching the analysis process. What if a case stumped me? How do I prepare for all possible cases that the students might bring to class? Of course, the fear was not well founded. I have been stumped—many times. However, these cases are not my responsibility; they are the student's responsibility. Maintaining this position reinforces the student's role as moral agent.

During my years in clinical practice, being perplexed by a particular patient situation was a predictor of an impending learning experience. Working toward understanding these perplexing circumstances frequently included input from my colleagues. Now that I have been using the case method for more than a decade, I start each class with excitement: Which case will stump me (predictor of a learning experience) during this class? When I am stumped in the classroom, I only need to be patient and a student will introduce, what is for me, a novel perspective to the topic that is key to bringing the group to an understanding of the particular case. It is crucial that the instructor seek these perspectives from the students and that the instructor credits the students for the successful problem solving. Student empowerment is as important in ethics instruction as it is in all professional education.

Teaching ethical analysis through a structured approach to analysis is helpful for both instructor and student. This approach allows the instructor to initially demonstrate the entire process to the student. The process is a series of information gathering and reflection points, with the outcome being a decision based on the narrative under discussion. Most of my students seem to be goal oriented and are more effective when they can see an overall approach and can anticipate an outcome. The structure also allows the student to know the answer to the question, "How do I know when my analysis is done?" In this approach, the answer is, "When you have completely, accurately, and thoughtfully answered all the questions in the moral brief." Some of these cases become seminal for the students and they will continue to reflect on them for a long time. As an example, I continue to work on a case that was first published in 1994.[16]

For the instructor, this structured approach provides a framework within which to instruct. This approach is particularly helpful when the ethics instructor gets lost in the process of analysis. For me, becoming lost in a case is not uncommon, particularly when the case is complex and the students become more active in class, offering multiple conflicting perspectives. The framework allows us to remind ourselves where we are in the process and to return to the correct step of the process. I use Nash's 11-question rules/principles moral brief as my framework to instruct students.[6] For another example of an ethics analysis framework, see Purtilo's book *Ethical Dimensions in the Health Professions*.[17]

The students are asked to write their moral brief using the questions as section headings. I have been frequently told that I request a lot of writing from my students. My experience is that writing slows the students down and creates a space for them to be more reflective. Reflection is crucial in clinical practice and writing enhances this aspect of expertise in practice.[18,19] A student then volunteers to orally present his or her preliminary analysis of the case study to the class. Initially, most students are hesitant to present their analysis to their classmates. However, by the end of the course students always offer the critique that I did not provide students with equal time to present their cases. These oral interchanges among the students clearly increase understanding of the student's own case and eventually leads to a better quality final write-up of the moral brief. I presume the better written the case, the better the case is understood by the student.

At the beginning of the analysis process, the student needs to understand the type of choices required by the particular case study. At times, the kind of problem we are facing is not clear. However, most frequently my students are facing a choice between good and bad or between two (or more) goods. When it becomes clear the choice is between good and bad, the ethical analysis should stop. (Referring to the Nash moral brief, this decision is made with Question 1 and/or Question 2.[6]) It is a prima facie ethical choice when the physical therapist selects good over bad. It is a prima facie unethical choice when the physical therapist selects bad over good. An indicator of a good choice is that choice which is in the patient's best interest. At this point, the work is to do the good and avoid the bad. The case is no longer an issue of

analysis but is frequently an issue of moral courage.[20] The moral agent needs to find the courage to act on the decision to do the good.

When the choice is between two or more equal goods, the student is involved in a classic moral dilemma. My experience informs me that clearly describing a moral dilemma can be quite a challenging task. It is common that cases initially presented as a choice between a good and a bad are actually a moral dilemma. I approach each case under the presumption a moral dilemma is present and needs to be uncovered. This step is critical in that all goods ought to be known prior to making a decision. If not, a patient good does not receive consideration prior to a decision being made about the case. If this step is inaccurate, all following steps are invalid.

The tragedy in a classic moral dilemma is that one (or more) patient good will not be served. This outcome can be distressing to some students. Likewise, it can be distressing when students determine, through their own analysis process, that their previous decision was an unethical choice. Initially, some students assume studying ethics means they will learn how to implement ideal actions. Although an ethical perspective may point to previously unrecognized positive alternatives in the case, usually ethics is about trying to make the best choice among commonly available possibilities. Presuming the analysis was well done, the instructor needs to remain focused and encourage students to follow through and plan to act on their classroom reasoning when they return to the clinic.

As students see the concrete nature of their ethical decision making, they are also concrete about why acting on their good reasoning will be difficult. Some entry-level students believe acting ethically will, as an example, "ruffle the feathers" of their clinical instructor (CI) thereby putting their affiliation grade at risk. Some postentry-level students believe acting ethically will, as an example, "cost me a physician referral source and I need that additional income to keep my daughter in college." These are all reasonable personal justifications. However, it would be difficult for these justifications to pass John Rawl's test of publicity.

The test of publicity asks if you would be willing to state your private justification publicly within your community. What physical therapist is willing to state publicly that she or he is knowingly acting unethically in a relationship with a patient to advance her or his own personal interests?

Regardless of the student's reaction to the idea of a test of publicity, the student is responsible for his or her case, including any actions taken related to that case. In the end, applying ethical analysis "to particular problems admit to no precision" but the student will need "to think out what the circumstances demand."[8] Even a well-written case and discerning analysis may not be sufficient to point to a clear decision. Although this can be frustrating to the moral agent, persisting in ethical analysis is a professional responsibility. Acting on the results of an ethical analysis can be particularly challenging if that decision would cause the student to act against the ethos of his or her clinical practice setting. The student will face the question, "Ought I to do the good thing or support the unethical way of being in our practice?"

Skepticism of Convention

I presume my students are, or want to be, good and do good acts. Some of these students are placed in difficult clinical circumstances that challenge their moral character. (Although I do not address the topic in this article, there are parallel challenges to the moral character of our students in the academic environment.) Are these students acting on what they believe or are they acting primarily on the traditions or conventions of the clinical environment within which they find themselves?

While presenting ethical concepts to a group of entry-level students, I had an intuitive sense the students were uncomfortable with some of my comments. Based on the context of the discussion, I asked, "If you have knowingly documented inaccurate information on a patient's billing form and/or medical record, please raise your hand?" Approximately half of the students raised a hand. I asked the students why they had behaved in this way. Their responses grouped into three themes, "Everybody does it." "I didn't want to

ruffle feathers." "My CI told me to do it." I have had similar discussions with individual students over the years; however, the response of the group was shocking.

The first response, that "everyone does it," comes from students with experience observing practitioners in a clinical environment where inaccurately documenting patient care is an accepted practice. The behavior may not be explicitly discussed, "everyone just knows" the expectation. However, these students ought to know "that everyone does it" is simply not accurate. The students using this justification held the evidence of their statements' inaccuracy. Of the students who participated in the described behavior, most had not done so during their prior affiliation. Their own experience disproves their proposed justification.

Some of these students may have been acting in a nonvoluntary or involuntary manner due to being uneducated, unaware, or uninformed that accurate documentation in the medical record is an expectation of physical therapists.[8] Presuming these students were being sincere in our discussion, some were ignorant of reality. It is important to consider if this ignorance was reasonable. If their ignorance is reasonable, their behavior is not blameworthy. For some of these students, their ignorance seemed reasonable as they lacked sufficient life experiences (wisdom) to be expected to understand their situation. For others, their apparent ignorance did not seem reasonable. These students appeared to lack the naiveté of their classmates and their behavior was blameworthy. Even if their justification, that "everyone does it," were accurate, the justification is not sufficient. Just because something is, does not mean it ought to be. However, moral justification in these situations is very complex and a CI ought not to place a student with limited experience and moral agency in this kind of a clinical situation.

The second student group did not want to "ruffle feathers" and felt a responsibility to "fit in" by behaving in a similar manner as the other practitioners in that particular clinical setting. To "fit in" can be a positive choice when good people doing good acts make up the clinical ethos in that "like activities produce like dispositions."[8] Under these conditions, passing on the character traits of the experienced practitioner to the novice practitioner is powerful and positive. Of course, the opposite is also true. When CIs involve students in unethical activities, such as fraudulent billing, they may be encouraging students to form habits resulting in a disposition to repeat these behaviors in the future.

Although similar to the prior situation, these students were explicitly instructed to carry out a specific act (e.g., "I know we only saw Mr. Smith for 30 minutes this morning but make sure to document 60 minutes—we need the units.") and they deferred to an authority figure, most frequently the CI. These students did not view the situation as requiring a choice between right and wrong. Rather, they viewed refusal of a directive from the CI to be disrespectful and ungrateful. They had voluntarily chosen the good act—respectfulness over disrespectfulness and gratefulness over being ungrateful. I presume here, although somewhat tentatively given the particular situation, that the CI is worthy of respect. From this perspective of respectfulness, I asked the students, "Can you imagine how you might maintain your respectfulness and gratefulness toward your CI while retaining your responsibility to be truthful?" Although they did not consider the possibility at the time, upon reflection, they now considered initiating a conversation with their CI at the beginning of their next affiliation. The imagined conversation would include a discussion of the student's past negative experiences, such as being pressured to document inaccurately, and a request that the CI assist them in avoiding such situations at this affiliation. These reflective discussions provide the student with the intellectual practice that may support a future proactive position to avoid engagement in unethical acts.

The final group attempted to justify their behavior by saying "My CI told me to do it." They knew documenting inaccurate information was wrong but they took the position that they had no choice in the situation. In reality, this group had a clear choice—document inaccurate information or refrain from documenting inaccurate information. When their choice was pointed out, they responded as though under compulsion, indicating the decision making was being done by someone else and seemed to experience no pain or pleasure associated with the situation—"It was not my fault."[21] This group also stated confidently that the behavior was due to their student status and the behavior would not continue after graduation. Their proposed justification of the behavior was seen as a current compromise to ensure passing the affiliation, thereby allowing them to graduate and serve patients in the future. This explanation may hold true for certain of these individuals. However, my past clinical experience informs me that this behavior of compulsion does not end for everyone at the time of college graduation. Rather, when some of these individuals' roles change from student to practitioner they simply shift responsibility for their acts to a different authority figure. Instead of "my CI made me do it," I have observed multiple incidences where the practitioner blames a different individual (a senior physical therapist, a physician, an administrator, or a third party-payer representative) for their behavior.

Some CIs seem not to appreciate the power they hold over many students, nor do they seem to appreciate the tendency some students have "to discredit [their] feelings, intuitions, and judgments" and therefore defer decisions to the CI.[17] The virtuous practitioner is characteristically trustworthy in relation to the patient; the patient can trust the physical therapist will act in their best interest. The virtuous CI is trustworthy in relation to their student; the student can trust the CI will act in their best interest. I presume all CIs and academic faculty believe fostering the student's ethical behavior is a fundamental responsibility (see APTA Guide for Professional Conduct, section 6.3.B).

Of the students who had not participated in the behavior, most said the topic of inaccurate documentation never came up in conversation during their affiliation. Others said it was discussed but they chose not to participate. The nonparticipating students did not experience any negative consequences of their choice not to participate in inaccurate documentation. When these students were asked why they resisted, they responded, "Because it is not the right thing to do. What they did is lying and I don't lie." These responses drew reactions from their participating classmates, indicating they had inaccurately documented but the action did not constitute lying. When asked to describe the difference between being knowingly inaccurate and lying, the participating students were unable to articulate a difference.

Students learn different lessons when they are all exposed to the same environment. They learn from both the explicit and implicit curriculum and accept a series of practices, attitudes, procedures, and customs, or what Nussbaum refers to as conventions.[21] Students who participate in conventions may learn habits that improve or harm their moral character. In the end, our curricula need to avoid harming students' moral character while providing them a benefit to be shared with patients. These benefits need to include expertise in certain knowledge of theory and manipulative skills and clinical decision making skills grounded in a moral character composed of such virtues as being compassionate, trustworthy, temperate, friendly, courageous, humble and just.[19] Individual practitioners speaking from such a moral character would certainly herald the end of moral silence.

✧ CONCLUSION

I concur with Aristotle's words, that "it is a matter of no little importance what sorts of habits we form from the earliest age—it makes a vast difference, or rather all the difference in the world."[8] My students do not qualify as being of "the earliest age" and therefore some might say my work as an ethics instructor is misdirected and futile. I believe the vast majority of my students enter my ethics course having inherently good moral habits. I hope during our time together that I successfully encourage my students to openly and actively express their moral character and diminish the professional moral silence. I am aware this encouragement may sound like an invitation to push Sisyphus's boulder up the mountain. Realistically, much about the current clinical practice environment gives little hope to many of my students that they will find a practice setting that will support their good moral character. Let me paraphrase a recent discussion with a past student: "You expect practitioners to be honest in documentation, to restrict their practice to areas in which they are competent and to do what is necessary to help patients become well again. I have been out there in the clinic for 2 years now. I haven't seen your ethics in practice. Your ideas are radical." My ideas on professional practice and on ethics may be radical. However, if these ideas are radical, the helping professions are in grave danger of no longer serving a societal purpose.

My intent as an ethics instructor is to continue being a gadfly—a persistent, provocative, perplexing, and when necessary, irritating stimulus for breaking the moral silence. Believing that language creates reality, I hope I am contributing in some small way, through this writing and my ethics instruction, to growing a robust ethical language that will refocus our helping professions on assisting citizens to remain well or become well again. Consider your language. Do you vigorously express your most heartfelt beliefs about how your clinical practice ought to be? Do you take responsibility for your thoughts, words, and acts? Can you resist the next act that you know is not in your patient's best interest? If you are successful at expressing your moral character, can you help others do the same?

Maybe we are at a historic moment in our professional journey and the path is diverging. I sense a number of my colleagues deciding to make a positive change on behalf of their patients and society. Should you stay on the same, well-traveled path or should you take a less familiar path based on the wisdom of Robert Frost?—"I took the path less traveled and it has made all the difference."[22]

References

1. Pellegrino ED: What is a profession? J Allied Health August:168–176, 1983.
2. McIntyre A: After Virtue. A Study in Moral Theory. University of Notre Dame Press, Terre-Haute, IN, 1984.
3. Soukhanov A (ed): The American Heritage Dictionary of the English Language. Houghton Mifflin Co., Boston, MA, 1996.
4. Drane JF: The Good Doctor. Sheed & Ward, Kansas City, MO, 1988.

5. Hursthouse R: On Virtue Ethics. Oxford University Press, Oxford, 1999.

6. Nash RJ: "Real World" Ethics: Frameworks for Educators and Human Service Professionals. Teachers College, New York, 1996.

7. Lee D: Plato: The Republic. Penguin Books, New York, 1955.

8. Thomson J: The Ethics of Aristotle: The Nicomachean Ethics. Penguin Books, New York, 1955.

9. Illich I: Medical Nemesis: The Expropriation of Health. Pantheon Books, New York, 1976.

10. Jonsen A: The New Medicine and the Old Ethics. Harvard University Press, Cambridge, MA, 1990.

11. Pattison S, et al: Do case studies mislead about the nature of reality? J Med Ethics 25:42–46, 1999.

12. Frankena W: Ethics. Prentice-Hall, Englewood Cliffs, NJ, 1973.

13. Coles R: The Call of Stories: Teaching and the Moral Imagination. Houghton Mifflin, Boston, 1989.

14. American Physical Therapy Association: APTA Code of Ethics and Guide for Professional Conduct. Available at: http://www.apta.org/PT_Practice/ethics_pt/pro_conduct. Accessed November 2003.

15. Beauchamp TL, and Childress JF: Principles of Biomedical Ethics, ed 4. Oxford University Press, New York, 1994.

16. Nalette E: Habits of thought: Truth-telling and deception, in practice. In Ethics in Physical Therapy. American Physical Therapy Association, 1998.

17. Purtilo R: Ethical Dimensions in the Health Profession, ed 3. WB Saunders Company, Philadelphia, 1999.

18. Schon DA: The Reflective Practitioner. How Professionals Think in Action. Basic Books, New York, 1983.

19. Jensen GM, et al: Expertise in Physical Therapy Practice. Butterworth-Heinemann, Boston, 1999.

20. Purtilo R: Moral courage in times of change: Visions for the future. J Phys Ther Educ 14(3):4–6, 2000.

21. Nussbaum M: A Classical Defense of Reform in Liberal Education. Harvard University Press, Cambridge, MA, 1999.

22. Frost R: The Road Not Taken. Holt, Rhinehart and Winston, New York, 1951.

24

Teaching and Learning About the Ethical and Human Dimensions of Care in Clinical Education: Exploring Student and Clinical Instructor Experiences in Physical Therapy

ELIZABETH MOSTROM, PHD, PT

Abstract

Clinical education experiences are essential components of professional education in physical and occupational therapy and are important "bridges" in the developmental trajectories of future therapists as they make the journey from being students in the classroom, to students in clinical practice settings, and ultimately to entering the profession. The focus of this chapter is to describe and explore student learning and development during clinical education experiences with special attention to their learning about the ethical and humanistic dimensions of care. My experience as a Director of Clinical Education in physical therapy programs for more than 20 years suggests that clinical education experiences are powerful teachers in and of themselves for physical therapy students. Yet such early practice experiences have the potential to erode or enhance ethical thought and practice in developing professionals; they can cultivate, expand, and deepen understandings of the importance of ethical thought and action (first touched on in academic environments) or diminish them and render such curricular content "useless," "impractical," and "unrealistic" in the student's view.

In this chapter, I draw on data from several qualitative investigations involving students and clinical instructors using reflective journals and interviews as data collection methods. I address the following questions: What are students learning about humanistic care during clinical experiences? How are they learning? When are they learning? From whom are they learning? What situations and experiences create ethical discontent or distress for students and instructors? What do instructors feel is important to teach in this realm? How do they teach it? What are perceived or real facilitators, barriers, or constraints to teaching and learning about the ethical and human dimensions of care in clinical settings? It is hoped that some of the answers to these questions can begin to elucidate and inform our work in ethics education in academic and clinical environments. By doing so, it will allow us to better create continuity and reflexivity between what students are learning in didactic and clinical curricula. Furthermore, to the extent that dissonance may still exist between what is taught in the classroom and what students experience in the clinic, we need to seek creative ways to help them anticipate, reflect on, and respond to such dissonance. The chapter concludes with some recommendations on how we might achieve these goals.

Clinical education experiences are essential components of professional education in physical and occupational therapy and are important "bridges" in the developmental trajectories of future therapists as they make the journey from being students in the classroom, to students in clinical practice settings, and ultimately to entering the profession. This is true for all aspects of professional learning and development including knowledge acquisition and extension, technical skill refinement, enhancement of sound clinical decision making and judgment, and perhaps most importantly, the development of reflective, ethical, and compassionate practitioners who are fully attentive to the humanistic dimensions of care. The focus of this chapter is to describe and explore this last dimension of student learning and development during clinical education experiences in physical therapy education. I do so by listening to and sharing the voices and stories of students and clinical teachers as they traverse these bridges together. Although my observations and experiences have been with physical therapist students and instructors, conversations with other rehabilitation professionals, including occupational therapists, suggest that the stories I share in this chapter are consonant with those of other therapy students and teachers.

My own experience as a Director of Clinical Education in physical therapy curricula for more than 20 years confirms that clinical education experiences are powerful teachers in and of themselves for physical therapy students. It is in clinical settings where theory, research, and text acquire contextual, relational, and personal meaning for health professional students. Curricular content and learning activities embedded in the didactic portions of professional preparation programs sow the seeds of care and ethical practice. The clinic is where these seeds are best nurtured and grow. Even so, my observations suggest that early practice experiences have the potential to enhance or erode ethical and humanistic practice in developing professionals; they can cultivate, expand, and deepen understandings of the importance of ethical thought and action (first touched on in academic environments) or diminish them and render such curricular content "useless," "impractical," and "unrealistic" in the student's view.

In this chapter, I use the term humanism to refer to the attitudes and actions of health care providers that demonstrate that human welfare is the central focus of concern. I draw on data from a variety of previous and ongoing qualitative investigations involving both students and clinical instructors. Using reflective journal and interview data I attempt to address the following questions so that we might better understand the nature of student and instructor beliefs, experiences, and learning about the ethical and distinctly human dimensions of care during clinical internships. What are students learning about humanistic care during clinical experiences? How are they learning? When are they learning? From whom are they learning? What situations and experiences create ethical discontent or discomfort for students and instructors during clinical experiences? What do instructors feel it is important to teach in this realm? How do they teach it? What are perceived or real facilitators, barriers, or constraints to teaching and learning about the ethical and human dimensions of care in clinical settings from both student and clinical instructor perspectives? The answers to these questions may elucidate and inform our work in ethics education in both academic and clinical environments. So let me now turn to some stories. First, I will present the voices of students as they complete clinical training.

✦ STORIES FROM THE FIELD: THE VOICE OF STUDENTS

The questions articulated above about student learning about the ethical and humanistic dimensions of patient care have been of interest to me for many years. They have been brought into even sharper focus during the past few years as the health care environment has become increasingly reimbursement focused, and health care and institutional policy and practice seem to have moved farther from humanistic aims. During this time, I, along with several of my colleagues who are regional clinical coordinators in our program, have attempted to explore and begin to answer some of these questions by carefully listening to the words and stories of students and clinicians involved in clinical education experiences as shared through (a) regional dialogue groups that meet monthly during clinical internships, and (b) student reflective journals written throughout clinical experiences.

The data I present in this section are drawn from the reflective journals of students. These journals are read by regional coordinators and myself as students complete internships. We respond to the journals in writing with our own reflections on what we have read about the experiences, thoughts, feelings, and insights of students. In this way we hope to create an ongoing private conversation in writing with the student. Concurrently, we analyze the journals for content categories and themes that emerge and change during the course of a final year internship. In addition, I draw on student reflective journal data collected by McGee, Ogger, and Triezenberg as part of their study aimed at identifying ethical issues encountered by physical therapist students during a semester-long clinical internship in the final year of professional preparation.[1]

Numerous authors and educational philosophers have emphasized the importance of engaging in dialogue and reflection in and on action to the learning and development of professionals in a variety of disciplines including physical therapy.[2-12] To advance professional learning, various forms of reflective writing, such as journals, diaries, and reflective summaries, have been suggested as strategies for fostering thoughtful examination of lived experience, and the ideas, questions, and insights that emerge out of those experiences.[13-18] With respect to the power of writing as a tool for reflection I share the words of Dr. Christopher Clark:

There is something special about writing. It forces me toward clarity in my thinking… It demands full attention to the content of the ideas I am trying to express … Writing moves me to remember, reinterpret, and reorganize what I know… Even with self as sole audience, writing often makes for uncomfortable confrontations with logical inconsistencies, confusions,

and contradictions that were otherwise quiescent and unconscious. Writing shines light into the corners of the mind easier left in darkness.[19]

So what are students writing about during clinical education and how are they making sense of their experiences? The answer to one of my previous questions, "Who are students learning from?" is clear. First and foremost, they learn about humanism in clinical care from their patients. This learning can then be supported and extended (or diminished) by clinical instructors and other staff who work with students. I first share a few of the lessons learned through encounters with patients and their caregivers and then those learned through or with clinical instructors or other health care professionals with whom students interact during the course of internships.

✧ LESSONS LEARNED FROM PATIENTS

In the following quote a student summarizes the opportunity afforded by clinical experiences, in contrast to the classroom, for learning about the human dimensions of care:

Working in the clinic has opened my eyes wider to the life of my patients. It's not like school when class is over and your [mock] patients are all better and able to go home and do whatever. These are real people with real problems who might not get better, or go home and cannot do just anything they want to. Some people may not be able to go back to work and support their family … they may not be able to go back to a job they have been doing for 20 years. Some people may not be able to play with their children or grandchildren. Some kids will not be able to play like their friends… Some of these people have lived with pain for almost their whole lives and sometimes no matter what you do you might not be able to make them better. I believe this is one of the hardest things about PT; there are some people you may not be able to help. It is very difficult to tell someone that … On the other hand there are other people you do help— for whom you can really make a difference in their lives.

Here, the student, while struggling with the realization that he may not be able to help all patients whom he encounters, clearly describes the distinctly human face of clinical practice and articulates a holistic view of the patient's experience of illness, impairment, or disability that has come into focus for him during his internship. Furthermore, he recognizes that in many cases the illness experience is not just the patient's own—it can have far-reaching effects relationally, socially, and occupationally.

In many cases, student learning about relationship building with patients and the human dimensions of care start with asking the right questions. One student writes:

> This last week I have wondered about my ability to comfort. I had a few patients who were very emotional this week—they were crying and understandably scared. Inside my heart feels for them, but outside do I show it enough? Do I sound sincere when I try to comfort them? Do they even want my comfort in the first place or do they want to be left alone? Am I saying the right things? Or the wrong things? Is humor good or bad [in these situations]? It's hard to know for sure—and it will be different for each patient. I suppose as long as I am recognizing their feelings in the first place, that's the first step, right?

Here, the student seeks affirmation and opens the door for conversation on this difficult topic. She goes on to try and at least partially answer her question:

> I think that trying to dismiss the emotion just because you don't know what to say or because you have to stay on schedule would be completely wrong. I am not seeking answers to all these questions right now. I know it will take time.

This student echoes a refrain reported by participants in studies of the clinical reasoning and practice of experienced occupational therapists and physical therapists.[11,20] The therapists observed and interviewed in those studies, seeking to achieve holistic and patient-centered care, often found themselves in conflict with institutional demands regarding the nature and extent of delivery of care or what "counts" as work. Fleming and Mattingly claim that the situation forced some therapists to go "underground" when attempting to reconcile this dilemma and continue to provide

compassionate care and treatment for "the whole person."[21]

In another instance, a student works to try and understand a challenging patient's anger, frustration, and unwillingness to engage in therapy by trying to step into the patient's and family's shoes. The patient had cancer with numerous metastases, was in a lot of pain, and according to the student had a personal skepticism and mistrust of the medical profession's many tests and treatments. The student writes:

> I figured it would be best and most productive to go at the patient's pace at first, in order to gain her trust and to prove to her, her capabilities. She is in her early fifties, the onset [of her problem] was sudden, and the prognosis is not very good. Her husband visits every night to bring dinner and her son was called home from college to visit his mother. I could only think—what if this woman was my mother and I received that call? How would I react to such news? How would my mother respond to this news? How would our family cope with a similar prognosis for our cherished mother? How would our family change as a result of such news? How would my life and current endeavors change?

The same student goes on to reflect on this patient's situation and those of other patients by continuing to ask important questions that lead her to a revelation about the importance of humanism in patient care:

> What do you say to this patient with metastases throughout her body and a poor prognosis when she asks, "Will I get strong enough to walk on my own again?" How do you provide comfort … to the wife of a patient in the ICU who sits by the bedside for hours everyday, with no apparent progress for weeks? These are some of the challenges that may seem at first outside the apparent and immediate scope of practice and patient care—but they are not. They can't be avoided and ignored—these questions, this distress, these social relationships are critical to quality of life for all involved with the patient and they must be addressed.

As physical or occupational therapists, because of the unique nature of rehabilitation professions, we are fortunate to often encounter and work with patients and their family members for extended periods of time as we journey with our patients through their rehabilitation. This helps us to be alert and attentive to the web of social relationships that infiltrate and surround a patient's illness experience. Consider this account of one student's learning through her patient's family:

One of my patients was a 34-year-old woman with multiple sclerosis. This case affected me the most of any other cases so far. I was most affected by her family; what they were going through, how they were coping, and what they shared with me as her physical therapist. First, her husband shared with me how her disease had progressed. He told me what his wife's functional capabilities were just a few years ago in comparison to what they are now. He shared with me how she had become more and more dependent on him. Before, she would only need his assistance for functional activities; now he has to do everything for her.

Then I spoke to her grandmother. She gave me a different perspective on how her granddaughter's illness is affecting the family. She told me how her granddaughter's children were being affected. She told me how sad they had been since their mother went into the hospital. She told me that every night the youngest child sleeps in his mother's favorite chair, hugging her favorite pillow. As I listened to my patient's family, I realized that there is so much more to treating patients than simply treating their illness. As a physical therapist, I must also address the concerns of my patient's families as well as those of my patients. I need to comfort and reassure them when I am able. I need to teach them and give them advice and information from a physical therapy perspective. Most of all, however, I need to listen to them and show genuine concern for what they say and for what matters most to them—their family member, the patient.[22]

Sometimes "asking the right questions" means asking hard questions of oneself in the context of personally and professionally difficult encounters with patients in the clinic. McGee and colleagues, in their study of ethical discomfort encountered by physical therapist students during internships, found that most ethical issues and discomfort encountered by students fell into four categories: (1) issues pertaining to professional role and responsibilities,

(2) issues pertaining to patients' rights and welfare, (3) issues pertaining to business and economic factors, and (4) issues pertaining directly to their identity and role as a student.[1] Of these four, the first two often arose in the context of interaction with patients or with other health care professionals around a particular patient. Consider this example of a student struggling with some personal fears and her professional responsibility "to provide adequate physical therapy services to all patients according to their need for care without regard to the patient's personal or social characteristics," which was the most frequently identified issue in category one.[1]

Despite my knowledge [of universal precautions] and safe actions, today I found myself overly cautious, almost to the point of paranoia, when treating a patient [with]… full-blown AIDS. When treating this patient today, I found myself thinking terrible thoughts to myself. For example, I thought—how did he become infected? How many other people has he transmitted this disease to? What if I got it? These thoughts consumed me and may have actually prevented me from providing the highest quality care I could provide. In the end, I don't think that my inner feelings were noticeable by (sic) the patient or anyone else … However, the fact remains they were present …[1]

This student recognized that her personal thoughts and fears, while understandable in her first encounter with a patient with AIDS, posed an "ethical challenge" and had the potential to, and in fact may have, interfered with delivery of compassionate and high-quality care.

There are many more lessons learned from patients that are articulated in students' journals. I conclude this section with three vignettes that echo some recurrent themes in student journals concerning their learning about the ethical and human dimensions of care. These excerpts describe student learning (a) about listening and what and who are important in patient-practitioner interactions, (b) through being the bearer of "bad news" (which has some similarity to physician learning through this experience),[23] and (c) through encounters with people with different cultural, ethnic, religious, or personal beliefs than their own.

One student, writing during her first final year internship, expressed a phenomenon observed in much of the journal data, that the ability to learn from patients can be a developmental phenomenon, one that requires a shift in focus from the student's own performance to full attention to the patient.

One of the most important lessons I have learned…is that I am not the center of the relationship between me and my patient.… Once I learned this, I stopped being so worried about my performance, or worried that I was missing some vital piece of information. I stopped thinking about myself, and started thinking about my patient first. This seems late in the game to have learned this, but alas, it is true. I stopped feeling so nervous, too. This helped immensely in learning to really listen, or to really feel or see what the patient was trying to show me.[22,24]

In another excerpt a student describes what she has learned from a patient and husband as they faced life-threatening illness together. In this case, the student had been one of the bearers of bad news. I'll call this patient Sarah. Sarah had come to therapy with a diagnosis of bilateral adhesive capsulitis and a complicated past medical and psychological history. In the course of the examination and early treatment sessions, the student became concerned about some serious neurological signs exhibited by the patient. She suspected amyotrophic lateral sclerosis (ALS) and referred the patient back to her physician for a neurology consult. Unfortunately, the student's suspicions were confirmed and a diagnosis of ALS of the bulbar type was made. The student committed herself to continuing to support the patient physically and emotionally during this difficult time. She writes about the experience of doing a home assessment with Sarah:

By now Sarah has been (officially) diagnosed. I visited her at her home last Wednesday… her husband welcomed me at the door… I entered their home, received hugs, looked at their collectibles. I saw the ice cream pail full of rice in the bathroom where Sarah did pulley exercises over the shower curtain bar. I saw her carefully constructed dolls which she had made in her craft room. I saw the oil painting he had been trying to finish only to be interrupted by his wife's medical needs… I was greatly encouraged by their… already emerging wisdom in regard to the truths ahead of them. He told me of their faith and of their belief that they would meet again one day soon, should they be separated for a while. She told me she wasn't afraid of dying.

This student, like many others, talked about how much she gained personally and professionally through her encounters with patients like Sarah. As she put it, "there are often things that I can give. But in the end I always feel that I gain more than I give."

A final example of student learning about working with culturally diverse clientele is a description found in Mostrom and Shepard.[22]

One student working in a diverse community in a large metropolitan area, wrote about her learning about working with individuals of Russian Orthodox Jewish background. Therapists and students alike in this clinic keep a Russian dictionary on hand and work hard to understand some of the language and beliefs of their clients, but much is learned about this in the course of therapy.

The other day I had my first experience [working with a patient who was of Russian Orthodox Jewish background]. When I went to introduce myself to this very pleasant gentleman dressed in black with his beard and black hat, I held out my hand to shake his. I quickly learned, by him informing me, that he does not shake women's hands. He is widowed and that is part of their religion. Then I had to ultrasound his shoulder so he had to take his jacket, shirt, prayer cloth (which I hadn't seen before) and undershirt off. Everything was fine but it just made me wonder if I couldn't shake his hand, how did he feel sitting there without a shirt on and having me work on his shoulder?

The student went on to further consideration of cultural and gender issues in therapy as a result of this encounter. In the context of this experience, she committed herself to (1) exploring more deeply her own cultural autobiography and beliefs, and (2) learning more about the beliefs and practices of this particular cultural group and how those might influence perceptions and outcomes in therapy.[22]

All of these excerpts from student reflective journals written during clinical internships illustrate some of the powerful lessons learned from patients and families about the highly contextual relational foundations and distinctly human dimensions of care. In the great majority of cases, the lessons learned from patients converge on students' emerging view of patients as people with complex and disrupted lives (hopefully temporarily) versus mere clinical problems to be diagnosed and managed. Such experiences, including writing about them, are rich resources for student learning about who and what they want to be as a clinician—and in some instances who and what they do not want to be.

✧ LESSONS LEARNED FROM CLINICAL INSTRUCTORS AND OTHER COLLEAGUES

What do students say about their learning from their clinical instructors and other professionals and staff? Students frequently discuss their learning about the ethical, relational, and human dimensions of care through observation of and work with their clinical instructors (CIs) and other staff members. As I have written elsewhere, "these individuals are important and powerful models for students as they guide and mediate student participation with patients during their clinical experiences."[22] The lessons can be both positive and negative. Students sometimes seek to emulate their CI's approach to patients; other times they reflect on differences between their preferred approach to patient care and that of their CIs or other professionals.

The following examples of journal entries echo recurrent themes in students' writing about learning from CIs. In this excerpt, a student comments on how an instructor's suggestion about listening to the patient's story has affected her work and, she believes, her outcomes with patients.

I am actually able to create a more comfortable environment for the patient by having them tell their story and by creating a conversation with them regarding their life as well as why they are in PT. This was a great suggestion that Wendy gave me to help increase the patient's comfort and trust in me as the provider of their care. It also helps bring out aspects of the patients' lives that I may not discover otherwise but which may affect their treatment or outcome.

Many authors, like physician Robert Coles, medical sociologist Arthur Frank, and anthropologist Cheryl Mattingly, who have studied the work of health care professionals for decades, have written about the importance of listening to and co-constructing patient's stories as we seek to understand the personal illness narratives of patients and create a healing environment.[20,25–28] In the experience of our students, many CIs helped them to understand the power of listening to and exchanging stories with their patients.

Another student wrote about a time when his CI engaged in a discussion about spirituality with a patient—a place the student feared to tread. In the end the student came to a realization that this is an important aspect of most human life and it may be one dimension that should not be considered taboo in interactions with patients. He writes:

A memorable situation occurred recently with a patient I was treating who had a stable cardiac arrhythmia and... decreased... strength and endurance. My CI was with me when we initiated treatment with her. As we began talking, she told me that her 40-year-old granddaughter with 3 small children had died the day before. She was asking why such a young person should have to die and why she, who was 92 years old, should still be alive when she would welcome death at this time. I began talking with her and trying to comfort her and my CI also came to discuss the issue with her. My CI asked some questions and shared some spiritual ideas... While I had certainly been thinking these things, I did not know if it was appropriate to discuss them... [I felt like] we should remain "neutral" in these situations and avoid giving advice or comfort from a religious basis.

The student went on to discuss how the conversation they had with the patient did seem to console and comfort her. In the end, he stated that "In the future, I think I will follow the patient's lead in these situations. If they mention heaven or other Christian themes, I think it would be acceptable for me to try and comfort them in religious terms." This student also noted, however, that this would be more challenging for him when working with a more diverse case load from religious beliefs and traditions other than his own.

In their writing, numerous students discuss the characteristics and behaviors of CIs who model humanism in their interactions with patients and frequently describe those characteristics they seek to appropriate and emulate. The most common descriptors include "genuine concern," "compassion," "active listening to patients," "incorporating patient needs and goals into therapy," "enthusiasm and love of their work," and "going out of their way to be an advocate for the patient." The following excerpt illustrates how observations of these attributes and behaviors are powerful teachers about humanism and moral agency in patient care.

My CI is always trying to do the right thing for patients. Throughout my internship I saw many episodes of kindness, compassion, concern, and empathy from my CI. He often sat down with patients if he noticed changes in their moods. He asked them how they were doing and what he could do to help... he allowed patients time to talk while he listened. One example is when a patient started crying during a treatment session. He allowed the patient to talk about her concerns about going home with a family member. Then my CI discussed the problems with the patient's team and the family member so the issues could be addressed before the patient went home. He often listened to the patients' concerns and altered the treatment for the day depending on their motivation, strength, energy, and level of anxiety or depression.... I know I will seek to be a more compassionate physical therapist because of his influence.

This excerpt clearly evokes the characteristics described in the definition of the core value of "compassion/caring" identified in a recent consensus conference on professionalism in physical therapy.[29]

As previously noted, many students learn about the concept of respect by observing respectful interaction between patients and therapists, between health care team members, and by being treated with respect by their CIs and team members. One student described his experience this way:

The staff are very respectful and caring toward each other and their patients. They work well as a team. Lines of communication are open and frequently used. The main focus for the team members is the well-being of the patients. They wanted to do everything they can to help their patients.... I did not see any attitudes, like 'I am better than you' or 'what do you know, you're just a PTA'... Everyone learned from each other. They all treated me with respect. They never looked down on me or thought I could not teach them something because I was a student. They were willing to go out of their way so I could learn as much as I could.

Inevitably, during the course of internships students also observe and experience interactions that are not respectful of them or others nor are they examples of humanistic care. Such experiences also become food for thought in written journal entries. Fortunately, we have found that what many students take from these experiences is a sense of what or who they don't want to be as a clinician or clinical instructor. One student wrote this about the way she was referred to by her CI:

Throughout the entire 7 weeks I was there, when speaking to colleagues and patients my CI only referred to me as 'the student.' This to me, was very impersonal and portrayed me as 'just a student.' I felt demeaned and very disrespected by this and at times, I wondered if my CI actually knew my name.

Such a loss of personal recognition and identity did not create a positive learning environment or experience for this student.

Another student, who was supervised by a visiting instructor during the time her primary supervisor was on vacation, noted that her alternate supervisor, "on day one... told me that he didn't like students and the only reason he was working with me that week was because he had no choice." This is most certainly not humanistic nor is it conducive to the creation of a respectful and nurturing learning environment!

Unfortunately, the study conducted by McGee and colleagues of ethical discomfort during clinical internships revealed that two of the most commonly reported ethical issues for students revolved around observation of CIs or other staff (1) not maintaining or protecting the patient's right to confidentiality, and (2) not respecting patients, other colleagues, and students, and not refraining from making derogatory or disparaging remarks about those individuals in a public forum.[1]

One incident regarding patient confidentiality involved a student's question to her CI about a patient she was treating. At the time of the question, the CI was "pulled away for an important phone call" and was unable to address the student's question. Later in the day, the CI approached the student while she (the student) was working with another patient in the therapy gym. The CI asked what and who her question was about. The student writes:

Instead of leaving the patient that I was treating and going into another room to discuss the earlier patient, we talked about it in the gym.[1]

In this journal entry, the student did recognize that the decision to leave the room and the current patient was a joint responsibility of the CI and the student. In the confusion of the moment, however, she deferred to the decision of the more experienced CI, who was the Director of the Rehabilitation Department. Later in the entry, the student identifies alternate courses of action that would have decreased her discomfort about confidentiality issues but would not have eliminated her concerns about not paying full attention to the patient she was currently treating.

I should have told my CI that I would speak to her later about it or I should have left the patient I was treating to go to another place to discuss the patient. Either course of action would have kept the patient's confidentiality intact, but what would the patient that I was treating think about my leaving in the middle of the treatment session to discuss someone else? And when would I have… another chance to ask my CI the question?

Although this moment of ethical distress may seem easy for more experienced therapists to overcome, it illustrates some difficulties and questions students might encounter due to their role and status as a student in the relationship with their instructors.

Many students in the McGee and colleagues study also reported overhearing or being the intended recipient of derogatory comments about other health care professionals by therapy staff members.[1] One of the more disturbing experiences for one student was to be an unwitting party to therapy staff demeaning a fellow student in his presence. This student described an episode where at the end of the day, he and other staff said "goodbye" to a student completing a clinical affiliation at the site. The student writes:

Despite their [the staff members] pleasant demeanor at that instant, it quickly changed when they were certain that he [the student] had left the floor and was out of sight. Immediately, staff members began to complain about this student's personality, his clinical skills, his dress style, as well as his sense of humor…[1]

Fortunately, this student was able to bring his discomfort with the situation to the attention of the staff and his CI by expressing the hope that they didn't talk about him in the same way when he was gone. In the end, the student reported that the CI apologized to the student for the staffs' comments and actions and recognized them as inappropriate.

As students proceed through their clinical experiences they gradually move from being peripheral participants in rehab team decision making to being accepted and integrated as full members of the team. In many cases this feeling of having their voice heard and being respected as a member of the community is a very positive experience. On the other hand, they become more aware of the difficult interactional dynamics of team decision making, especially when there is dissension among participants. One student described an experience in a team meeting where she felt respect for the patient, the situation, and other team members fell by the wayside. The discussion revolved around a discharge determination for a patient whose wife had recently passed away and who did not have family in the area. The patient had been determined not to be a candidate for rehabilitation by occupational and physical therapy. The student writes:

When this patient came up for discussion during weekly rounds, the nurse practitioner's response was to throw her arms and head down on the table and state, 'I don't care anymore what we do with this patient. I just want him out of here.' I was appalled by her comment and actions.

The student reported that the nurse continued by disparaging the therapists who had determined that this person was not a reasonable candidate for acute rehabilitation services.

Not surprisingly, students also often experience difficulty during clinical experiences as they begin to assume responsibility for supervision of and delegation to support staff such as physical therapist assistants (PTAs) and aides. They struggle with being a "student" while being asked to supervise "more experienced" staff and they often express some concern about the quality of care being delivered by this student/PTA team. But for several students, the most disconcerting issue around working with support staff had to do with the patient's right to informed consent about the qualifications of the individuals providing therapy services. The students had learned to always identify themselves as a student PT so patients would be informed of their qualifications and have the right to refuse treatment by a student. Their concern arose when they did not see the same information forthcoming from support staff regarding their qualifications and role.

Every time I have seen this PTA introduce herself, she says 'Hi, my name is [blank] and I am from physical therapy.' I have yet to hear her explain exactly who she is and what her role is. Granted many of the patients really don't mind who they are working with or if it is a PTA or a PT, but I just feel there are ethical issues behind just saying 'I am from physical therapy.' Surely she is not identifying herself as a physical therapist, but she is also NOT identifying herself as a physical therapist. I have been trying to reflect on why this bothers me. I really don't think it is a competence issue… It is more that I feel that the patient's rights aren't being respected—they aren't well informed and maybe there will be questions they have that might be better directed to their physical therapist rather than the PTA.

Fortunately, in this particular case, the student went on to discuss this issue with her clinical instructor and a reiteration of policy regarding identification of rehabilitation staff credentials to patients was the result.

The following is a final excerpt from a journal where a student learned by negative example what respectful interaction and humanism is not. Here a student describes a situation where a patient (whom she and her CI had seen before) came in for his appointment, but that day he was scheduled to be seen by another therapist due to a scheduling conflict. The CI was standing near the check-in area when the patient arrived for therapy. The student writes:

The man came in and Jack was standing there leafing through some papers, never [looking up or] acknowledging the patient. So, finally the patient said, 'Hi, Jack,' to which Jack replied 'I am not working with you today, you are on Dave's schedule.' The man then replied, 'Oh, is that why you're acting like I am not even here?'

In this case, the student also observed the patient's displeasure with, and reaction to, the way he had been treated by the therapist. She committed herself to a different mode of interaction with her own patients.

Following such observations, students sometimes discussed these events and their feelings with their CIs, although they did not always feel able to do so because of power and status differentials and the evaluative nature of CI-student relationships. When they described and discussed such situations in their journals, however, they often sought to explore how things could be different in a way that would express respect and honor the humanistic dimensions of caring for patients. In addition, the reader of the journal was invited into the discussion. In this way, we could also try to help the student make sense of the event, encourage them to discuss their feelings about it with CIs, and affirm their commitment to respect and humanism.

❖ MORE STORIES FROM THE FIELD: THE VOICE OF CLINICAL EDUCATORS

Now I turn to the voice and stories of clinical instructors, drawing on data from talking with, and listening to, hundreds of physical therapy clinical educators in one-to-one conversations and in regional dialogue groups over the past decade. In addition, they are drawn from two other sources: (1) a focus group interview specifically directed at addressing some of the following questions: What are clinical educators' beliefs about their role as teachers of the ethical and human dimensions of care? What do they feel is important to teach? How do they teach these things? What do they see as facilitators and impediments to teaching and learning about humanism in clinical practice? and (2) one-on-one interviews with individuals who have been recognized as exceptional clinical educators by students and colleagues and were recipients of an "Outstanding Clinical Instructor" award given annually by the Michigan Physical Therapy Association. The latter data are part of an ongoing investigation of expertise and mastery in clinical education.

Clinical Educator Focus Group

The nine participants in the focus group were physical therapists who work at a community hospital complex that provides a broad array of outpatient rehab services and inpatient subacute, geriatric rehab, and long-term care services. This was a purposive sample of physical therapy clinical educators; over the years, I had observed what I perceived to be a sustained dedication to modeling and teaching about respectful interaction and humanistic care in the work of these staff members with students. The participants' years of experience as physical therapists ranged from 2.5 years to 23 years with a total of 73.5 years of practice. Collectively, these individuals had been involved in clinical education (either as CIs or as Center Coordinators of Clinical Education) for a total of 53 years, with a range from 1 to 15 years. During the past 5 years, they reported that they had worked with a total of 47 students, with a range from 1 participant (the newest therapist) who had only had 1 student to date and another participant who had worked with 14 students during that time. Thus, collectively this group had extensive experience in practice and clinical education in a variety of settings.

In talking about how they and others try to exhibit respect and enact humanism in their care with patients, these therapists focused on the following features of interaction with their patients: soliciting patient perspectives and goals and building therapy around those, listening to patient stories and trying to gain a holistic view of their lives and problems, and respect for patient autonomy, choice, and personal dignity. This is what Mattingly and Fleming have described in occupational therapy as taking an anthropological or phenomenological approach to interactions with patients or "treating the lived-body."[20] For example, one therapist in the focus group stated that she was:

...very conscious of how I interview people... [trying] to glean a holistic perspective... and targeting my questions to the patient's life and home situation and their goals for themselves. That's a big part of our task—wanting to know what the patient's goals are and trying to achieve them.

Another therapist stated that he always tries: "... to respect the patient's wishes. Because [in this setting] patients... are a kind of captive audience... so still trying to maintain the patient's ability to choose [when I go in their room]. And then always focus on what the patient's goals are—not necessarily just what our goals are for the patient.

One therapist who primarily treats patients with vestibular dysfunction described how the patients who come to her have often seen numerous professionals but as she stated:

...nobody has really listened to their stories. And it's usually quite an extensive history. So I make sure I schedule extra time... because I know that they really need to tell me their whole story.

Finally, one of the physical therapists who works with patients with mild brain injury and uses manual and soft tissue techniques (involving close personal contact) to help with their problems and pain, makes sure to give thorough descriptions of what he is going to do and why he is going to do a procedure, including showing the patient illustrations of the procedure or technique. According to this therapist, he does this so patients can decide if they are uncomfortable with a procedure and decline participation if they might feel that their personal space, privacy, or dignity would be threatened by the intervention. In this way, he is seeking to respect the patient's autonomy.

When asked about their own definitions of humanism in patient care, the descriptions from members of the focus group can largely be summed up in one therapist's definition. She said:

It's honoring the patient by being sensitive to and respectful of the unique qualities of the individual. Having a composite and holistic picture, to the extent possible, of their values, cultural and personal beliefs, lifestyle, family context, relationships, interests, faith perspective, outlook, goals and concerns. It's continually evaluating the subtle clues that provide better understanding [of the patient] as you interact and form a relationship with them.

This final statement is an important one—all of these therapists viewed the human dimensions of care as being about developing relationships—they saw their work with patients as an interactional, transactional, and relational endeavor.

They did not, however, suggest that this is always an easy endeavor. They described encounters with extremely challenging patients—patients with whom, given the choice, they would not choose to engage with in the community—but felt that conveying respect and being humanistic involved continually seeking glimpses of the person that went beyond the immediate, sometimes angry and disturbing, presentation. As one therapist put it, it involves:

… setting apart your own values and preferences and bringing the patient to the foreground— knowing that your job here is as their advocate— setting aside your personal reactions to them—and putting on the hat of being the patient's advocate no matter what.

Assuming and modeling the role of the PT as patient advocate is a frequent refrain from clinical educators when they describe what they try to be as a clinician and what they try to teach their students. For these therapists, being an advocate for their patients was a moral obligation—one that they hoped their students would also claim.

As might be expected, most CIs I have encountered, including the participants in the focus group, suggest that modeling is the primary strategy they use to "teach" students about the relational and human dimensions of care. One therapist stated:

I use modeling a lot. Because I think if you see respectful interactions day in and day out, you establish a standard for care… How you need to interact

with the patient and what your role is as that patient's advocate. I don't know how much talking I do about it—I think it's more just showing it…. It is just woven throughout all episodes and aspects of care.

As suggested by the descriptions above, the values, attitudes, and behaviors these therapists sought to model for students specifically were, in one therapist's words:

… approaching each patient as an individual, being careful not to be judgmental or make assumptions, engaging the patient in collaborative problem solving and goal setting, serving as a patient advocate, and involving family members early in the rehab course according to the patient's wishes.

One therapist described a situation in which such modeling of patient advocacy led to some conflict between rehab team members, and yet she felt it was important to do what she did. In this case, as a method for behavior modification and anger management, a team member had suggested taking away a patient's electric wheelchair. According to the therapist, this wheelchair was the patient's only means for mobility and his only source of freedom. The therapist felt that this particular method would be one that would deny one of the patient's basic human rights. And so she spoke out. Such actions, of course, provide fertile ground for student learning about patient advocacy and moral agency through observation. These therapists felt that such learning could be enhanced by discussion prior to, and after, such situations. They saw the inevitability of discrepancies of opinion among team members as an opportunity for a student and CI to come up with creative alternatives or recommendations and to develop "diplomatic" strategies for presenting their suggestions to others. All of these therapists agreed that modeling humanism is not just about respectful interaction with patients and family members—it is also critically important to model respectful interaction among team members and other professionals and as one therapist put it, "with people in general." So situations like the one described above provide an opportunity to demonstrate how to advocate for what you feel is in the patient's best interest but to do it in a way that is not disrespectful or denigrating of the team member with whom you have a difference of opinion. It is worth noting how this approach to team decision making and interaction differs from that described by a student earlier in this chapter.

In fact, the therapists in this focus group felt that they more often engaged in explicit instruction (what they described as "formal" or "up-front" discussion) about patient advocacy and humanism when they anticipated or encountered more difficult situations. They described these as situations that encouraged or required what they called "teaching ahead of time" or "setting the scene." Some examples they gave of such situations include: (a) discharge planning and preparation when not all members of a family or the rehab team are in agreement about an appropriate course of action, (b) when reimbursement issues and scarcity of resources become determinants of decisions about care versus what they perceive as the patient's best interests, (c) when the patient bears some responsibility for their current medical and rehabilitation problems, or (d) when patients (or family members) are angry or emotionally labile or have cognitive impairment that interferes with their ability to express their needs or goals.

One of the therapists described a strategy that he likes to use to assess student recognition of, and learning about, humanism when confronting such difficult situations that aren't anticipated. When both he and the student have witnessed a disturbing interaction, he likes to:

> ... wait and see if the student initiates a discussion about it... Waiting to see if they initiate a discussion or make a comment about it is a way to assess where they are in terms of recognizing humanistic care [or lack of it].

Many therapists in this group also reported that assessment of generic abilities as described by May and colleagues has been a valuable tool for evaluation of interpersonal interaction skills and for teaching about the relational and ethical dimensions of humanistic care in clinical settings.[30]

When asked about constraints or barriers to teaching about humanistic care during clinical education experiences, these therapists tended to describe impediments that could either be classified as external or internal constraints. Among the key external constraints identified were resource allocations or reimbursement issues and payment systems, time constraints and productivity expectations, and other administrative or institutional policies or procedures that seem to detract from the humanistic aspects of care. In many cases, all three of these constraints were linked. For example, one therapist discussed a payment issue:

> We want to let the patient choose and participate [in decision making about therapy services]—but when you're in the last day of a [rehab] window to make a payment category—you might be a little more persuasive than you would've been otherwise.

Likewise, therapists felt ineffective and powerless when they watched patients be discharged who they truly believed were not ready to leave. In this case, their feelings of success as a patient advocate are diminished because of reimbursement requirements that seem to take precedence in discharge decisions. Like the nurses described by Varcoe and Rodney, these therapists sometimes feel a sense of futility and constrained moral agency in the face of what they see as overly complicated and multilayered regulations and policies that do not put the patient's best interests at the forefront of decision making about care.[31] The therapist's descriptions of these external constraints also point to the tension between three realms of ethics discussed by Glaser and Hamel—the individual, the institutional or organizational, and the societal, and described in Glaser's chapter in this book.[32] On numerous occasions, I have listened to therapists in a variety of settings describe how their ideals of being patient-centered and humanistic in their care are threatened by the kinds of external constraints identified by the therapists in this focus group.

Some types of internal constraints or barriers to teaching and learning about humanism that therapists reported are: the life experience and prior learning of the student, the past experience and feelings of the therapist, and personal attributes and characteristics of the student. For example, one therapist echoed others when she stated:

Sometimes the life experiences that your student comes to you with can either be a help or a hindrance... Some students really haven't had a lot of inter-cultural or inter-generational experiences... and aren't comfortable with older adults or people with other beliefs and practices [unlike their own]. So, they may have some preconceptions or judgments that couldn't be otherwise. Then we have to work to open their eyes and expand the window of their experiences to change them.

In another case, one therapist described his difficulty modeling and enacting characteristics of humanistic care for students when patients are persistently late, inconsistent in their attendance at therapy sessions, or are nonadherent with therapy programs. Although this therapist explores and seeks to understand the reasons for these behaviors in his patients, he finds it hard not to feel and show frustration with the patient and the situation.

Finally, one therapist reported that she had encountered a student with, in her opinion, such limited interactional skills and "no notion of the concept of respect" that she felt she just could not teach these things. As she put it:

I think that some things can't be taught. I think there is a certain type of person and personality that does well working in a health care profession. I can think of one student that I had that was not that type of personality and I don't think there is anything I could've done to teach him how to be caring and humanistic. And believe me, I tried. [Head nods all around]

Outstanding Clinical Instructors

Finally I turn to the voices of a small sample of individuals who have been identified and recognized as exceptional clinical teachers by their students and professional colleagues. During interviews with these individuals, I asked the following questions: "In the course of clinical experiences, many CIs and students encounter everyday ethical distress or discomfort. Can you identify some times in your experience working with students like this? How do you approach such situations when working with students? What are you trying to teach in these situations?"

Like the therapists in the focus group, the response of these CIs to the question about the type of situations they encountered that were sources of ethical distress fell primarily into four areas: (1) restrictions of or constraints on services (deemed necessary by the therapist) for patients because of reimbursement and resource issues (including time); (2) struggles between patient autonomy and the therapists' duty of beneficence; (3) observations of disrespectful interaction with patients or outright mistreatment and negligence, and (4) inappropriate utilization of support personnel.

In the first category, one example involves when services for patients with chronic wounds (that require long-term intervention) are no longer being covered by insurance. In this case, the therapist describes his ethical distress accordingly:

So... can I live with myself? Can I close my eyes and not provide that service [that is still needed]? Generally the answer is 'no, I will do what I have to live with.'...I provide services above and beyond because I just have to.

This therapist chose to provide pro bono services for this type of patient when such situations arose. He discussed his sources of discomfort and decision making process with students and hoped that it would help them make well-considered decisions in similar situations in their future career.

In the second category, one therapist described the ethical discomfort he feels when he has committed himself to a patient-centered approach and yet finds himself in situations when he is unable to realize this ideal—for example, when he tries to involve patients and family members in collaborative decisions about care (or in this case discharge) and the family then makes a choice that he feels will result in great risk and potential harm to the patient (i.e., going home alone). In the typical language of principle-based ethics this would be described, as it is above, as a struggle between patient autonomy and the duty of beneficence. Yet the description of this therapist's struggle shows that it is much more complicated than such labels convey because of the highly contextual and interactionally negotiated nature of the relationship between therapist, patient, and family that has developed over the course of rehabilitation. In describing what he tries to help students take from such experiences, he said that he tries to model a caring and information-giving approach:

I tend to approach the situation…with the patient and family. I let them know the benefits of them making their own choices and doing what's going to make them happier, but at the same time I outline very clearly the risks and what my recommendations are and my rationale [for those recommendations]… But ultimately, I do leave it up to the patient and the family with the exception of one or two [cases] where there were issues regarding competence…

In the third category, one therapist described a heart-wrenching observation of negligence and lack of humanistic care. This therapist and his student were treating a patient near the end of her life. The patient was only occasionally responsive, had no family in the area, and would probably soon be moved to hospice care. One afternoon, when the CI and student went to see the patient, they found that

…she had somehow slipped in the bed and had her head caught between the bars and the railing and her nose had a cut on it—it was stuck in the bar. We helped her get straightened out and went up to talk to nursing to inform them of what had happened. The comment from the nurse was 'well, she's going to die anyway.' So I asked when was the last time somebody was in there? 'Oh, probably this morning sometime.' It was very, very hard for me not to blow up.

He went on to describe his own and his student's feelings and response to the situation, which in the end involved joint discussions with the nurse, supervisors, and other appropriate personnel:

…when we were in there trying to untangle this patient, you could see that both of us felt so bad, we were ready to cry, we felt so bad for this person. They couldn't do anything for themselves really and then to hear the comment that we did. It was very hard… It was not patient care, it was patient abuse. And so the student and I talked a lot about what is considered quality care with somebody and what do you do when you run into a situation like this and what are the levels [through which you need to proceed]. Obviously, we have to go farther than just talking to her [the nurse] because somebody else needed to know that this had occurred. So that was a learning experience for both [of us] because that was the first time I had ever really run into that.*

In this case, then, the student traveled the path of patient advocacy with the CI in territory where he had never been.

✧ HOW CAN ACADEMIC AND CLINICAL FACULTY EXPAND AND ENHANCE OPPORTUNITIES FOR TEACHING AND LEARNING ABOUT THE ETHICAL AND HUMAN DIMENSIONS OF CARE IN CLINICAL SETTINGS?

So what do the voices of students and clinical instructors and these stories tell us? In making these concluding recommendations I draw on the voices and stories shared in this chapter, my own experiences, and literature in the areas of educational psychology and professional learning and development.

First and foremost, we must treat students with respect and be interested in them as individuals and learners. In some, but not all ways, we might think of them as we do our patients. Inquire about their past life and professional experiences, their learning styles and needs, their hopes and goals for clinical experiences, and then use this knowledge in constructing learning experiences for them. Yes, modeling is extremely important—and this modeling does not occur just in our encounters with patients—we must be respectful and thoughtful people, teachers, and clinicians.

Furthermore, we must recognize that clinical teaching is not just an individual effort. Instead, it is a profoundly social and relational endeavor influenced moment to moment by the collection of experiences created for and with students by numerous individuals, the culture of the institution or agency (nested in the culture of the prevailing health care system and society), and professional attitudes and interactions. Patients, professional staff, co-workers, and other health care team members are all an important part of the learning experience for students. To the extent that we can create a culture of respect and humanism in our clinical settings, the more successful we will be in nurturing future professionals who are humanistic.

This is no small task! We should start with a critical examination of our own practice and that within our departments, and then move on from there. Work to change local cultures, if not the institutional culture or the culture of the health care system as currently configured. The latter is a monumental charge. But if we do not respond or act when edicts from administration or third-party payers or the federal government threaten our capacity to provide humanistic care, such lack of action suggests at least apathy, if not complicity. This is not the kind of baggage health professionals need nor is it what we want to model for future professionals. As Purtilo has suggested, these challenges and moments are opportunities for exercising moral courage.[33]

As we model and teach about humanism, we must recognize what we are teaching and explore how we can teach most effectively. What and how we are teaching has been described, in part, through the voices and stories you have heard in this chapter. We are teaching about and through personal values, characteristics and qualities, our behaviors, and the enactment of moral commitments and virtuous practice as we interact with patients, families, students, health care professionals, and other staff. We do this frequently through implicit or informal instruction (modeling) or occasionally through more formal and explicit instruction. Both are powerful teachers and are methods we can use as we shape our work with students.

While there is no question that modeling is a powerful teacher about the humanistic dimensions of care, perhaps we can and should engage in explicit teaching about this critical aspect of care more often. For example, as Branch and the voices and stories in this paper suggest, we might more actively seek out and seize upon "teachable moments" or what Branch referred to as "seminal events" in clinical education.[23] Open the door to and facilitate discussion with students about such events—in some cases before the event or situation (when possible) and in other cases after the event as the clinical instructors in this paper have suggested. Alternatively, we can anticipate or create such moments—some authors have called this latter strategy "intentional serendipity."

The excitement and the exigencies of clinical practice provide numerous chances for student learning about humanism and the ethical dimensions of practice. I contend that such learning can go undeveloped or unrealized if we do not build in opportunities for students to regularly engage in deliberate and critical reflection and dialogue in and on action. As Jensen claims, such opportunities can help students and practitioners cultivate "mindful practice."[34] These opportunities can be created through the structure and requirements of the academic program's didactic curriculum, the program's clinical education model and curriculum, or through the structure and requirements of the clinical center's program for clinical education. As you have heard, in our own program, we do this by ensuring that there are multiple avenues and opportunities to engage in both private and public reflection and communal dialogue with students and faculty during clinical internships.

Private dialogue (one-on-one) with academic faculty members during internships is achieved through written exchanges in the form of reflective journals (or e-mail messages) and face-to-face meetings during the course of each internship. Public dialogue about clinical learning experiences occurs at several levels: (a) when students in defined regional geographic groups come together on a monthly basis to discuss some of their questions and experiences with each other and a faculty member, and (b) through web-based asynchronous discussions that can occur at a regional group level or with the entire class of clinical interns. In these ways we try to create a connected community of teachers and learners long after students have left the university campus. And because of the diversity of experiences and individuals, each participant has something to offer the other. These types of discourse communities can be created at clinical centers as well.

Burbules in his book, *Dialogue in Teaching*, describes a typology of dialogue that clinical and academic faculty alike may benefit from as they seek to enhance student learning regardless of what they are teaching about.[3] Drawing on the work of educational philosophers and writings from the field of hermeneutics, Burbules uses the term dialogue to "refer to a particular kind of pedagogical communicative relation: a conversational interaction directed toward teaching and learning."[3] He argues that there are four more or less "distinct genres or approaches to dialogue suitable to different teaching styles, different students, and different subject matters." He calls these genres: (a) dialogue as conversation, (b) dialogue as inquiry, (c) dialogue as debate, and (d) dialogue as instruction[3] (Fig. 24.1).

He further classifies these genres based on four distinctions: Dialogue can be primarily convergent or divergent. Convergent dialogue assumes that participants can eventually come to consensus around a "correct answer" or point. Divergent dialogue assumes a plurality of viewpoints that may not converge toward a single view.[3]

Finally, dialogue can be inclusive or critical (see Fig. 24.1). This dimension refers to the stance or orientation of participants toward their partners. In inclusive dialogue, we take and accept at face value what the other participants say and then seek to understand what led that person (or persons) to that position or belief. A critical orientation is more skeptical and questioning; what is said will need to be tested against evidence and examined for its logic and consistency.

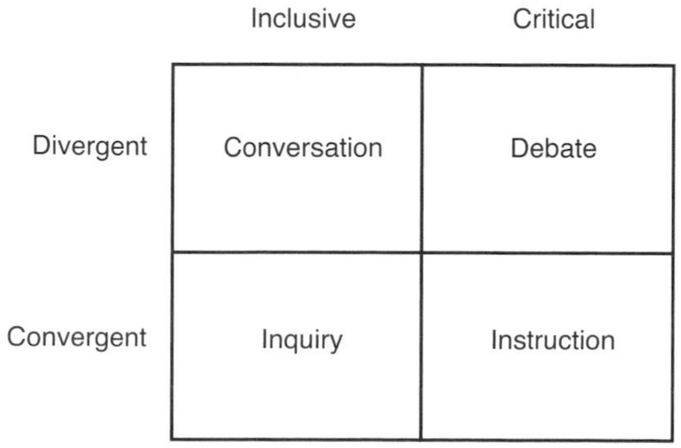

I suggest that three of these four genres of dialogue can be very useful for facilitating student learning in clinical settings. Dialogue as conversation is inclusive and divergent; it is characterized by cooperation, a tolerant spirit and openness, and is directed toward mutual understanding, though not necessarily agreement or reconciliation of differences. Using conversation early in clinical experiences with students can convey respect and create a "climate of humanism" and genuine interest in a way few other forms of dialogue can.[23] It can also serve to model the types of humanistic engagement we seek with our patients in our encounters with them.

Dialogue as inquiry "aims toward the answering of a specific question, the resolution of a problem, or a reconciliation of a dispute."[3] It is inclusive and convergent. It is inclusive insofar as it invites the proposition of many ideas and potential answers or solutions on its way to rest in consensus. Many of our individual and collective activities around clinical problem solving or trying to answer the question of "What should we do next?" involve this kind of dialogue. In fact, it often starts out divergent (as in "brainstorming") and then becomes convergent. This is a form of dialogue I have observed and used repeatedly in regional group meetings and web-based discussion boards as students puzzle over some of their more challenging patients and clinical situations and try to come to consensus on how the patient or situation might best be handled. Because it is inclusive, it is a wonderful form of dialogue to use with students and it invites their participation and respects their input as a starting point for the discussion. Furthermore, it is a form of dialogue well-suited to health care team deliberations and decision making.

Finally, dialogue as instruction is critical

	Inclusive	Critical
Divergent	Conversation	Debate
Convergent	Inquiry	Instruction

Figure 24.1 ✧ Typology of dialogue. (From Burbules NC: Dialogue in Teaching: Theory and Practice. Teachers College Press, New York, 1993.)

and convergent. Here the use of questions or other statements move the discussion toward a definite conclusion. Think of this as a "leading" form of dialogue as in the Socratic method or in the way educational researchers have written about "reciprocal teaching," or what others have called "scaffolding instruction."[35–37] This form of dialogue uses questioning (and then confirmation) to help students climb the ladder, if you will, to new insights and understanding without telling them so. In not telling them, they come to own the new knowledge more than if they had been told what to do or say; in addition, they have been led through a dialectic process of learning that they may then appropriate and use internally in other situations.

I believe that many academic and clinical educators use these forms of dialogue as they go about their work with students. I encourage all of us to more consciously, actively, and frequently use and practice them to foster the habits of reflection, learning, and development of our students and future health care professionals especially in this most critical area—teaching about the relational, ethical, and humanistic dimensions of care in clinical settings. We will all be better for it.

References

1. McGee BJ, Ogger J, and Triezenberg HL: Journaling of ethical considerations during the clinical internship year [unpublished master's thesis]. Central Michigan University, Mt. Pleasant, MI, 2000.
2. Boud D, Keogh R, and Walker D: Reflection: Turning Experience into Learning. Kogan Page/Nichols Publishing, New York, 1985.
3. Burbules NC: Dialogue in Teaching: Theory and Practice. Teachers College Press, New York, 1993.
4. Dewey J: How We Think: A Restatement of the Relation of Reflective Thinking to the Educative Process. DC Health, Lexington, MA, 1933.
5. Harris IB: New expectations for professional competence. In Curry JF, Wergin and Associates, (eds): Educating Professionals. Jossey-Bass, San Francisco, 1993, pp 17–52.
6. Schon DA: The Reflective Practitioner. How Professionals Think in Action. Basic Books, New York, 1983.
7. Schon DA: Educating the Reflective Practitioner. Jossey-Bass, San Francisco, 1987.
8. Mezirow J, et al. Fostering Critical Reflection in Adulthood: A guide to Transformative and Emancipatory Learning. Jossey-Bass, San Francisco, 1990.
9. Saylor CR: Reflection and professional education: Art, science, and competency. Nurse Educ 15(2):8–11, 1990.
10. Zeichner KM, and Liston DP: Teaching student teachers to reflect. Harvard Educ Rev 57(1):23–48, 1987.
11. Jensen GM, et al: Expertise in Physical Therapy Practice. Butterworth-Heinemann, Boston, 1999.
12. Shepard KF, and Jensen GM: Physical therapist curricula for the 1990s: Educating the reflective practitioner. Phys Ther 70(9):566–577, 1990.
13. Gandy J, and Jensen GM: Group work and reflective practicums in physical therapy education: Models for professional behavior development. J Phys Ther Educ 6(1):6–10, 1992.
14. Jensen GM, and Denton B: Teaching physical therapy students to reflect: A suggestion for clinical education. J Phys Ther Educ 5(1):33–38, 1991.
15. Lukinsky J: Reflective withdrawal through journal writing. In Mezirow J (ed): Fostering Critical Reflection in Adulthood: A Guide to Transformative and Emancipatory Learning. Jossey-Bass, San Francisco, 1990, pp 213–234.
16. Perkins J: Reflective journals: Suggestions for educations. J Phys Ther Educ 10(12):8–13, 1986.
17. Tryssenaar J: Interactive journals: An educational strategy to promote reflection. Am J Occup Ther 49(7):695–702, 1996.
18. VanManen M: Researching Lived Experience: Human Science for an Action Sensitive Pedagogy. Althouse Press, London, Ont., Canada, 1990.
19. Clark CM: Hello learners: Living social constructivism. Teaching Educ 10(1):89–110, 1998.
20. Mattingly C, and Fleming MH: Clinical Reasoning: Forms of Inquiry in a Therapeutic Practice. FA Davis Co, Philadelphia, PA, 1994.
21. Fleming MH, and Mattingly C: The underground practice. In Mattingly C, and Fleming MH (eds): Clinical Reasoning: Forms of Inquiry in a Therapeutic Practice. FA Davis Co, Philadelphia, PA, 1994, pp 295–315.
22. Mostrom E, and Shepard KF: Teaching and learning about patient education. In Shepard KF, and Jensen GM (eds): Handbook of Teaching for Physical Therapists. Butterworth-Heinemann, Boston, 2002, pp 287–320.
23. Branch WT, et al: Teaching the human dimensions of care in clinical settings. JAMA 286(9):1067–1074, 2001.
24. Mostrom E, and Shepard KF: Teaching and learning about patient education in physical therapy professional education: Academic and clinical considerations. J Phys Ther Educ 13(3):8–17, 1999.
25. Coles R: The Call of Stories: Teaching and the Moral Imagination. Houghton Mifflin, Boston, 1989.
26. Frank AW: At the Will of the Body: Reflections on Illness. Houghton Mifflin, Boston, 1991.
27. Frank AW: The Wounded Storyteller: Body, Illness and Ethics. The University of Chicago Press, Chicago, 1995.
28. Mattingly C: Healing Dramas and Clinical Plots: The Narrative Structure of Experience. Cambridge University Press, Cambridge, UK, 1998.
29. American Physical Therapy Association: Report on the Consensus Conference on Professionalism. American Physical Therapy Association, Alexandria, VA, 2003.
30. May WW, et al: Model for ability-based assessment in physical therapy education. J Phys Ther Educ 9(1):3–6, 1995.
31. Varcoe C, and Rodney P: Constrained agency: The social structure of nurses' work. In Bolaria BS, and Dickinson HD (eds): Health, Illness and Health Care

in Canada. ed 3. Nelson, Toronto, Ont., Canada, 2002, pp 102–128.

32. Glaser JW: Three Realms of Ethics. Sheed and Ward, Kansas City, MO, 1994.

33. Purtilo R: Moral courage in times of change: Visions for the future. J Phys Ther Educ 14(3):4–6, 2000.

34. Jensen GM: Exploration of critical self-reflection in the teaching of ethics: The case of physical therapy. Paper presented at: American Educational Research Association Annual Meeting; April 21, 2003, Chicago.

35. Palincsar AS: The role of dialogue in providing scaffolding instruction. Educ Psychol 21:73–98, 1986.

36. Palincsar AS, and Brown AL: Reciprocal teaching of comprehension-fostering and comprehension-monitoring strategies. Cognition Instr 2:117–175, 1984.

37. Cazden CB: Classroom Discourse: The Language of Teaching and Learning. Heinemann, Portsmouth, NH, 1988.

25

Mock IRB: A Teaching Case

JAN BRUCKNER, PHD, PT

The need for allied health professionals to have a better background in bioethics has been documented in the literature for the past two decades.[1–7] Allied health accrediting bodies require coursework in bioethics.[8] Despite this situation, however, the level of ethics education appears to be fairly low. No consensus on curricular content has emerged. Elder and Andrew surveyed allied health deans and found that they rated ethics as the most important of 14 content areas, but rated philosophy, of which ethics is a part, the lowest.[3] Geddes, Finch, and Larin devoted a page or less to 12 ethical issues facing physical therapists and devoted two-thirds of their book, *Ethical Issues Relevant to Physical Therapy*, to reprinting four codes of ethics without comment or discussion.[9] Triezenberg found that 13 out of 16 ethical issues arising out of clinical practice were not covered in professional curricula.[4]

At a time when increasing numbers of allied health professionals are getting doctoral degrees and doing research, governmental citations for ethical misconduct in science and concern for protection of human subjects are also increasing.[10–15] The National Institutes of Health Office of Protection from Research Risks (OPRR) sees education as an inexpensive and effective way of protecting research subjects, but the current textbooks on allied health research provide procedural material on completing institutional review board (IRB) forms.[16,17] No literature could be found discussing substantive issues confronting allied health researchers.

My own experience in the classroom reflects the views in the literature. Students in my research courses tolerate presentations on codes of ethics and institutional review but they are not engaged in substantive discussions about protection of human subjects, confidentiality, conflicts between researchers and clinical care providers, or dilemmas about withholding treatment from control group subjects. This teaching case describes a way to engage students in substantive ethical discussions through an exercise akin to moot court in a law school setting that I call "mock IRB." The example used here, based on my own research, involves the dilemma of obtaining informed consent to be a research subject from elderly individuals with mental retardation and developmental disabilities who were asked to participate in a study to develop a tool to identify people who were at risk for falls.

✦ SETTING THE STAGE

I use the Portney and Watkins text in my classes so I require that students read Chapter 3, "Ethical Issues in Clinical Research."[17] In lecture format, I present some historical material about the Nazi medical experiments,[18] the Willowbrook hepatitis study,[19] the Tuskegee syphilis study,[20,21] and the Gelsinger case.[22] I give an overview of procedures and documents protecting human research subjects, including the

Nuremberg Code, the Belmont Report, the latest OPRR statements, and our own university's IRB forms and procedures. I tell the class that they will play the institutional review board and that I will play the researcher requesting permission to do my study. At the end of the class, they will vote whether to let me do my study or not.

✦ THE CASE

Any research study can be used in the mock IRB exercise, but I chose to use a real case that has an ethical dilemma about informed consent.[23] The case concerns elderly individuals with mental retardation and developmental disabilities who live in the community and attend day programs. A number of these individuals started getting frail, became unsteady on their feet, and began falling. As the number of incident reports began growing, staff in the group homes and day centers wanted something done. The physician in charge of the day programs asked the occupational therapist associated with the programs to screen all of the appropriate clients to identify individuals at risk for falls. The occupational therapist searched the literature for an appropriate screening tool and found none. She approached a physical therapist to assist her with the problem and they both decided to investigate whether a modified version of the Get Up and Go Test could be used with this population. Together, the occupational therapist and the physical therapist developed a protocol to test the reliability and validity of the Get Up and Go (GUAG) test. They discussed the study with the physician and the day program staff. Everyone agreed that the study was necessary.

At this point in the class, I demonstrate the standard GUAG test. The test involves having a person start by sitting in a chair in front of a 10-foot walkway. When a person with a stopwatch says "Go," the subject must rise out of the chair, run down the walkway, turn around at the end, run back and sit down. The whole process is timed. Each subject gets three trials. In the actual case we added two additional conditions: a walker condition and a personal assistant condition. Subjects repeated the same procedures but had to use a rolling walker for the walker trials and held the hand of a personal assistant for the personal assistant trials. In class, students can ask questions about the technical details of the GUAG instrument and its modified version. All questions about the facts of the case get answered. I establish that the actual test is noninvasive, not using sensitive material, not burdensome in terms of time demands, and generally low-risk procedurally.

✦ ISSUES OF INFORMED CONSENT

After the technical questions are answered, discussion turns to matters of informed consent. All of the subjects are elderly, chronologically 55 years or older, and none has a parent involved in his or her case. Most of the subjects have been institutionalized all of their lives so few have family members involved with their care. Under state law, these individuals are considered emancipated adults so they have no legal guardians. All persons have been evaluated by a psychologist so we know that their cognitive ages are less than 12 years of age. Usually, moral agency is granted to people who are 21 years or older with the assumption that the individuals possess an eighth-grade reading level or higher. My first question to the class is: Would you consider these subjects to be adult moral agents who can give consent to participate in the study?

The ensuing discussion focuses on the issue of moral agency. Can you be a moral agent if you cannot read? Can you be a moral agent if you are younger than 18 years of age? Or younger than 16 years of age? What about individuals who are intellectually mature at 12 years of age or individuals who are immature at 21 years of age? What does it mean to be "cognitively an adult"? Who makes this determination and how certain are we of it? Can moral agents make "bad" or morally wrong decisions and what do we think about this? Who grants or determines moral agency? Could the subjects be considered moral agents and be given the right to grant informed consent and sign the consent forms? If the subjects are not moral agents and cannot sign the forms for themselves, who can give consent?

Fundamental to the concept of informed consent is the idea of weighing the benefits against the risks. Will the individual be able to understand what benefit he or she will derive from participating in the study? In the modified GUAG study, no one will benefit directly since the study's goals are to establish the validity and reliability of the assessment tool. Will the individuals understand the risks involved in the study? The study involves the physical risk of falling during the test, but we took care to have sufficient numbers of assistants to guard against anyone falling. A bigger possibility of risk exists in the psychological realm. Many individuals in this population get stressed when their daily routine is disrupted or when they have to confront people who they do not know. The research team engaged staff who knew the individuals well to participate in subject recruitment and to assist during the actual testing. Whether the subjects experienced short-term or long-term psychological stress from the testing situation was difficult to assess. Members of the mock IRB are challenged to explore the possibilities.

At this stage in the discussion, I introduce a model of community consent developed by Thomasma.[24] Thomasma's model is based on the ethical principle of beneficence and claims that every person has an obligation to improve society. This obligation applies to vulnerable individuals so they can be expected to participate in research studies along with everyone else. Thomasma asks who benefits from the research. If the individuals taking part in the study will also be beneficiaries of it, Thomasma is more inclined to let them participate. He also asks about the risks involved in the study. It is more reasonable to include vulnerable subjects in low-risk, high-benefit studies than in high-risk, no-benefit studies. Thomasma then examines moral agency and the issue of competency. The question here hinges on whether the individual may become competent or had been competent and what the individual's wishes were during the period of competency. To oversee the process, Thomasma proposes the formation of a research community that comprises members of the subject class, advocacy groups, researchers, and any other interested parties. The research protocols would be submitted to

this research community and they could give consent for vulnerable subjects to participate. Thomasma's guidelines are that in minimal-risk studies surrogate-consent models can apply. In moderate-risk or unknown-risk studies, the research community–consent model could apply. High-risk studies should not be done because of the possibility of abuse.

I ask my students to examine Thomasma's model. Does it seem reasonable? What dangers do they see in using a community consent approach? How can we determine the level of benefit to the subject? How do we determine competency and what are the areas of possible abuse? Who determines the amount of risk in a study and what safeguards are in effect for ensuring appropriate ranking? Do they like the community-consent model?

Finally, I introduce the students to an autonomy-based model grounded in a Piagetian approach.[25] Piaget described four stages of intellectual development. Stage 1, the Sensory Motor Period, goes from birth to the onset of language at approximately 18 months of age. During this period, the individual is developing a sense of object permanence, eye-hand coordination, and basic knowledge about the physical world. Stage 2 is called the Preoperational Period and involves the individual learning communication skills, mathematical concepts, basic scientific ideas, and early aspects of socialization. It lasts from 2 to 6 years of age. Stage 3, the Concrete Operational Period, corresponds to the time that individuals start formal schooling, 7 to 12 years of age. Individuals in this stage understand cause-and-effect relationships and have a more sophisticated view of how actions can influence results. Piaget's final stage, Formal Operations, begins about 12 years of age and lasts through adulthood. In this stage individuals can understand abstract concepts and hypothetical constructs. In our study with the elders with mental retardation and developmental disabilities, we excluded individuals whose psychological profiles placed them in the sensory motor period since these individuals were nonverbal and conveying the risks and benefits of the study proved too difficult. Informed consent forms were written at the remaining three levels: preoperational, concrete operational, and formal operational. We used the psychological profiles to match individuals' cognitive functioning with the appropriate form and explained the study using words appropriate to the cognitive level. This approach gave the subjects an understanding of the study in a language that they could understand and then they were able to agree or decline to participate.

I ask the students in the mock IRB what they think of the Piagetian autonomy approach. The class discusses what happens when researchers start accepting individuals who are functioning cognitively below the current standards for moral agency. In what ways can we best safeguard the risks against abuse when cognitively impaired individuals are granted autonomy in decision making? Which approach, Thomasma's beneficence model or the Piagetian autonomy model, seems most reasonable for studies being done by allied health professionals?[24,25] Can we develop a better model?

✧ FINAL REFLECTIONS

Kuczewski called on bioethicists to begin examining the ethical dilemmas that occur in rehabilitation settings.[26] I agree that it is time to begin rigorous examination of the ethical issues unique to the allied health fields. While I welcome any assistance, I think that allied health professionals are better equipped to research the ethical dilemmas that confront allied health professionals rather than leaving the task to philosophers who know little about our clinical problems, our patients, and our research subjects.

We have little consensus on what ethical issues should be taught in professional curricula and our literature uses a more procedural rather than a substantive approach to the material. Misconduct in science is increasing and OPRR is getting increasingly concerned about the safety of research subjects. To address the need to engage students in substantive discussions about ethical dilemmas in allied health research, I developed an exercise called a "mock IRB." The mock IRB exercise encourages student engagement with substantive issues and the examination of ethical issues that confront

allied health researchers. Philosophers, who know little about our clinical problems, our patients, and our research subjects, cannot have the sole or even the primary responsibility for analyzing the ethical dilemmas that confront allied health professionals. Allied health professionals and students must learn how to use a focused, philosophically based approach to ethical questions. The mock IRB process gives students a way to move beyond a procedural approach and begin to confront the kind of ethical problems they will face in clinical practice and research.

References

1. Purtilo R: Ethics in allied health education: State of the art. J Allied Health 12(3):210–220, 1983.
2. Glazer-Waldman HR: Perceptions of patient-provider relationships in allied health education textbooks. J Allied Health 13(2):104–111, 1984.
3. Elder OC, and Andrew ME: Important curriculum content for baccalaureate allied health programs: A survey of deans. J Allied Health 21(2):105–115, 1992.
4. Triezenberg HL: The identification of ethical issues in physical therapy practice. Phys Ther 76:1097–1107, 1996.
5. Brown K, and Griffiths Y: Confidentiality dilemmas in clinical education. J of Allied Health 29(1):13–17, 2000.
6. Ekelman BA, Goodman G, and Dal Bello-Haas V: Inclusion of medical-legal issues in entry-level occupational and physical therapy curricula. J Allied Health 29(1):36–40, 2002.
7. Lesh SG, et al: Perceptions of change in the health care industry. J Allied Health 30(1):11–19, 2001.
8. Layman E: Ethics education: Curricular considerations for the allied health disciplines. J Allied Health 25(2):149–160, 1996.
9. Geddes EL, Finch E, and Larin H: Ethical Issues Relevant to Physical Therapy. McMaster University School of Rehabilitation Science, Hamilton, Ontario, Canada, 1999.
10. Kraemer LG, and Lyons KJ: Research productivity of allied health faculty in academic health centers. J Allied Health 18(4):349–359, 1989.
11. Associated Press: Regulators suspend Chicago Hospital's Human Research. Associated Press State and Local Wire. November 19, 1999.
12. Hilts PJ: U.S. Halts Human Research at Alabama. *New York Times*. January 22, 2000, sect A:12.
13. Matthews J: Father's complaints shut down research: U.S. Agencies act on privacy concerns. *Washington Post*. January 12, 2000, sect B:7.
14. Marwick C: Protecting subjects of clinical research. JAMA 292(6):516–517, 1999.
15. Woodward B: Challenges to human subject protections in U.S. medical research. JAMA 282(20):1947–1952, 1999.
16. Ellis GB: Keeping research subjects out of harm's way. JAMA 282(20):1963–1965, 1999.
17. Portney LG, and Watkins MP: Ethical Issues in

Research. ed 2. Prentice Hall Health, Upper Saddle River, NJ, 2000.

18. Annas GS, and Grodin MA: The Nazi doctors and the Nuremberg Code: Relevance for modern medical research. Med War 6(2):120–123, 1990.

19. Krugman S: The Willowbrook hepatitis studies revisited: Ethical aspects. Rev Infect Dis 8(1):157–162, 1986.

20. Corbie-Smith G: The continuing legacy of the Tuskegee syphilis study: Considerations for clinical investigation. Am J Med Sci 317(1):5–8, 1999.

21. White RM: The Tuskegee syphilis study. Hastings Cent Rep 32(6):4–5, 2002.

22. Gelsinger P: Jesse's intent. Bull Med Ethics 179:13–20, 2002.

23. Bruckner JS, and Herge A: Assessing the risk of falls in elders with mental retardation and developmental disabilities. Top Geriatr Rehab 19(3):206–219, 2003.

24. Thomasma DC: A model of community substituted consent for research on the vulnerable. Med Health Care Philos 3:47–57, 2000.

25. Phillips JL: The Origins of Intellect: Piaget's Theory. WH Freeman and Co., San Francisco, 1969.

26. Kuczewski MG: Disability: An agenda for bioethics. Am J Bioethics (3):36–44, 2001.

Reflections on the Ethics of Teaching

AIMEE J. LUEBBEN, EDD, OTR, FAOTA

Abstract

Although I am fascinated with the teaching of ethics, this is not a chapter on ideas, strategies, or methods to teach ethics. (In writing this chapter, I was heartened by finding continuing growth in a substantial knowledge base on the teaching of ethics, written primarily since the early 1990s in the teacher education field.) The area in which I am more interested is a recombination of words—the ethics of teaching—because of my background and experience; before entering school to become an occupational therapist, I completed professional training to be a teacher.

Dewey and Schön both have extolled the value of reflection to resolve complex issues.[1-4] To resolve the complex issue of the ethics of teaching, I have invoked Dewey's spirit and used Schön's guidance to write a reflective chapter on various aspects of the ethics of teaching: the *what* (content), the *how* (method or the art), and the *why* (assessment or the science). Demonstrating various aspects of the ethics of teaching, for this chapter I have threaded components of a self study, which for me is a continuum ranging from any informal investigation into teaching practice at one end to the other end—the formality of action research, which provides evidence-based documentation comparing one iteration to another within the evolution of a course. My self-assessment, a critical self-reflection nested within this overall reflective chapter, examines the evolution—across four iterations—of a course in pathophysiology, a content area common to both occupational therapy and physical therapy.

Reflection, according to Dewey "involves running over various ideas, sorting them out, comparing one with another, trying to get one which will unite in itself the strength of two, searching for new points of view, developing new suggestions; guessing, suggesting, selecting, and rejecting."[2] Describing reflection as a type of thinking, Dewey wrote, "The function of reflective thought is, therefore, to transform a situation in which there is experienced obscurity, doubt, conflict, disturbance of some sort, into a situation that is clear, coherent, settled, harmonious."[1] For me, the terms *obscurity, doubt, conflict,* and *disturbance of some sort* characterize what I call *ethical dilemmas* and what Purtilo terms *ethical problems* or *ethical issues*.[5] The value of reflection, particularly in ethical situations, is evident. Indeed, without reflection, many current and historical ethical decision making models could not have existed. Differentiating between *knowing-in-action* and *reflecting-in-action*, Schön—whose dissertation on Dewey's theory of inquiry and subsequent life work sparked interest of new generations in the master—wrote about the value of reflection for a practitioner.[3,4] Because problems do not present themselves to the practitioner as givens in real-world practice, Schön has advocated moving away from technical rationality that emphasizes what I term the *science* of professional practice—a process of problem solving—toward reflection-in-action that emphasizes the art of professional practice—a process of defining decisions to be made, ends to be achieved, the means which may be chosen.[3] In the spirit of Dewey and with the guidance of Schön, this is a reflective [notice *reflexive*, an often misused word that is actually the antithesis of *reflective*, is not used*] chapter on the ethics of teaching. Although the teaching of ethics (which now has a substantial knowledge base, especially in education), is a worthy subject, this chapter is a reflection on some aspects of the ethics of teaching: the *what* (content), the *how* (method or the art), and the *why* (assessment or the science). This is the reflection* of a teacher-turned-therapist who now happily blends both professions at the higher education level.

Even though I use the terms *teach* and *teaching* in a generic sense, I am careful how I use *teacher* (the *who*), a word that I know from personal experience requires a professional credential, which indicates successful completion of specialized didactic education, one or more internships, and certification. In other words, for me, not everyone who teaches is a teacher. The focus of this chapter is therefore not on the teacher, but on the purposeful activity or the *doing* (occupational therapists call this *occupation*) of teaching, clearly the purview of the person who teaches, rather than *learning* (another occupation), the *doing* of people on the receiving end of information. By concentrating on the occupation of teaching, I sidestep the whole *teaching* versus *learning* debate that continues to rage in education. Dancing around the larger conflagration allows me to bypass a smaller debate beginning to enflame the education profession. Just as the occupational therapy profession uses the term *client-centered* and the physical therapy profession speaks of *patient-focused* to ensure that our practice is firmly grounded in the people we serve, professional teachers are in the midst of debating the terms

learner-centered and *learning-centered*.* In another reflection on various terminology debates, I chose not to engage in this chapter in the multiple millennial-long, transdisciplinary argument of *ethical* versus *moral* (or any other derivations of those two words). A classical language teacher by training, I tend to become mired in the etymological aspects of words.†

◆ OPENING REFLECTIONS

To entice the flow of my beginning reflections regarding the ethics of teaching, I started by searching the literature of my second profession, occupational therapy (within the larger context of health care and medicine). Heartened by a sizable number of articles on a recombination of words—the teaching of ethics—but little on my interest here—the ethics of teaching—I moved quickly into the literature of my first profession, teaching. I found that the occupational therapy and physical therapy professions are not alone: according to Goodlad, Soder, and Sirotnik, ethical practice of teaching remains largely neglected in the teacher education literature.[6] For the dearth of information on the ethics of teaching, Swartz blamed the "positivist-behaviorist, management-oriented perception" of the teaching profession, "requiring certainty and measurable outcomes," whereas Huebner found fault with educational language (e.g., accountability, alignment, quality control, rigor, and standards)—in vogue at the time—that tended to address problems that could readily be solved technically.[7,8]

---

*Although I have seen the term *reflexive* often used in conjunction with qualitative research, I posit that *reflexive* (as the adjective form of the noun reflection) was coined by researchers whose education lacked grounding in classical languages. Employing *reflexive* to modify reflection—and using *reflective* and *reflexive* interchangeably—unfortunately has become common usage.

*For a rich description and history of reflection in teacher education, please see Fendler (2003).

† I started my professional career as a Latin teacher almost four decades ago and I found a history professor willing to tutor me in classical Greek close to 10 years ago. As a result, "I have listened to words in two languages that are considered 'dead' by many people, but are very much alive to me" (Luebben, 2003, p 10). Etymology is a passion for me, and I love to debate words from a definitional, historical, and common practice standpoint. I have decided to refrain from my passion here: for consistency, I have used the word *ethics* throughout this chapter because of my twist on words—ethics of teaching—for my subject matter as well as my title.

"Teaching is an inherently moral activity because it involves interactions between people and purposeful activities."[9] Reflecting on the ethics of teaching related to the rationale of Anderson as well as others that teaching is a moral activity, I am struck that what is identified as *faculty* (a role in the occupational therapy profession) and *education* (a role in the physical therapy profession) may occur in one of the most ethically complex settings of our professions.[10–15] I use three ethical identity periods—which Purtilo described and identified as consecutive—simultaneously to describe the ethical complexity faced on a daily basis by occupational therapists and physical therapists who are educators.[16] For unlike university faculty in a purely academic curriculum, professional program educators walk a three-ply ethical tightrope with the first two braided strands being the educational institution (period of patient-focused identity—reinterpreted, perhaps, as *student-focused* identity in the academic setting) and the profession (period of self-identity). The third interwoven ply in the ethical tightrope is the public (period of societal identity), "part of the extended duty of the educator because the public is the ultimate recipient of services."[17] Put another way, we concurrently provide a service resulting in monetary exchange (contractual obligations) in the universities that employ us, initial competence for therapists entering our fields (in preparation for fiduciary obligations), a gatekeeping function within our professions (socializing new generations, yet weeding out marginal students), and a duty to protect society from harm.

Anderson continued, "Within this dynamic interactive process, teachers exercise considerable authority and autonomy over what and how curriculum is presented for learning."[9] Though some teachers may exercise considerable authority and autonomy, this may not be true of professional educational program faculty who until recently have been driven from the top down. Society drives credentialing agencies (professional program accreditation and individual practitioner certification), which in turn drive university administration. The department chairperson is then driven by society,

credentialing agencies, and university administration whereas the faculty member is driven by society, credentialing agencies, university administration, and the department chairperson. A recent bottom-up twist in professional training has squeezed faculty into a middle position as a result of more students making educational demands coupled with threats of malpractice—extending professional liability to educational malpractice. The complexity of the dynamic interactive process of teaching is difficult enough without adding various aspects of the ethics of teaching to the mix.

To demonstrate various aspects of the ethics of teaching, I have threaded components of a self-study, which Zeichner credited as the single most significant development ever in the field of teacher education research.[18] According to Kosnik and Beck, self-study is "neither self-indulgent nor unduly sentimental, but a serious attempt to understand one's teaching with a view to improving it."[19] To substantiate his point, Zeichner presented examples of self-assessments conducted by teachers who investigated their practice to expose gaps between what they thought they were doing and the experiences of their students.[18] For me, self-assessment is a continuum that ranges from any informal investigation into teaching practice at one continuum end to the other end—the formality of action research, which provides evidence-based documentation comparing one iteration to another within the evolution of a course.

My self-assessment, a reflection nested within this overall reflective chapter, examines the evolution—across four iterations—of a course in pathophysiology, a content area common to both occupational therapy and physical therapy. I begin this self-assessment with some background information. When I was hired in 1992 to create an entry-level occupational therapy program at the University of Southern Indiana, my first tasks included developing the curriculum and hiring faculty. Before distributing courses to faculty, I had assumed I would have my choice of classes as well as my choice of offering times. I was naïve; I ended up with leftovers—classes and time offerings other faculty did not want. The pathophysiology course is a primary example; with no other faculty available, I taught the class (a content area not among my favorites) for almost a decade before reassignment to a new faculty member. The course had merit: the absence of deep devotion to content allowed me to change those components I deemed undesirable, try new approaches I had found in my professional reading, and generally keep improving the course until I was somewhat saddened when another person began teaching the class.

✧ REFLECTIONS ON THE *WHAT* OF THE ETHICS OF TEACHING

Although I was the only faculty member for almost a year, my administrative duties of designing the curriculum and developing courses absorbed my time until suddenly the pathophysiology course needed an instructor. I have to admit that I succumbed at first to what Anderson called "inertia of tradition" and emphasized content, the *what* aspect of the ethics of teaching. In this case, I am speaking about preset, teacher-determined content—information from the textbook, a few selected references I made available, and some lectures.[9] Please realize these were the days before ready access to the Internet.

The first change in my thinking about the *what* aspect of the ethics of teaching came after reading Bork, who reported that more than half of what he had learned in his entry-level professional education program (approximately 30 years before) had been modified by new findings or even rejected.[20] Indeed, the explosion of new and applied knowledge coupled with the proliferation of technology since Bork's writing has resulted in health profession content with an estimated shelf life of 3 years.[20] For occupational therapy and physical therapy, both post-baccalaureate professions with educational programs that are at least 5 years in total length (preprofessional plus professional components), this shelf life almost becomes a half-life: the *what* students learn at the beginning of professional training has a high probability of needing more current information by graduation.

To the question, asking if I advocate that occupational therapy and physical therapy programs not teach content, my response is a vehement, "No." After all, where would our professions be without our unique knowledge bases—content? To enhance the *what*, I advocate recognizing the dynamic aspect of *what* to allow ongoing change and modifying the *how* aspect of the ethics of teaching in a way that promotes continuing competence and lifelong learning.

✧ REFLECTIONS ON THE *HOW* OF THE ETHICS OF TEACHING

I may use method (the art)—the *how* of the ethics of teaching—atypically, compared with many occupational therapy and physical therapy faculty, because I was trained as a teacher nearly a decade before becoming an occupational therapist. I entered my second profession, having studied that the movement from so-called Socratic learning to transmittal of information occurred when the teacher read aloud (the word *lecture* comes from the Latin "lego, legere, legi, lectum": read) a book, which was copied verbatim by students to make sure everyone had the same text. (Before the invention of the printing press, there was often only one textbook.) That "college teaching is probably the only profession in the world for which no specific training is required" probably explains why even now, hundreds of years after the printing press was invented, lecture format seems to rein supreme in higher education. I, on the other hand, agree with Dewey and Vygotsky and others eschewing traditional teaching techniques such as lecture.[21-23] One of my favorites, Mortimer Adler wrote, "All genuine learning is active, not passive. It involves the use of the mind, not just the memory. It is a process of discovery, in which the student is the main agent, not the teacher. ..."[24]

Even the first iteration of the pathophysiology course never consisted of lecture alone—I used what I called *diagnosis referrals* to stimulate students' higher order cognitive skills: application, analysis, synthesis, and evaluation.[25] The method, diagnosis referrals, came from a realization that seasoned therapists are excited to receive referrals of patients or clients who have new or rare diagnoses. I told students I wanted them to be as excited as "real" therapists about receiving referrals with unfamiliar diagnoses—hence the teaching strategy, diagnosis referral (see Table 26.1 for a diagnosis referral example used in iterations 1 and 2), which consisted of just the minimum—name, age, diagnosis, and location. At that time, I divided diagnosis referrals within a category (e.g., cardiac) among small groups of students, who provided information on their set of diagnoses back to the class in lecture format. During graduate study in my first profession, I found that my *how* had a name: *constructivism*, which is predicated upon the student putting together (constructing)* knowledge by converting information through active engagement in educational events. Since that time I have found that National Academy Press publications related to how people learn are resources rich in substance and ideas.[26,27]

Some years later, when I devoured the January/February 1999 *American Journal of Occupational Therapy*, a special issue on faculty development that catapulted me into the professional literature on small group learning, I realized I had been using cooperative and collaborative learning in the pathophysiology course. In this first course of the professional curriculum, I moved away from individualistic toward cooperative and collaborative learning to accomplish a goal that was secondary to solving problems related to diagnoses: I wanted students to realize that ambiguity may be good, perfectionism is not always healthy, and multiple answers can all be correct.

I admitted in the previous section that I succumbed to Anderson's "inertia of tradition" by emphasizing the *what*: preset, teacher-determined content.[9] After 2 years of having textbooks that were not adequate and realizing the

shelf life of health care information, I decided a second iteration was in order. With the same diagnosis referrals in place, I changed the emphasis on the *what*—by moving away from teacher-determined content to teaching students research strategies to seek and evaluate current information—to promote continuing competence and lifelong learning and address the health profession content shelf life issue. Students continued to provide information on their set of diagnoses within a category back to the class in lecture format.

The third iteration of the pathophysiology course came 2 years later, after my professional reading became focused on case-based and problem-based learning. At this time, I worked to "flesh out" what used to be referral diagnoses into thumbnail-sized descriptions of people with actual problems (see Table 26.1 for a case-based problem example used in iterations 3 and 4). Although students were dealing with idiosyncrasies of people—requiring more in-depth higher order cognitive skills—they still worked in collaborative groups on a smaller subset of diagnoses within a category, learning the remaining diagnoses (coupled with the initial case-based problems) from their classmates.

The fourth and current iteration resulted when rereading Nolinske and Millis returned me to collaborative learning literature.[28] During this reading, I found that my method of dividing a category (e.g., cardiac)—first by diagnosis referrals, then by problem-based case studies—and having each student group bring information back to the class to fit like a puzzle piece into a whole category had a name: *jigsaw*.[29] I decided another change was in order after watching students actively engaging in completing their own group's set of diagnoses and disregarding information their classmates provided when information was jigsawed together. After 6 years of groups completing tasks in jigsaw fashion (the first three iterations), I decided to investigate how students' learning was effected if each group completed the whole puzzle—all case study problems—rather than just one jigsaw piece.

By this point, my reflection may have raised questions for some readers regarding

---

*For me, helping occupational therapy and physical therapy students construct knowledge brings both professions full circle. After all, close to a century ago, occupational therapists and physical therapists began as two classes of reconstruction aides. In the educational setting, we are continuing our tradition of "building" minds and lives.

outcomes of these four iterations; after all, I provide only pedagogical strategy descriptions in this *how* of the ethics of teaching section. Other readers may immediately classify this self-study as an example of the scholarship of teaching and learning.[30] Readers will find the course's iteration outcomes in the next section, the *why* of the ethics of teaching, and a commentary on various classifications of scholarship, including the scholarship of teaching and learning, in the parting reflections section.

✦ REFLECTIONS ON THE *WHY* OF THE ETHICS OF TEACHING

The *why* of the ethics of teaching is ongoing assessment that provides evidence either to support continued use or to make modifications resulting in better practices (notice the term *best practices** was not used). Although content of courses comprises the science of a particular profession, assessment—the *why*—involves the science of teaching. To show changes in the evolution of this pathophysiology course, my self-assessment remained near the informal end of the self-assessment continuum for the first three iterations, and then moved to action research (at the formal end of the self-study continuum) to compare changes made in the fourth iteration with those in the third iteration. Rather than engage in yet another terminology debate (this time between the terms *case-based* and *problem-based* learning), I have chosen to use Harden and Davis's "range of options" in an 11-step educational strategy continuum.[31] See Table 26.1, which synthesizes Harden and Davis's information into a graphic organizer, delineating educational approach, student emphasis, and general examples.[31] A fourth column pro-

vides examples from iterations 1 and 2 and also iterations 3 and 4 in the evolution of this pathophysiology course.

The first two iterations were very similar. Since even the first iteration (diagnosis referrals, collaborative groups, and jigsawed content) did not consist of lecture alone, the pathophysiology course bypassed Harden and Davis's first step (theoretical learning) altogether, and started at the second step—problem-oriented learning.[31] The difference between the first and second iterations was a change primarily in *how* the *what* was delivered, from teacher-determined to student-driven content. The remaining components of the second iteration's *how* (diagnosis referrals, collaborative groups, and jigsawed content) remained the same. Although this modification promotes continuing competence and lifelong learning by teaching students research strategies to seek and evaluate current information, the *how* changed little so the second iteration remained at Harden and Davis's second step, problem-oriented learning.[31]

The third and fourth iterations were characterized by evolutionary—almost revolutionary—changes compared with the first two iterations. Even though some of the *how* (collaborative groups and jigsawed content) of the third iteration remained the same, the big change was in redesigning what used to be referral diagnoses into thumbnail-sized descriptions of people with actual problems. This radical change in the *how* of the ethics of teaching moved the pathophysiology course seven steps higher on Harden and Davis's continuum—from the second step, problem-oriented learning, to the ninth step, problem-centered discovery learning.[31]

I did not expect the fourth iteration to show a change in Harden and Davis's continuum because the final two steps involve generalization that happens during simulations in labs (10. problem-based learning) or occurs in real-time in clinical settings (11. task-based learning).[31] After 6 years of groups completing tasks in jigsaw fashion (the first three iterations), I used action research, at the formal end of the self-study continuum, to investigate the effects of student learning when each of the collaborative groups completed all problems

---

*To describe practice, I prefer using the comparative adjective *better* to argue that continuous improvement is always possible rather than the superlative adjective *best*, which indicates perfection. (After all, practice probably would not be called *practice* if perfection were expected at all times—the phrase *best practice* may just be an oxymoron!)

Table 26.1 ✧ Information-Oriented–Problem-Based Learning Continuum

STEP	EDUCATIONAL APPROACH	STUDENT EMPHASIS	GENERAL EXAMPLES	PATHOPHYSIOLOGY COURSE EXAMPLE
1	Theoretical	Acquiring information	Traditional lecture, textbook	
2	Problem-oriented learning	Acquiring information in a format relevant to practitioner	Lectures with practical slant, including intervention protocols or management guidelines	Diagnosis referral (see last row)*
3	Problem-assisted learning	Acquiring information in a format relevant to practitioner with planned opportunities to apply knowledge in practical setting	Lecture followed by practical experience in a lab or clinical setting	
4	Problem-solving learning	Solving problems, but not learning information related to problems	Case histories provided with problems to solve, followed by case discussions	
5	Problem-focused learning	Using a 3-step process: (1) subject (topic, vocabulary, key principles), (2) problem, (3) review principles and concepts already learned for applicability to the problem in new context	Introductory lecture followed by case histories, ending with discussions to generalize new information	
6	Problem-based, mixed learning	Starting either by (a) solving the problem, then moving to mastery of underlying principles, or (b) concentrating first on information, then solving problems	Students opt for either information-based or problem-based learning strategies	
7	Problem-initiated learning	Encountering beginning problems designed as triggers that arouse students' interest	Problems are used just at the beginning to interest students in a topic	
8	Problem-centered	Solving problems with less emphasis on learning issues and students finding information	Text provides a series of problems followed with information to solve problems	
9	Problem-centered discovery learning	Solving problems while simultaneously learning issues and finding information	Students meet to identify learning issues related to problems and then derived principles from their work	Case-based problem (see last row)**

(Continued)

Table 26.1 ✧	Information-Oriented–Problem-Based Learning Continuum *(Continued)*			
Step	Educational Approach	Student Emphasis	General Examples	Pathophysiology Course Example
10	Problem-based learning	Generalizing knowledge derived from solving problems while simultaneously learning issues and finding information	Information from one problem is generalized to another under simulation circumstances	
11	Task-based learning	Generalizing knowledge derived from solving problems while simultaneously learning issues and finding information	Generalization occurs in real time in the clinical setting	

*Diagnosis referral (Iterations 1 and 2)
• Name: Clara Timson
• Age: 89 years
• Diagnosis: Pneumonitis
• Location: Sunnyvale Home

**Case-based problem (Iterations 3 and 4)
A well-loved resident of Sunnyvale Home for 10 years, Clara Timson, is an 89-year-old woman with a diagnosis of pneumonitis. She never married, choosing to take care of her parents until they died while she supported the family by working as an accountant. In her facility, she is the coordinator of all social events, active on the residents' rights committee, and takes care of the unit animals.

Harden RM, and Davis MH: The continuum of problem-based learning. Med Teacher 20:317–322, 1998.

instead of just a component. Notice that one *how*—collaborative groups—was not modified in any iteration; this teaching strategy has a strong basis of evidence in the literature and students demonstrated competence through testing on an individual basis.[28,32–34]

To test the difference between the two conditions of the independent variable, no jigsawing in the fourth iteration versus jigsawing in the third iteration, I used an independent measures research design with students' pathophysiology final examination scores as the dependent variable. Although demographics of students and testing format were similar enough in the third and fourth iterations to provide an argument for matched samples (and a repeated measures t-test), I chose a more conservative approach and used an independent t-test to compare the last two iterations in the evolution of the pathophysiology course. I found that what I had seen in the first three iterations (students actively engaging to complete their own group's set of diagnoses and disregarding information their classmates provided) was, in fact, true. Fourth iteration students

(M = 96.73, SD = 3.34) who completed all components of assignments (no jigsawing) scored significantly higher in content competence (as measured by pathophysiology final examination scores) than third iteration students (M = 89.08, SD = 5.59) who had jigsawed content, $t(57) = +6.082$, d = 1.368, p < .001. I concluded from this action research study that I was justified in removing jigsawing, used in the first three iterations of the course. I found that students who completed all assignment components demonstrated a marked improvement in assessment of content mastery, both in the improvement in mean exam grade—from a B-level to an A-level of performance—and in the size of Cohen's effect size (d), which may be interpreted as large.[35]

✧ PARTING REFLECTIONS

For occupational therapists and physical therapists who are faculty, the *what* of teaching (content) often seems of primary importance; however, for those who wish to engage in the ethics of teaching, the *how* (method or the art) of teaching and the *why* (assessment or the science) of teaching are of importance equal to content. If the *what*, *how*, and *why* of the ethics of teaching have similar importance, then occupational therapy and physical therapy faculty must resolve two difficulties: (1) the *where* to accomplish the *how*, and (2) *when* to complete the *why*. Before addressing the *where* to accomplish the *how* and *when* to complete the *why*, I offer a short commentary on scholarship, particularly the scholarship of teaching and learning.

A movement sweeping across many university campuses, the scholarship of teaching and learning, is an outgrowth of the Carnegie Foundation for the Advancement of Teaching. The movement began when Boyer, Carnegie Foundation President at the time, proposed that scholarship be differentiated into four types: scholarship of discovery (conducting traditional, basic research), scholarship of integration (writing textbooks, synthesizing literature reviews), scholarship of application (providing professional services or outreach), and scholarship of teaching.[36] In a publication often called the sequel to Boyer, Glassick, Huber, and Maeroff modified scholarship terminology and proposed six standards to evaluate any type of scholarly work: clear goals, adequate preparation, appropriate methods, significant results, effective presentation, and reflective critique.[36,37] A year later, in 1998, the Carnegie Foundation for the Advancement of Teaching launched the initiative, Carnegie Academy for the Scholarship of Teaching and Learning (CASTL). At the higher education level, CASTL aims to advance the development of a scholarship of teaching and learning that will:

1. Foster significant, long-lasting learning for all students;

2. Enhance the practice and profession of teaching; and

3. Bring to faculty's work as teachers the recognition and reward afforded to the other forms of scholarly work.[38]

Colleges and universities have responded to the Carnegie Foundation for the Advancement of Teaching scholarship of teaching and learning initiative in various ways. Some higher education institutions have embraced the concept, creating centers for teaching/learning excellence for faculty and rewarding faculty who provide evidence of the scholarship of teaching and learning in terms of tenure, promotion, and merit. Other institutions, though interested in demonstrating evidence of student learning (particularly to accreditation agencies), have offered little support (related to time and opportunities* as well as to decisions of tenure, promotion, and merit) for faculty scholarly products related to teaching and learning. Still other colleges and universities look at the scholarship of teaching and learning as the ugly stepsister of basic science research, offering neither assistance nor recognition of products.

Scholarship, in general, and the scholarship of teaching and learning, in particular, are related to *where* to accomplish the *how* and *when* to complete the *why*. To resolve the difficulty of *where* to accomplish the *how* of the ethics of teaching, occupational therapy and physical therapy faculty must first understand that "despite the similarities between clinical and educator activities, 'doing therapy' and 'teaching therapy' are not synonymous activities."[39] Nevertheless, occupational therapists and physical therapists who have no teaching background are likely to enter higher education in the midst of Anderson's "inertia of tradition."[9] Nolinske forewarned that "the professional education of occupational therapy practitioners and future faculty must encompass more than training: it must also be linked to scholarship that includes research and teach-

---

*Interestingly, the word *scholarship* has an interesting derivation and history, and at one time was intricately intertwined with the concepts of leisure and having time available. The Greek feminine noun σχολη (transliterated as schole), a root word of scholarship, means *leisure, rest, ease* as well as *learned discussion,* whereas the neuter noun σχολαστηριον (transliterated as scholasterion), means *devoting one's leisure to learning, academic, theoretical.* To me, the verb σχολαξω (transliterated as scholaxo), which means *to have leisure time, to have nothing to do,* and also *to have time or opportunity,* is the most fascinating derivation because scholarship for many faculty has come to signify just the opposite: there is neither time nor opportunity.

ing."[28] Unfortunately, the majority of occupational therapy and physical therapy educational programs are not yet at that stage. In many professional training programs today, occupational therapy and physical therapy faculty consist primarily of practitioners who have moved directly from clinics to universities with little transition or training in the new—and many times alien—setting. Most occupational therapists and physical therapists enter this new setting thinking that keeping current in the *what* (content) is their primary responsibility. Still, as in any new setting, occupational therapy and physical therapy faculty are ethically responsible for becoming competent in the delivery of services. Competence in the delivery of services in the academic setting is related to the *how* of the ethics of teaching. To accomplish the *where* of the *how*, occupational therapists and physical therapists who teach can follow Nolinske's recommendation that even though "many faculty in professional training programs do not have formal instruction in teaching and learning, they can take advantage of literature within the field of education."[28] Finding creative teaching ideas may be as simple as entering key words or terms (e.g., *collaborative groups*) into search engines of professional literature databases and implementing new teaching strategies in the classroom, or tapping into the vast (and often underutilized) resources offered by centers for teaching/learning excellence implemented by many universities as a result of the Carnegie Foundation for the Advancement of Teaching scholarship of teaching and learning initiative. Contrary to Milton and Shoben's declaration, teaching at the university level no longer needs to be the only profession in the world for which no specific training is required.[21]

Resolving *when* to accomplish the *why* of the ethics of teaching may be more difficult because the academic setting is highly complex and imposes inconsistent demands in terms of time. Although occupational therapy and physical therapy faculty are ethically obligated to deliver evidence-based services, finding time (and university support and recognition that the scholarship of teaching and learning is a valid form of inquiry) to conduct the *why*—ongoing assessment that provides evidence

either to support continued use or to make modifications resulting in better practices of teaching—may be hard to accomplish in the educational setting. To resolve the difficulty of *when* to complete the *why*, I recommend capitalizing on the complexity of the academic setting by combining at least the first two components of what I call the *academic trinity*: teaching, scholarship, and service. (Please note: the components of the academic trinity are likely to have a different priority order, depending on a university's mission and Carnegie classification.) Crepeau, Thibodaux, and Parham promoted, "Capitalizing on the interrelationships among teaching, research, and service allows each to reinforce and inform the other."[40] Establishing a research agenda that is separate from teaching—an agenda based in Boyer's *scholarship of discovery*—is noble; however, the time involved in accomplishing both is likely to compromise teaching, scholarship, or both.[36] In addition, research conducted outside the *why* of the ethics of teaching, though likely to add to the knowledge base of the profession, will neither enrich the practice of teaching within the academic setting nor improve the competence of practitioners making the transition from the clinic to the classroom. Crepeau and colleagues provided further support for combining scholarship and teaching, "during the academic year, expert scholars blend research and teaching into their schedules."[40]

To the question asking if I advocate concentrating on Boyer's scholarship of teaching and learning, my answer is equivocal.[36] Before labeling products as scholarship of teaching and learning, I recommend faculty check the university's mission, Carnegie classification, and general attitude about the scholarship of teaching and learning. As I indicated earlier, colleges and universities have responded to the Carnegie Foundation for the Advancement of Teaching scholarship of teaching and learning initiative in various ways. My response to faculty who work in universities that have embraced the scholarship of teaching and learning at the highest levels, is yes—label all scholarly products related to teaching and learning as such. To faculty in an institution that offers little or no support for the scholarship of teaching and learning, I advocate using terminology the university considers appropriate rather than completely ignoring the scholarship of teaching and learning.

In an earlier section, I wrote that educational self-assessment exists for me in a continuum that ranges from any informal investigation into teaching practice at one end to the formality of action research, which provides evidence-based documentation, at the other end. For me, the informal end of the self-assessment continuum can generate information related to the scholarship of teaching and learning. If not readily publishable, information generated through the scholarship of teaching and learning may be suitable for professional presentations, annual performance review portfolios, and promotion and tenure dossiers. Action research at the formal end of the self-assessment continuum is an example of Boyer's scholarship of integration and Glassick, Huber, and Maeroff's scholarship of synthesis.[36,37] Not only is this type of scholarship readily publishable, the data generated through action research will enrich the practice of teaching and learning within occupational therapy and physical therapy educational programs, improve competence of faculty at multiple points in their educational careers, and ease the clinic-to-classroom transition for occupational therapists and physical therapists.

Using evidence to build the body of knowledge systematically, thereby showing evidence of effectiveness, has become a goal of occupational therapy and physical therapy. Occupational therapy and physical therapy educators must also use evidence to build the teaching and learning body of knowledge, showing the effectiveness of teaching and learning in both professions. Before sharing some concluding reflections, I feel strongly the need to reflect first on evidence—especially the present level of the majority of current evidenced-based research studies in health care. To me, the state of so-called evidence-based information in occupational therapy today—with a preponderance of determining hypothetical mathematical averages of aggregate data—has become jammed in the middle of a four-level evidence hierarchy developed by forensic scientists. Forensic science moved from the first level, classifying (determining the category of an unknown substance), in the mid-1800s to the second level, identifying (classifying within a category), in the 1900s. Some group comparison studies (classifying within a category) in occupational therapy, to me, provide evidence that forensic scientists were considered cutting-edge more than 100 years ago, whereas other investigations are at the third hierarchical level, differentiating (breaking down into component parts), a predominantly positivistic, linear approach. I believe action research has potential to move health education evidence to the highest point of the four-level evidence hierarchy—individuating (tracing to single entities), the level to which forensic scientists moved in the 1960s. Most of us deal with individuated evidence; the problem comes when we share our findings. McLean stated the strength and weakness succinctly: "action research is, at the same time, the most valid and the least valid research about classroom practice."[41] Individuated evidence produced through action research provides a high level of internal validity; however, reengineering that same evidence from the highest hierarchical level downward provides a low level of external validity. To me, this means that the teaching and learning scholarly products I generate have the most meaning in my own classes.

Action research, even with low external validity, still produces information that has ramifications for generalization beyond individuation. Because external validity of any type of research design steadily improves with an accumulation of replicated studies, occupational therapy and physical therapy faculty need only to look for patterns in research investigations that are similar to their own teaching situations, and then replicate the research study. For example, although the focus of this chapter is on the ethics of teaching, my self-study's action research component that investigated changes made in the fourth iteration has generalized beyond the pathophysiology course to effect change in the area of that recombination of words—the teaching of ethics, which I have incorporated into each of my courses (professional code of ethics issues in the first-year orientation course and ethical dilemmas in the communication, evaluation, research, and leadership courses). Whereas in the past I used jigsawed content within collaborative groups as the *how* of the teaching of ethics, once I found that jigsawing was not an effective *how* in the pathophysiology course, I eliminated this teaching strategy from all of my courses. For any area of content, students must now complete the entire puzzle rather than just a jigsaw piece.

Shulman stated, "The scholarship of teaching makes the private public and the clandestine observable. Once the work of teaching is public, new ethical dimensions arise."[42] Ethical issues arising within the ethics of teaching can involve power and authority in the classroom, use of student work, and also aspects related to university units that oversee human subjects research (institutional review board—IRB—in many universities) including informed consent, risk/benefit ratios, and anonymity/confidentiality. Pritchard provides insight into the ethics of educational research, using a fascinating metaphor that involves a troll (the IRB) who resides under a bridge (research), exacting tolls (paperwork and time) from travelers (researchers).[43]

Related to educational inquiry, I am fortunate in the fact that receiving approval to conduct studies of this kind at my university is not difficult. An expectation in annual performance review, promotion, and tenure guidelines is that faculty will engage in scholarly inquiry resulting in constant revision of courses and curricula. The university committee that reviews proposals for faculty and student research projects involving human subjects has determined that investigations into normal educational practices are exempt from review. In fact, at the time of this writing, my university's IRB regards the process as educational assessment, not research, and does not require a research study application. Kosnik and Beck cautioned that not all faculty are as fortunate; some IRBs are resistant to classroom research proposals.[19] They warned that, stemming primarily from unfamiliarity with self-study methodology, some human subject committees question student experimentation and challenge whether self-study constitutes "real" research. IRBs and researchers alike would be well advised to heed Pritchard's noteworthy recommendations, called "concrete improvements in the roadbed

of research" in his captivating metaphor.[43] Before conducting any investigation into the ethics of teaching, I highly recommend that occupational therapy and physical therapy faculty seek permission with appropriate supervisors and human subjects committees to determine how a particular university regards continuous improvement of educational practices. Both professions can benefit from Hutchings's viewpoint, "ethical issues are not simply occasions for caution but windows into our values and aspirations as teachers and scholars of teaching."[44]

✧ CONCLUSION

Reflection, according to Schön, "gives rise to on-the-spot experiment. We think up and try out new actions intended to explore the newly observed phenomena, test out tentative understandings of them or affirm the moves we have intended to change things for the better."[4] Through reflection along the self-assessment continuum, occupational therapy and physical therapy faculty can fulfill their ethical responsibility for becoming competent in the delivery of services in the educational setting. As Dewey stated, "The function of reflection is to bring about a new situation in which the difficulty is resolved, the confusion cleared away, the trouble smoothed out, the question it puts answered."[1] Not only will emphasis on the ethics of teaching have the potential to resolve difficulties, clear confusion, smooth troubles, and answer questions, faculty reflection along the self-assessment continuum will enrich the practice of teaching within occupational therapy and physical therapy educational settings by systematically accumulating evidence of effectiveness through the scholarship of teaching and learning.

References

1. Dewey J: How we Think: A Restatement of the Relation of Reflective Thinking to the Educative Process. DC Heath and Co., New York, 1933.
2. Dewey J: Essays in Experimental Logic. The University of Chicago Press, Chicago, 1917.
3. Schön DA: The Reflective Practitioner. How Professionals Think in Action. Basic Books, New York, 1983.

4. Schön DA: Educating the Reflective Practitioner: Toward a New Design for Teaching and Learning in the Professions. Jossey-Bass, San Francisco, 1987.
5. Purtilo R: Ethical Dimensions in the Health Profession. ed 3. WB Saunders Co., Philadelphia, PA, 1999.
6. Goodlad JI, Soder R, and Sirotnik KA (eds): The Moral Dimensions of Teaching. Jossey-Bass, San Francisco, 1990.
7. Swartz GE: Teaching as vocation: Enabling ethical practice. Educ Forum 63:23–29, 1998.
8. Huebner D: Ethics of inquiry: Issues in the scholarship of teaching and learning. J Curr Superv 11:267–275, 1996.
9. Anderson A: The moral dimension of teaching physical education. Phys Educ 56:49–56, 1998.
10. Corrigan SA, and Tom AR: The moral dilemmas of teacher educators. Educ Forum 63(1):66–72, 1998.
11. Gordon W, and Sork TJ: Ethical issues and codes of ethics: Views of adult education practitioners in Canada and the United States. Adult Educ Q 51(3):202–218, 2001.
12. Mathiasen RE: Moral education of college students, faculty and staff perspectives. Coll Student J 32(3):374–377, 1998.
13. Ramler S: Teaching and learning in a global society. Independent Sch 61(3):100–106, 2002.
14. Tom AR: Teaching as a Moral Craft. Longman, New York, 1984.
15. Winston RB, and Saunders SA: Professional ethics in a risky world. New Dirs Stud Serv 82:77–94, 1998.
16. Purtilo RB: A time to harvest, a time to sow: Ethics for a shifting landscape. Phys Ther 80(11):1112–1119, 2000.
17. Kanny EM, and Kyler PL: Are faculty prepared to address ethical issues in education? Am J Occup Ther 53(1):72–74, 1999.
18. Zeichner KM: The new scholarship in teacher education. Paper presented at: AERA Division K Vice-Presidential Address (revised version). 1998, San Diego, CA.
19. Kosnik C, and Beck C: Who should perish: You or your students? Dilemmas of research in teacher education. Teacher Educ Q 27:119–135, 2000.
20. Bork CE: Introduction: An invitation. In Bork CE (ed): Research in Physical Therapy. JB Lippincott Co, Philadelphia, PA, 1993, pp 1–6.
21. Milton O, and Shoben EJ: Learning and the Professor. Ohio University Press, Athens, OH, 1968.
22. Dewey J: Democracy and Education. Macmillan, New York, 1916.
23. Vygotsky LS: Educational Psychology. (R. Silverman, trans.). CRC Press, Boca Raton, FL, 1997, (1926 Original Work).
24. Adler MJ: The Paideia Proposal. Collier Books, New York, 1982.
25. Bloom BS, et al (eds): Taxonomy of Educational Objectives: The Cognitive Domain. McKay, New York, 1956, No. 1.
26. Bransford JD, Brown AL, and Cocking RR (eds): How People Learn: Brain, Mind, Experience, and School. National Academy Press, Washington, 2000.
27. Donovan MS, Bransford JD, and Pellegrino JW (eds): How People Learn: Bridging Research and Practice. National Academy Press, Washington, DC, 2003.
28. Nolinske T: Preparing and developing faculty through faculty development initiatives. Am J Occup Ther 53:9–13, 1999.
29. Clark J: Pieces of the puzzle: The jigsaw method. In Sharon S (ed): Handbook of Cooperative Learning Methods. Praeger, Westport, CT, 1999, pp 34–50.
30. Hutchings P, and Schulman LS: The scholarship of teaching: New elaborations. Change 31(5):11–15, 1999.
31. Harden RM, and Davis MH: The continuum of problem-based learning. Med Teacher 20:317–322, 1998.
32. Johnson DW, and Johnson RT: Learning Together and Alone, ed 5. Allyn and Bacon, Boston, 1999.
33. Sharan S: Handbook of Cooperative Learning Methods. Praeger, Westport, CT, 1999.
34. Slavin RE: Cooperative Learning. ed 2. Allyn and Bacon, Boston, 1995.
35. Cohen J: Statistical Power Analysis for the Behavioral Sciences. ed 2. Lawrence Erlbaum Assoc, Hillsdale, NJ, 1988.
36. Boyer EL: Scholarship Reconsidered. Carnegie Foundation, Princeton, NJ, 1990.
37. Glassick CE, Huber MT, and Maeroff GI: Scholarship Assessed: Evaluation of the Professoriate. Jossey-Bass, San Francisco, 1997.
38. Hutchings P: Preface. In Hutchings P, Babb M, and Bjork C (eds): The Scholarship of Teaching and Learning in Higher Education: An Annotated Bibliography. The Carnegie Foundation for the Advancement of Teaching, Menlo Park, CA, 2002.
39. Crist P: Career transition from clinician to academician responsibilities and reflections. Am J Occup Ther 53:14–19, 1999.
40. Crepeau EB, Thibodaux L, and Parham D: Academic juggling act: Beginning and sustaining an academic career. Am J Occup Ther 53:25–30, 1999.
41. McLean JE: Improving Education Through Action Research: A Guide for Administrators and Teachers. Corwin Press, Inc, Thousand Oaks, CA, 1995.
42. Shulman L: Preface. In Hutchings P (ed): Ethics of Inquiry: Issues in the Scholarship of Teaching and Learning. The Carnegie Foundation for the Advancement of Teaching, Menlo Park, CA, 2002.
43. Pritchard IA: Travelers and trolls: Practitioner research and institutional review boards. Educ Researcher 31(3):3–14, 2002.
44. Hutchings P: Ethics of Inquiry: Issues in the Scholarship of Teaching and Learning. The Carnegie Foundation for the Advancement of Teaching, Menlo Park, CA, 2002.

27

Applying the Scholarship of Teaching and Learning to Ethics Education in Occupational and Physical Therapy

AMY MARIE HADDAD, PHD

Abstract

The purpose of this chapter is to suggest possible ways to apply the scholarship of teaching and learning (SoTL) to critical inquiry about ethics education in the health sciences. A general overview of SoTL is provided. The impetus for and design of a specific SoTL project in the context of a pharmacy ethics course is discussed. The SoTL project in pharmacy ethics is but one example of the kind of inquiry into ethics education that could be applicable to other health science disciplines. Ideas for further inquiry in occupational therapy and physical therapy ethics education are proposed using three key questions concerning what works in ethics education, what is possible and what is really happening when students learn.

Consider the following fictionalized vignettes of instruction in occupational and physical therapy and what they tell us about student learning and understanding in the area of ethics.

Vignette One

A physical therapy student meets with the instructor of record for the ethics course in the PT program. The student has been struggling the whole semester with the written requirements of the course, which includes case analysis. The student has had special difficulty in applying ethical principles to problems. As the instructor and student go over the steps of a normative decision making model as applied to a case, the student remarks, "Well, I know what the ethical problem is since the case is in the chapter that deals with patient autonomy."

The instructor replied, "That's a good place to start, of course, but what other principles might apply to the case?"

"Other principles?" the student responded. "You mean all of these principles could apply to this case?"

Vignette Two

It is late in the semester and time seems to be running out in the occupational therapy ethics course. The instructor of record does a quick calculation and finds that she will not get through the textbook if they keep going at this pace even though the students are reading a chapter a week. She decides to eliminate the content on ethical theories and a debate on Medicaid policy. She knows that she will have to push to cover the remaining content in lecture.

Vignette Three

During a clinical rotation, an occupational therapy student encountered a situation in which a patient's confidentiality was breached by an occupational therapy technician. The student could have intervened to prevent the violation, but stood by and did nothing. When the clinical instructor found out about the violation of confidentiality and the student's unwillingness to stop it, he asked the student, "Didn't you learn about this in your ethics course? Didn't you know what the tech was doing was wrong?"

The student replied, "We did learn about confidentiality and I could probably still give you a definition but so much of what we learned in ethics was so abstract. It didn't seem to have much to do with clinical practice."

Vignette Four

The term "active learning" really describes what occurs in an ethics course in a physical therapy program. Students are involved in role-playing exercises, case study analysis, term papers, and discussion boards on the Internet. Each week, the students scanned the lay press for articles that dealt with ethical issues and wrote commentaries. The final assignment, a group paper and presentation, addressed the most pressing ethical issues in physical therapy and proposed actions to resolve them.[1]

Before we criticize the teacher in the second vignette for rushing to cover content or relying too much on lecture as a teaching mode and before we praise the instructor in the fourth vignette for using a variety of active learning strategies, let us look more deeply at what each vignette tells about teaching and learning. Most faculty members, like the instructor in the first vignette, have experienced the feeling that there is too much content and not enough time in a course to cover it. What drives the instructor's decision to cut certain content and to push to cover other topics in a course? What do students really learn and retain through this "forced march" approach that many faculty adopt near the end of a course? The second vignette is one that many faculty members can identify with regardless of the subject matter being taught. An initial reaction to the student's statement about the applicability of ethical principles to clinical problems might be, "Where has this student been all semester?" Why has this student missed one of the most basic approaches to ethics? The student's misunderstanding of this basic concept raises bigger questions about what this student and other students in the class really understand about the process of ethical decision making. The third vignette focuses on the application of knowledge beyond the classroom and into clinical practice. The student could still recall a definition for a concept learned in ethics, but did not recognize the principle at work in practice. Could it be that the student did not have enough opportunities to apply these abstract concepts to real-world situations? Finally, vignette four presents the preferred teaching approach of the hour, an activity orientation, in which students participate in a wide variety of experiences related to ethics. Yet, the variety of activities does not guarantee that the students are learning what is most important about the discipline of ethics. What are the ends of all of this activity? What are the big ideas in ethics and the skills necessary to act on these ideas in professional practice? How would we know if our students understood the ideas we deem most important and whether or not they possess the skills to act?

The scholarship of teaching and learning (SoTL) is one approach to help unravel the problems that these vignettes suggest. Furthermore, SoTL provides a way to answer the larger question: What is (are) the most appropriate way(s) to teach ethics in physical and occupational therapy?

✧ THE SCHOLARSHIP OF TEACHING AND LEARNING

The jury of higher education is still out as far as reaching an agreement on a singular definition of the scholarship of teaching and learning. However, there appears to be growing consensus on what the scholarship of teaching and learning should entail. Shulman provides a comprehensive definition: "A scholarship of teaching will entail a public account of some or all of the full act of teaching—vision, design, enactment, outcomes, and analysis—in a manner susceptible to critical review by the teacher's professional peers and amenable to productive employment in future work by members of that same community."[2]

McKinney contrasts the more traditional roles of being a good teacher as well as a scholarly one with the SoTL. "SoTL goes beyond being a good teacher (facilitating significant student learning) and beyond being a scholarly teacher (reading the pedagogical literature, attending teaching development activities, etc.). It involves systematic reflection on teaching and/or learning and the public sharing of such work."[3]

Not all faculty members will pursue this type of scholarly inquiry into their work as educators. Some will continue with their disciplinary research with occasional forays into the area of SoTL; others will opt for SoTL as their primary work.

The purpose of this chapter is to suggest possible ways to apply SoTL to ethics education in the health sciences. The guiding principle for the chapter is that there is no single best method or approach for conducting the SoTL.[4] A general overview of a specific SoTL project in the context of a pharmacy ethics course is provided. The SoTL project in pharmacy ethics is but one example of the kind of inquiry into ethics education that could be applicable to other health science disciplines. Ideas for further inquiry in occupational therapy and physi-

cal therapy ethics education are proposed using three key questions developed by Bass.[5]

Case in Point

Even though ethics is regarded as an essential component of pharmacy education, methods to teach ethics and evaluate the abilities of students are not well developed. In question are the abilities to:

1. Recognize ethical issues in a clinical context
2. Propose resolutions to identified problems
3. Use the tools of ethics such as principles and theories
4. Justify proposed resolutions
5. Anticipate arguments to proposed resolutions
6. Cope with the uncertainty and emotional nature of ethical issues commonly encountered in clinical practice

Numerous teaching and evaluation methods have been used in pharmacy ethics education such as true/false and multiple-choice examinations, essay examinations, role-playing, group discussion, case study analysis, and instruments that measure moral reasoning.[6,7]

Most instruction in ethics has been geared toward ethical analysis of case studies, i.e., the student is asked to read a case, identify the ethical issues verbally or in writing, propose different resolutions supported by principles and theory, and select the best course of action. It is safe to say that these teaching strategies are employed in most health science ethics courses and perhaps other nonhealth professions, such as law and engineering.

Cases can be used to teach philosophical ethics. As Veatch notes, "The first step is to recognize an ethical problem when it is encountered. It also involves understanding major alternative theories. Students should know the difference between a virtue theory and an action theory, between utilitarianism and deontological ethics, between value theory (axiology) and a theory of right action, between *prima facie* duty and duty proper, and between rule-based and situation-based theory."[8]

Yet, case analysis will only take us so far. Written case analysis is an unlikely route to developing skills in coping with the uncertainty and emotional nature of ethical issues commonly encountered in health care. There is clearly a difference between reading a text about ethical issues and interacting with a real patient, peer, or another health professional.

When a student reads a case and writes a response to the ethical problem(s) encountered therein, he or she is involved in "third-person ethics." Even though the student might identify with the people in the case or feel sympathy for the situation the principals find themselves in, the student is not really involved in the case. Students can view ethics from a distant, more objective position. In reality, ethics is up close and personal. "The clinical encounter is an encounter of agents who discern and act in the first person."[9] So, a teaching and learning method that gets closer to "first-person" ethics is desirable.

An additional question regarding methods of teaching ethics is: How much of what a student learns in an ethics course translates to actual clinical practice? In other words, once the student has completed the ethics course and embarks on the final year of clerkships (that is the traditional model in pharmacy education) how much, if anything, of what the student learned in ethics will be used in clinical practice? In occupational therapy and physical therapy, faculty may wonder how and if the students use what they learn in ethics during clinical rotations that occur earlier in the professional program than in pharmacy. These questions steer us in the direction of a teaching method and course design that gets as close to real-life practice as possible—clinical simulations.

The primary research question for this project was: What impact do clinical simulations involving standardized patients (SPs) have on student learning regarding resolving ethical problems in a pharmacy ethics course? Specifically, what impact do clinical simulations have on third-year students in a Doctor of Pharmacy program in a required, three-semester-hour ethics course?

Secondary questions were also developed:

✦ Is there a relationship between critical

thinking and the ability to analyze ethical problems?

✦ Is there a relationship between moral development and ability to resolve ethical problems in SP interactions?

✦ Could SP interactions improve cognitive moral development scores?

✦ Do interactions with SPs have an effect on ethical sensitivity?

✦ Does critical self-reflection about interactions with SPs have an effect on ethical decision making?

✦ Do interactions with SPs have an effect on self-efficacy in identifying and resolving ethical problems in clinical practice?

✦ Do interactions with SPs have an effect on the quality of written work (ethical analysis) as demonstrated on exams, critical self-reflection, and other writing assignments?

For the purposes of this chapter, preliminary findings to these research questions will not be presented. Rather the focus of the chapter is on how these questions (and others) were developed using a SoTL approach to finding answers.

Since it is not possible to predict when students will encounter an ethical issue in clinical practice, clinical simulations can be used to approximate what they will likely encounter in actual practice and gets us closer to "first-person" ethics. It should be emphasized that SP encounters or clinical simulations are not a substitute for direct patient contact in clinical settings.[10] Standardized patient methods, one type of clinical simulation, have been used to give students practice for many clinical skills, most often physical assessment, in a realistic and safe environment. SP encounters are designed to supplement student experience and allow practice of clinical skills, such as recognizing and resolving ethical problems. The lion's share of the work with SPs has been in medical education with a focus on patient assessment and the psychomotor skills it involves.[11] However, SPs have been used for other types of learning in pharmacy and other health science programs to help students improve communication skills and patient education.[12–15] There are even a select few examples in the literature of the use of standardized patients and ethics in medical education.[16]

SPs are laypeople who are given a detailed case history and trained to portray an individual in a health situation. SPs are not given a script but background information regarding the important clinical, or ethical, components of a case as well as several prompts to move the interaction forward. SPs not only portray patients, but peers and other health professionals as well. SPs are often used for evaluation purposes; that is, as part of a single interaction coupled with a writing assignment or drug calculation (called a couplet) or multiple "stations" with numerous SPs and case histories (called an OSCE).[17] SPs were used in this SoTL project in pharmacy ethics education as a teaching, assessment, and professional development tool rather than a "high stakes" examination or evaluation tool.

The context of the SoTL project in pharmacy ethics is a required, three-credit-hour course in ethics at a private midwestern school of pharmacy. We know from specialists in education and interpersonal dynamics that students need repeated experiences to practice these new and complicated ways of working with others that are a part of resolving ethical problems in clinical settings.[18] Thus, the students in the pharmacy ethics course have four opportunities during the semester to interact with SPs in four different clinical simulations that focus on commonly encountered ethical issues in pharmacy practice. The clinical simulations are but one component of a complicated course design that includes opportunities for the students to develop in the six facets of understanding proposed by Wiggins and McTighe.[1] Students have opportunities to: explain, build and test their own theories through self-reflection writing assignments; develop their own interpretations and appreciate other interpretations of the same event; apply principles to realistic situations including planning, troubleshooting and reflection; appreciate multiple views of the same issue; confront experiences to develop empathy and develop self-knowledge through structured reflection. As Bass notes, not only does SoTL require looking at teaching and learning differently, but the means by which we determine or

assess learning should reflect this change in focus as well:

> It takes a deliberate act to look at teaching from the perspective of learning. Actually, it takes a set of acts—individually motivated and communally validated—to focus on questions and problems, gather data, interpret and share results The range of questions can take many forms. The nature of the data may be quantitative or qualitative; it may be based on interviews, formative assessment instruments, test performances, student evaluations or peer review, or any combination by which the "multiples of evidence" may be obtained.[19]

Preliminary findings regarding the primary research question include: clinical simulations have a multifaceted impact on student learning particularly in the areas of developing confidence, recognizing ethical problems in realistic clinical situations, demonstration of understandings of ethics and insight into their own professional development.

✧ FURTHER INQUIRIES IN SoTL IN ETHICS EDUCATION

The questions and problems about what is the best way to teach ethics to students in occupational therapy and physical therapy or how to facilitate their development as moral health professionals are really scholarly research questions, not merely matters of technique and classroom strategies. Randy Bass, a Carnegie Scholar, recently presented three basic but complex questions that described the path he has traveled in trying to understand how his students learn. The three questions Bass poses provide a helpful way to organize further inquiry into the teaching and learning of ethics in physical and occupational therapy.[5]

What Works?

Most faculty members begin with the "What works?" type of questions in their quest to figure out what is going on in their classrooms and their students' minds and hearts. Questions like, "Do my students learn better this way?" fall into this category.

Participants at the Fall 2003 Leadership in Ethics Education Conference were invited to brainstorm regarding the kinds of questions they might ask in this category. Here is a sampling of the types of questions the participants proposed, all of which could be developed into a SoTL project: Does problem-based learning (PBL) enhance student learning in ethics? How do we prepare students to engage more effectively in self-regulation re: whistle-blowing? Do student generated case studies work differently than instructor generated cases?

What is Possible?

Design questions fall into the "What is possible?" category. The participants at the Leadership in Ethics Education Conference offered the following questions: What is the best course/curriculum design to facilitate students' synthesis of past learning? Is it possible to develop learning activities that facilitate student moral roles outside of patient relationships? What is the best placement of the ethics course in the curriculum? What learning activities encourage development of moral courage?

What Is?

This final category of questions deals with what is actually going on when our students are trying to learn. What are the component activities or skills of ethical decision making in clinical practice? What do the students need to do well to be successful at recognizing and resolving ethical problems? Here are examples of questions from participants at the Leadership in Ethics Education Conference that fall into the "What is?" category: What is the nature of face-to-face interaction between clinical instructors and students? What is the "ah-ha" moment when students "get it"?

Through critical inquiry with students, collaborative and interdisciplinary work, and the critical eye of SoTL, we can identify these component parts of working through ethical problems and what it means to help shape the development of students into ethical health professionals.

References

1. Wiggins G, and McTighe J: Understanding by Design. Association for Supervision and Curriculum Development, Alexandria, VA, 1998.
2. Shulman L: Introduction. In Hutchings P (ed): The Course Portfolio: How Faculty Can Examine Their Teaching to Advance Practice and Improve Student Learning. American Association of Higher Education, Washington, DC, 1998.
3. McKinney K: Applying the scholarship of teaching and learning: Can we do better? Teaching Professor 17(7):1, 2003.
4. Hutchings P: Approaching the Scholarship of Teaching and Learning. In Hutchings P (ed): Opening Lines—Approaches to the Scholarship of Teaching and Learning. The Carnegie Foundation for the Advancement of Teaching, Menlo Park, CA, 2000.
5. Bass R: Personal communication with Randy Bass, Ph.D., regarding presentation on evidence of his journey in search of his scholarship of teaching. Paper presented at: 2001–2002 Carnegie Scholars Summer Meeting, 2002, The Carnegie Foundation for the Advancement of Teaching, Menlo Park, CA.
6. Haddad AM, et al: Report of the ethics course content committee: Curricular guidelines in pharmacy education. Am J Pharm Educ 57(Winter Suppl):34S–43S, 1993.
7. Rest JR, and Narvaez D: Defining Issues Test 2. Center for Research in Ethical Development, Minneapolis, MN, 1998.
8. Veatch R: Case analysis in ethics instruction. In Haddad A (ed): Teaching and Learning Strategies in Pharmacy Ethics. ed 2. The Pharmaceutical Products Press, New York, 1997.
9. Bishop JP: Creating narratives in the clinical encounter. Med Humanities Rev 14(1):10–24, 2000.
10. Ainsworth MA, et al: Standardized patient encounters: A method for teaching and evaluation. JAMA 266(10):1390–1396, 1991.
11. Barrows HS: An overview of the uses of standardized patients for teaching and evaluating clinical skills. Acad Med 68(6):443–451, 1993.
12. Monaghan M, et al: Student attitudes toward the use of standardized patients in a communication course. Am J Pharm Educ 61(Summer):131–136, 1997.
13. Yoo MS, and Yoo IY: The effectiveness of standardized patients as a teaching method for nursing fundamentals. J Nurs Educ 42(10):444–448, 2003.
14. Teutsch C: Patient-doctor communication. Med Clin North Am 87(5):1115–1145, 2003.
15. Logan HL, et al: Using standardized patients to assess presentation of a dental treatment plan. J Dent Educ 63(10):729–737, 1999.
16. Singer PA, et al: Performance-based assessment of clinical ethics using an objective structured clinical examination. Acad Med 71(5):495–498, 1996.
17. McGuire C: Perspectives in assessment. Acad Med 68(2):S3–S8, 1993.
18. Mentkowski M, et al: Student and Alumna Learning in College and Beyond: Perspectives from Longitudinal Interviews. Alverno College Institute, Milwaukee, WI, 1998.
19. Bass R: The scholarship of teaching and learning: What is the problem? Inventio 1(1):7, 1998.

Index